The
Psychoanalytic
Study
of the Child

VOLUME FORTY-THREE

Kindly submit five copies of new manuscripts to

Albert J. Solnit, M.D.
Yale Child Study Center
P.O. Box 3333
New Haven, CT 06510

The
Psychoanalytic
Study
of the Child

VOLUME FORTY-THREE

New Haven
Yale University Press
1988

Designed by Sally Harris
and set in Baskerville type.
Printed in the United States of America by
Vail-Ballou Press, Inc., Binghamton, N.Y.

Library of Congress catalogue card number: 45–11304
International standard book number: 0–300–04341–4

The paper in this book meets the guidelines for
permanence and durability of the Committee on
Production Guidelines for Book Longevity of the
Council on Library Resources.

2   4   6   8   10   9   7   5   3   1

Contents

FREUD AND THEORY BUILDING

Trauma or Drive—Drive and Trauma

A Reading of Sigmund Freud's Phylogenetic Fantasy of 1915

ILSE GRUBRICH-SIMITIS

I

IN LONDON, IN 1983, A HITHERTO UNKNOWN MANUSCRIPT FROM FREUD'S pen was discovered among papers in Sándor Ferenczi's literary estate. It proved to be the draft of the twelfth metapsychological essay of 1915, an "Overview of the Transference Neuroses." The German edition, with a facsimile, was published in 1985; the English language version two years later.

On July 28, 1915, Freud had sent the manuscript to his friend and colleague Sándor Ferenczi, for his opinion. In the accompanying letter he left it up to him to throw the draft away subsequently or keep it as he wished. In the same letter Freud emphasizes that the fair copy follows the draft "sentence for sentence, deviating from it only slightly" (Freud, 1985a, p. xvi). With the newly discovered manuscript we thus acquire, for the first time, detailed information about the twelfth metapsychological essay—the keystone in that major theoretical structure that Freud had created during World War I as a series of twelve interconnected metapsychological papers. Originally he had intended to publish the collection in book form after the war, under the title *Preliminaries to a Metapsychology (Zur Vorbereitung einer Metapsychologie)*, but as he later declared: "The attempt remained no more than a torso; . . .

This essay is an expanded version of the Thirty-seventh Freud Anniversary Lecture, held on April 28, 1987, at the invitation of the New York Psychoanalytic Institute, in the Academy of Medicine. The German text appeared in *Psyche*, 41:992–1023, 1987.

I would like to thank Veronica Mächtlinger for her translation.

the time for theoretical predications of this kind had not yet come"
(1925, p. 59). In the *Internationale Zeitschrift für ärztliche Psychoanalyse*
Freud published singly—between the years 1915 and 1917—only five
of the twelve papers: basic classical psychoanalytical texts (1915a–
1915c, 1917a, 1917b). He later discarded the remaining seven manuscripts, although they too had been virtually completed. One assumes
that he destroyed them—at least no trace of them has been found to
date. The reemergence of the draft of the final essay is therefore all the
more of a surprise.

I want here to draw the reader's attention to the *second* part of the
manuscript, to that strange, highly imaginative passage that Freud
called his "phylogenetic fantasy."[1]
We know from Freud's letters that essays on the three transference
neuroses—anxiety hysteria, conversion hysteria, and obsessional neurosis—were included among the seven lost papers (Strachey, 1957, p.
106). As the title implies, Freud planned in the twelfth essay to provide
an overview, a synthesis. For the first part he chose six familiar psychoanalytic points of view from which he wanted to compare and contrast
the three transference neuroses on a high level of abstraction: repression, anticathexis, substitute and symptom formation, relation to the
sexual function, regression, and finally disposition. It is in dealing with
disposition, the sixth point of view, that Freud seemingly abruptly
launches into a breathtaking speculative flight of fancy—his phylogenetic fantasy, in which along with the transference neuroses he
includes the "narcissistic neuroses," in his usage the psychoses.
It is not possible here to describe the phylogenetic fantasy in detail.
Its richness and variety can naturally only unfold in a reading of the
entire text. However, Freud himself has given us a succinct summary
of his argument, once again in a letter to Sándor Ferenczi on July 12,
1915,[2] a few days before he wrote the draft:

> Dear Friend
>   In my preparations for the "Overview of the Transference Neu-
> roses" I am beset by fantasies that disturb me and are hardly likely to
> find public expression. So pay attention:
>   There is a chronological sequence in the occurrence [of the indi-
> vidual psychoneuroses] in patients as follows:

1. In a letter to Ferenczi on July 18, 1915 (quoted in Grubrich-Simitis, 1985, p. 80).
2. Previously published by Ernest Jones (1957, p. 330). In order to facilitate comprehension of this very condensed letter, I have added a few comments in square
brackets.
Translator's note: The letter has in part been newly translated. This applies equally to
many of the following Freud quotations.

Anxiety hysteria—conversion hysteria—obsession—dementia prae-cox—paranoia—melancholia-mania. [Freud wants to say here that the transference neuroses can occur relatively early in childhood; the psychoses, in contrast, first in puberty or in adulthood.]

The libidinal dispositions [of the psychoneuroses] in general run in the *opposite* direction, that is to say, the fixation in the first-named group [the transference neuroses] is to be found in very late [ontogenetic] developmental stages, in the latter group [the psychoses] in very early ones; a statement that does not always hold true.

On the other hand, the sequence seems to repeat—phylogeneti-cally—a historical course of events. What are now [psycho]neuroses were once evolutionary stages of the human species.

Under the impact of the privations during the Ice Age, men [who, Freud assumed, had until then lived happily and still uncivilized in a friendly, paradisal world] became *anxious*, they had [in their now threatening environment] every reason to transform libido into anxiety. [Anxiety hysteria defends against a return of the condition prevailing in this stage.]

Having learned that propagation was now [as a result of the shortage of food] the enemy of [self] preservation and must be restricted, they became—still speechless—hysterical [in the sense of conversion hysteria].

In the hard school of the Ice Ages man—essentially the males—developed speech and intelligence. Subsequently they formed primal hordes governed by the primal father's two prohibitions; their love life was forced to remain egoistic and aggressive. Obsessional neurosis defends against a return to this stage. The [psycho]neuroses that followed belong to the new epoch and were acquired by the sons.

To begin with they were forced [by the primal father's prohibition] to relinquish sexual objects altogether, possibly they were robbed of all libido by castration: dementia praecox. [In the draft Freud presupposes the *reality* of castration, at least as far as the elder sons are concerned.]

Having been driven out by the father, they then learned to organize themselves on a homosexual basis. Paranoia defends against this stage. Finally, they overpowered the father in order to achieve an identification with him, triumphed over him, and mourned him [this characteristic mood-sequence returns in]: mania-melancholia. [In the draft Freud speaks bluntly of the actual killing of the primal father—he thus proposes a variation on the great theme of the murder of the primal father, of the origin of the sense of guilt and of civilization, broached in *Totem and Taboo* (1913a).] . . .

With heartfelt greetings,

Freud

On reading this phylogenetic fantasy for the first time—and then in this highly condensed form—one might be tempted to exclaim, as did

Richard von Krafft-Ebing, when he heard Freud's 1896 lecture on the etiology of hysteria: "It sounds like a scientific fairy tale" (Freud, 1985b, p. 184). At the very least one could speak of an aberration in view of the fact that Freud, only a year before, had observed with satisfaction that he had learned to "restrain [his] speculative tendencies" (1914, p. 22). It is well known that in characterizing his psychoanalytic method of research he liked to stress its empirical nature: "I am timid rather than courageous and gladly sacrifice much for the feeling that I am on solid ground" (1971, p. 187f.). Nevertheless he who had once described himself as having a "conquistador's temperament" (1985b, p. 398), in a tense polarity throughout his life, was also a bold systematist, who especially in metapsychology conceded a place of first importance to speculation and fantasy in his creative process.

In 1915, in the midst of his work on the metapsychological papers he had, in a letter to Ferenczi on April 8, described the "mechanism" of scientific creativity as a "succession of daringly playful fantasy and relentlessly realistic criticism" (quoted in Grubrich-Simitis, 1985, p. 83). By naming the sequence of ideas in the second part of his twelfth metapsychological essay a "phylogenetic *fantasy*,"[3] he openly acknowledged its fantasy character. He emphasized that he would burden the reader with "a number of hypothetical intermediate links" (Freud, 1985a, p. 13) and put forward "unconfirmed ideas . . . simply because they are stimulating and open up perspectives" (p. 11). But ultimately after he had subjected his daringly playful phylogenetic fantasy to relentlessly realistic criticism, he discarded it. *He did not publish and would never ever have published the phylogenetic fantasy.*

In spite of Freud's devastating judgment, I think that this document of failure is not only of great historical interest to us but has topical relevance as well. One could interpret it in many ways: as a rare example of a draft, an inbetween product, an étude from Freud's creative process; as a revealing autobiographical daydream; as a treatise on the origins of religion; as a reflection on the relationship between violence, privation, and the development of civilization; as a guide should we want to imagine a new man-made Ice Age, and think in psychoanalytic terms about the consequences of a nuclear winter, etc.

In this essay I want to read the phylogenetic fantasy in a different way again. I will try to show that with it Freud reverts to a central problem of his work in the 1890s when he developed the paradigm of psychoanalysis in a dialogue with Wilhelm Fliess—or more precisely, when he switched from the trauma model to the drive model in the

3. My italics.

etiology of the neuroses. My thesis is that Freud, in his phylogenetic fantasy, once again made an effort to integrate theoretically the traumatic aspects of pathogenesis into the drive model—a task with which we are still confronted today.

II

But why should Freud in 1915, 20 years later, with his phylogenetic fantasy, revert to a theme that had occupied him in his pioneer days? In fact, quite concretely, merely because of a number of outer and inner parallels he was reminded of the Fliess period. Shortly after he had sent the draft of the "Overview of the Transference Neuroses" to Ferenczi, he admitted, in a letter to Lou Andreas-Salomé, that he "often" felt "so alone," as "in the first ten years, in the desert" (1966, p. 35). As a result of the war his international relationships had shrunk or been cut off completely, his colleagues had been drafted. Only few of his patients were in a position to continue their analyses; in his "splendid isolation" in the '90s he had also occasionally complained about a decline in his practice. And, as was the case then, in a state of enforced idleness he was troubled by feelings of despondency and presentiments of death. So he fled from the misery of everyday life into soaring thoughts about his far-reaching metapsychological papers.

It is true that Freud's isolation in both of these highly creative phases was mitigated by his relationship with an exceptional discussant and correspondent: earlier, the friendship with Wilhelm Fliess, in 1915, with Sándor Ferenczi. Fliess, as Freud had told him in 1894, was the indispensable "only other" (1985b, p. 73); and he assured Ferenczi 20 years later: "You are now really the only one to remain working at my side" (quoted in Grubrich-Simitis, 1985, p. 77). As the surviving letters prove, in Freud's later friendships it is only the mutuality with Ferenczi that matches the intimacy and inspiring intensity of his relationship with Fliess. Both Fliess and Ferenczi were brilliant, fascinating, endangered personalities, deeply concerned in a boldly speculative manner, with questions of general biology. Fliess (1906) wanted to lay the "foundations of exact biology"; Ferenczi searched for a "metabiology" or "bioanalysis." From the one as from the other, Freud had hoped for help in constructing the biological basis for his deductions drawn from the psychical material of his patients. What he wrote to Fliess, on December 17, 1896, he could similarly have imparted to Ferenczi: "I can only gather facts in the psychic sphere, as you do in the organological one; the in-between area will require a hypothesis" (1985b, p. 215).

This "in-between area" was and still is today the domain of metapsychology which Freud, in the same letter to Fliess, calls his "ideal and problem child" (p. 216). And in fact, the term appears for the first time in the letters to Fliess (p. 172). Freud wanted to use it for his currently developing "psychology that leads behind consciousness" (p. 301f.), whereby with respect to the unconscious he always envisaged a biological dimension in depth. The most important metapsychological text at that time—the seventh chapter of *The Interpretation of Dreams* (1900)— also originates from the turn of the century. Thereafter, it was not until 1915 that Freud in the twelve metapsychological papers again devoted himself fully to his "budding metapsychology" (1985b, p. 324), that is, to the development of his theoretical ideas on the highest level of abstraction, a process in which he saw "the consummation of psychoanalytic research" (1915c, p. 181). It is therefore not farfetched to look at the newly discovered draft in terms of a resolute decision to take up once more certain themes contained in his revolutionary theorizing during the '90s.

In order to support my argument I must divert the reader's attention for a while to the Fliess documents, that unique log book on the origins of psychoanalysis. Here we can follow Freud, poised between anguish and joy, trying in bursts of creativity to approximate the goal he once set himself: "to throw light upon unusual, abnormal or pathological manifestations of the mind—that is to say, to trace them back to the psychical forces operating behind them and to indicate the mechanisms at work" (1936, p. 239). He is searching for "the key that unlocks everything, the etiological formula" (1985b, p. 45f.).

We have become accustomed to read two basic, consecutively developed etiological models in the Fliess documents: the trauma model and the drive model.[4] The trauma model in its extreme form corresponds to the so-called seduction theory, whereas the drive model represents the psychoanalytic etiological theory proper. As a reminder, the main characteristics of the two models will be sketched in a somewhat schematic manner.

In the mid-90s, Freud had frequently heard about experiences of child seduction in his clinical work. This led him to modify the

4. The term "drive model" referring strictly speaking to a later phase of Freudian theorizing is thus predated. It is true that the word "drive," used separately and in compound words such as *"drive* life" (1985b, p. 99), *"drive impoverishment"* (p. 102), "sexual drive" (p. 80), already appears in the Fliess documents; but there are as yet no fixed definitions, although the elements of the drive model are tangible in many passages.

etiological formula that he had developed with Josef Breuer—a formula which, in the tradition of Charcot's theory of hysteria, already acknowledged the influence of traumatic experiences, but with the emphasis being placed on those occurring in youth and adulthood. Step by step, in the Fliess documents,[5] one can follow the process by which Freud henceforth attributed ever greater significance to *sexual experiences in childhood* in the causation of neuroses. According to Freud's at that time thoroughly conventional conception, the sexually immature child is incapable of specifically sexual excitations, feelings, and ideas, and thus is "innocent." If a child is the victim in a sexual scene with an adult or an older child, this experience cannot be assimilated psychically. The child is terrified. When, with the process of sexual maturation in puberty, a further experience follows, which by associative connection is capable of reviving the memory of the earlier event and of investing it with the impact of sexual meaning, the mechanism of repression is set in operation—as it were *after the event,* following a latency period.[6] This means that overstimulation, this time induced endopsychically by the memory, necessitates the defense. Looked at from this point of view, the memory triggered off after the attainment of sexual maturity—"having a greater releasing power" (1985b, p. 163)—is incomparably more arousing, and in this sense more traumatic than the event occurring prepubertally. As long as the defense can be maintained, the condition still more or less approximates that of mental health. It is only when the defense fails, as the result of later conflict, that the path of psychoneurotic symptom formation proper is opened up.

This means that Freud, even in this relatively early transformation of his etiological formula, did not conceive of the pathogenic effect as being the spontaneous result of a simple stimulus-response mechanism. Rather he describes a diphasic pathogenesis at the center of which—alongside the sexual seduction—repression is to be found. That is, even the trauma model in the form of the seduction theory postulates a complex causal interrelationship in which external and

5. One could equally well reconstruct the seduction theory on the basis of Freud's published, i.e., official etiological papers of the time, especially the important texts of 1896a and 1896b. In these, somewhat different pathogenic assessments and temporal allocations can occasionally be discerned when compared with the Fliess documents—which do, of course, represent the more rudimentary and cruder original version of the emerging theory.

6. Freud occasionally emphasizes that in cases of sexual precocity, the arousal of the memory and the subsequent process of repression can occur as early as 8 to 10 years of age.

internal, that is to say, social, psychic, and somatic conditions, are variously intertwined.

Freud, however, soon had his doubts. Analyses were broken off in spite of technical innovations. To Fliess, he admitted: "I do not yet know everything after all about the mainspring of the matter" (p. 243), and gradually the insight grew, "that there is no indication in the unconscious of what is real, so that one cannot distinguish between truth and affect-cathected fiction" (p. 264). As he then, on closer investigation, discovered that his patients' reports of sexual seduction in childhood corresponded only partially to real events, he had the inner strength in spite of his disappointment, at this critical moment in his theorizing, not to push the fantasy products of his patients aside and regard them as lies, but to accord them the same rank as material reality. These repetitive fantasy configurations were taken to instigate a further and fundamental transformation of his etiological formula. He was prepared for this step because in the meantime two of his until then relatively independently pursued research activities had flowed into the mainstream of his thinking about the etiology of the neuroses: his revolutionary investigation of dreaming and his self-observation which had intensified into a rigorous self-analysis.

Against the background of a widening concept of sexuality, Freud now laid bare the facts of the intensive sexual life of children, the different phases of libidinal development with their corresponding erotogenic body zones and the structure of the oedipus complex. That is, he had launched the scientific survey of man's unconscious inner world. Because psychoneurosis betrays more of the rules of unconscious mental life and the hitherto strongly warded-off early stages of ontogenesis than normal adulthood does, it proved to be the access hatch into a new general psychology embracing normal *and* pathological phenomena: psychoanalysis. In other words, the etiological formula for the psychoneuroses widened itself unexpectedly to an anthropological formula for a fundamentally new understanding of the human condition.

The letters to Fliess show how surprised Freud himself was by the expansion of his findings. On the one hand, he was delighted, as "the barriers suddenly lifted, the veils dropped, and everything became transparent—from the details of the neuroses to the determinants of consciousness" (p. 146); to Fliess he declared: "I cannot convey to you any idea of the intellectual beauty of this work" (p. 269). But he was also horrified because most certainly his discoveries did not correspond to his thoroughly bourgeois—conventional taste. At the time he would probably spontaneously have preferred to cling to the cliché of an inner childhood paradise, of the undisturbed harmony of the parent-child relationship, and especially to the comforting notion of a sharp contrast between mental health and psychopathology.

The early trauma model would have permitted this: the seduction theory is concerned with those relatively *few* unfortunates—exceptions—whose parents, siblings, or other relatives or caretakers had assaulted them as children, as it were against all the rules of nature, and so introduced the possibility of an aberration in their psychic development. After all, long before Freud, it was well known that such attacks occur.[7] With his seduction theory, he had merely dared to focus attention on the pathogenic consequences of such assaults. By contrast, the drive model was—and still is—outrageous because it refers *to each and every one of us* and brings home the undeniable facts of our own archaic infantile love and death wishes, of the ineluctable needs of our biologically anchored drive nature, and of our lifelong endangered psychic structure, which, owing to its complex early development, ineradicably carries the seeds of neurosis, psychosis, and perversion.

Freud was under no illusion about the repellent effect of the findings on which the drive model was based. "In my case I can very well account for people's resistance in terms of the misgivings emanating from the theme" (1985b, p. 420). Indeed his own disgust reverberates in his joking references to Fliess about his researches in connection with anality, as his "smut" (p. 289), his "theory of the inner stench" (p. 288), or indeed his "Δρεκκology" (p. 290).[8] During this period he may have been constantly tempted to revert to his trauma model. In my opinion, by henceforth exaggerating the truly considerable difference between his two etiological conceptions into an either-or opposition,[9] he created for himself an intellectual bulwark against this emotionally consuming temptation; as early as 1897 when discovering the pathogenic effect of fantasies, one of the major components of his drive model, he speaks in a letter to Fliess of this "collapse of all values" (p. 266), but later, too, in his official accounts of the history of psycho-

7. See Freud's own references to contemporary publications on this subject (1896b, p. 207).

8. Derived of course from *Dreck,* but especially from the identical stark Yiddish expression (Rosten, 1971, p. 104).

9. "After I had made this correction, 'infantile sexual traumas' were in a sense replaced by the 'infantilism of sexuality' (1906, p. 275)—Freud does not write "complemented." How powerful this disjunctive attitude of Freud's was can be judged by its repercussions, e.g., in the fact that even Ernst Kris, an outstanding authority on the history of psychoanalysis, quite naturally perpetuated it in his commentaries on the first edition of the Fliess documents (Freud, 1950).

analysis, he bluntly disqualifies the seduction theory as plain "error" (1925, p. 33).[10] In this way, by catapulting himself with the help of a strong anticathexis away from the allegedly totally false trauma model, he succeeded in attaining the momentum in his creative economy to further approach his drive model against strong inner resistance.

But it is not in fact a question of two antagonistic models. Rather, what we have here are two successive versions of Freud's etiological formula:[11] the one—the trauma model—accentuating the obvious external factors; the other—the drive model—focusing on those invisible internal factors which tend over and again to elude our apprehension. Throughout his life Freud held the opinion that a sexual seduction in childhood, together with subsequent repression, could prove decisive in pathogenesis. Roughly 20 years after the alleged "collapse" of the seduction theory, he wrote: "There are cases in which the whole weight of causation falls on the sexual experiences of childhood, cases in which those impressions exert a definitely traumatic effect and call for no other support than can be afforded them by an average sexual constitution and the fact of its incomplete development" (1916–17, p. 364). However, he now knew that the external assault alone need not necessarily be a determining condition in falling ill. This could occur equally as a result of primarily internal causes.

Already in the '90s Freud had used his two etiological conceptions to supplement one another. It is therefore by no means inconsistent when, in the Fliess letters—even after the discovery of the pathogenic force of fantasy—he again and again returns to the traumatic etiology, depending upon which perspective he chooses to view the clinical phenomena. As he once said in another context: "The work . . . proceeds in loops" (1985b, p. 246), winding its way as it were between the trauma model and the drive model. While his further investigation of the traumatic aspects of pathogenesis is carried out quietly in the background, the exploration of the drive factors, especially the influence of the oedipal fantasy configurations and libido fixations, is emphasized and constantly discussed in the foreground.[12] It is as though Freud

10. See, however, the more balanced judgment in a footnote, added in 1924, to 'Further Remarks on the Neuro-Psychoses of Defence' (1896a, p. 168).

11. The succession also took place less abruptly than the words "collapse of all values" might lead one to suppose. As early as in one of the main papers on the seduction theory he considers: "But have we not a right to assume that even the age of childhood is not wanting in slight sexual excitations?" (1896a, p. 202).

12. However skeptical one might be with regard to the value of statistical statements in such a context, it might be of interest to mention the frequency with which the terms "drive" and "trauma" are distributed in Freud's psychoanalytic writings. In the *Concor-*

had to be continually on guard lest the latter should once more fall into that oblivion from which he had rescued them with such enormous intellectual and emotional strain. He pledged his followers and himself, so to speak, to maintain the dark inner world of man with its strange and unfamiliar laws, which he had discovered, unswervingly at the center of attention, even at the cost, if necessary, of neglecting the external factors.

III

In 1915, Freud wrote his metapsychological papers in the shadow of extreme, traumatic, external events, the catastrophe of World War I.[13] We must also remember that in November 1914, just a few months before he conceived his phylogenetic fantasy, he had finished his case study of the "Wolf-Man," in which a real seduction is central to pathogenesis. "The old trauma theory of the neuroses . . . had suddenly come to the front once more" (1918, p. 95). Both sets of impressions may have induced him when further differentiating his etiological formula to place the traumatic factors once more at the center of his theoretical efforts, as he had done in the mid-90s.

And if one compares the Fliess documents with the draft of the twelfth metapsychological essay, one is in fact astonished by the similarity of the main themes: now as then, he deals with structural comparisons among the psychoneuroses,[14] with the chronological sequence of their appearance in the life-cycle, with questions concerning the choice of neurosis, and with the problem of heredity. Heredity especially, in the '90s as in 1915, proves to be a cardinal point. As late as 1893 Freud, in a manuscript sent to Fliess, still supports the hypothesis that he had developed with Josef Breuer: "every case of hysteria that is

---

dance of the Standard Edition (Guttman, 1980) there are roughly 2,600 entries referring to "instinct"/"drive" (including derivatives such as "instinctive," "instinctiveness," "instincts," and "drives") and about 600 references to "trauma" (and its derivatives such as "traumas," "traumatic")—a frequency ratio of about 4 to 1—that, on the one hand, reflects the extent to which Freud had indeed placed the drive factors at the center of his researches; but which also, on the other hand, emphasizes with perhaps surprising clarity how much he nevertheless retained a lifelong interest in the traumatic aspects.

13. He explicitly expressed his thoughts on the long-term traumatic sequelae of this war in two papers: 1915d and 1916 (especially p. 307).

14. In the Fliess documents Freud mainly compares hysteria, obsessional neurosis, and paranoia, whereas the draft, as has been mentioned, is at first concerned with the parallels among the three transference neuroses (anxiety hysteria, conversion hysteria, obsessional neurosis) and then with the inclusion, alongside paranoia, of dementia praecox and melancholia-mania.

not hereditary is traumatic" (1985b, p. 40). When he shortly afterward raised the traumatic causation to its position as the main etiological factor in his seduction theory, he simultaneously reduced the weight thus far attributed to heredity. It is therefore not surprising that, in the famous letter of September 21, 1897, in which he writes of the "collapse" of the seduction theory and discusses its consequences, Freud regretfully stresses: "with this the factor of a hereditary disposition regains a sphere of influence from which I had made it my task to dislodge it—in the interest of illuminating neurosis" (p. 265). From the context one could add that the word "illuminating" refers both to the theoretical clarification of etiology and to the question of curability of the neuroses. Thus Freud in 1897 had to acknowledge that he had come up against an apparently immovable barrier.

It is precisely at the point at which he, 20 years later, deals with the factor of hereditary disposition in the twelfth metapsychological essay, that he tries to break through this barrier by stating with Lamarckian conviction: "When the constitutional factor . . . comes into consideration, acquisition [is] not eliminated thereby; it only moves into still earlier prehistory, because one can justifiably claim that the inherited dispositions are residues of the acquisitions of our ancestors. With this one runs into [the] problem of the phylogenetic disposition behind the individual or ontogenetic [one]" (1985a, p. 10).

Subsequently Freud reconstructs those events and acts that he held to have been laid down genetically in the constitutional factor. I will once again outline the phylogenetic fantasy narrative:

In the final resort, Freud ascribes the hereditary disposition to the transference neuroses to the radical environmental alterations with which our ancestors were confronted when the climatic change in the Ice Ages overwhelmed them and put an end to their paradisal, still uncivilized existence.[15] In order to survive they were compelled to produce fundamental innovations in their affective reactions, sexual habits, and ego capacities—characteristics that Freud, in a modified form,[16] thought were revived in the symptoms of his patients suffering

15. As Freud mentions (1985a, p. 13), he felt stimulated by Ferenczi (1913) in pursuing the idea of an influence of "the geological fate of the earth" or, more specifically, the "exigencies of the Ice Age" on the development of civilization. However. it was also an idea that preoccupied him constantly in a more abstract form—that of the relationship between outer privation and inner coercion toward sublimation. Time and again he spoke of "the pressure of vital needs—Necessity ('Ανάγκη [Ananke])"—which he called "a strict educator" that "has made much out of us" (1916–17, p. 355).

16. "The pictures naturally cannot coincide completely, because neurosis contains more than what regression brings with it. It is also the expression of the struggle against this regression and a compromise between the primevally old and the demands of the culturally new" (1985a, p. 13).

from transference neuroses. As a phylogenetic link to the affective storms and the ego alterations in the psychoses, he postulates schematically[17] a succession of violent acts in the primal horde, which had formed toward the end of the Ice Age as a primitive social structure under the leadership of the primal father; in order to maintain his dominance, that is, his absolute personal power and his right of disposal over the women, the jealous primal father, who had become ruthless under the extreme conditions of the Ice Ages, persecuted his sons and castrated at least the elder ones. The sons fled, organized themselves on a homosexual basis as a fraternal clan, and finally killed the primal father.

There are naturally many good arguments which can be advanced to reject Freud's reconstruction or, rather, construction[18] as unscientific. I would like to mention at least two of these which might lead us too quickly to declare the phylogenetic fantasy as unworthy of our serious attention: First, there is—even today—no conclusive proof of a Lamarckian mode of inheritance; an organism's environmental experience can at best produce modifications, i.e., changes in the phenotype; it is unable, however, to transform the genotype. In other words, information from the environment cannot, as it were, be directly formulated into the DNA. With reference to Freud's construction, this means that castration and patricide in the dawn of mankind cannot have led in any straightforward manner to a hereditary predisposition to psychosis.[19] Second, as we know, behavior does not petrify and therefore cannot be found in fossil form (e.g., Mayr, 1974, p. 702). It is thus a waste of time to ponder the question whether real castration and actual patricide were common patterns of behavior occurring over a longer period of time in prehistory, in an epoch which has left only meager symbolic traces.

These objections would not have surprised Freud. After all he knew that the biology of his time refused "to hear of the inheritance of

17. "The story is told in an enormously condensed form, as though it had happened on a single occasion, while in fact it covered thousands of years and was repeated countless times during that long period" (Freud, 1939, p. 81).

18. Freud himself emphasized over and again the hypothetical nature of his view of the primeval history of the human family by calling it a "construction," e.g., in the *Moses* book, in which he, however, likewise insists that it is not merely a figment of the imagination. "But anyone who is inclined to pronounce our construction of primaeval history purely imaginary would be gravely under-estimating the wealth and evidential value of the material contained in it." And after presenting such evidence he summarizes: "There is nothing wholly fabricated in our construction, nothing which could not be supported on solid foundations" (1939, p. 84).

19. See references to the more recent discussion in the realm of evolutionary biology in Grubrich-Simitis (1985, p. 101f.).

acquired characters by succeeding generations" (1939, p. 100). But this did not prevent him, at the end of his twelfth metapsychological essay, from fantasizing in a Lamarckian train of thought the solution to an enigma which continued to plague him. The question might be put as follows: What, in the last analysis, are the origins of the pathogenic terror of the threat of castration, the inextinguishable glow of oedipal love and death wishes, and the force of the associated guilt and anxiety which operate unabated in each generation anew? And, a closely related question: What is the origin of the sluggish pace of the psychoanalytic process?[20]

Perhaps Freud, in all the intervening years, did not cease to wonder at the *reality quality* of man's unconscious inner world that he had discovered in the '90s and with which he remained in daily contact in his clinical work. He stressed that he was accustomed to working with the unconscious "as though it were something palpable to the senses" (1916–17, p. 279). Brought up on the physicalism of the nineteenth century, he might have thought: something as undeviating and massively effective must in the last resort be rooted, or at least once have been rooted, in the external material world.

In the concepts of libidinal development and erotogenic body zones Freud had in his drive model, from the beginning, accorded unconscious fantasies a somatic foundation. With the reinstatement of the concept of hereditary disposition, he added a genetic base. In other words, the body—that transitional sphere between inside and outside, between subjectivity and objectivity, that inner-outer reality—was given a central position in his drive model. He did not deny that, in doing so, he surrendered part of his etiological formula, so to speak, to the darkness of biology, which even his friends Fliess and Ferenczi, experienced biologists, could not illuminate. When thinking in this border area, Freud had no choice but to use prescientific concepts when necessary. It is well known that he spoke of the drive theory expressis verbis as "so to say our mythology" (1933a, p. 95) or, about the nature of the process of excitation in the psychic systems, as of the "great X," which in the meantime, in the absence of more sound knowledge, he would have "to carry over into every new formula" (1920, p. 31).

20. A third question that might also have stimulated Freud, that convinced Darwinist, to develop his phylogenetic fantasy could be formulated as follows: Did conditions once prevail in the primeval history of man, such that behavior, which we under present-day circumstances call neurotic and psychotic, was perhaps of value in ensuring the survival of the species? "I have repeatedly been led to suspect that the psychology of the neuroses has stored up in it more of the antiquities of human development than any other source" (1916–17, p. 371).

At the end of his twelfth metapsychological essay Freud supplements the somatic and genetic foundation of his drive model with an extensive etiological reflection on the phylogenetic disposition that becomes apparent behind the ontogenetic one. On the ontogenetic level, up to this point the concept of hereditary disposition had served to emphasize the final anchoring of drive impulses and fantasies in the body substrate. On the phylogenetic level he now uses this same concept in order, at least theoretically, to loosen this anchor, as it were, to detach it from biology; in his rigorous research into the origins he takes a further step back and investigates the inception of these bedrocks of human nature.

How did these ineluctably effective, compulsive, stereotyped programs enter into the body substrate in the first place? He surmises that they are, so to speak, somatically fixed and transgenerationally inherited traces of environmental changes and social acts which really occurred in the external world and overwhelmed our ancestors in primeval times. Indeed, Freud, in the phylogenetic fantasy, imagines these events and acts as having been traumatic: radical changes in climate, existential threat through cold and hunger, persecution, expulsion, and castration by the primal father, and, ultimately, the killing of the primal father.

Evidently he is trying here to underpin his drive model with elements from the trauma model. In Freud's construction of the experiences of primal man, sexual seduction no longer plays a primary role, however, as once in the seduction theory. The trauma concept is a broader one. In the new transformation of the etiological formula that can be read into the phylogenetic fantasy, the drive model no longer appears disjunctive to the trauma model; instead they are brought together. Expressed schematically: no longer trauma *or* drive, but rather drive *and* trauma.

Nonetheless we should not overlook the fact that Freud placated his latent fear that the trauma model might endanger the drive model, by predating the traumatic factor back in phylogenesis; he separated it from contemporary psychoneurotics by a buffer of hundreds of thousands of years.[21] And let us also not forget that he accentuates un-

---

21. A few years after writing the phylogenetic fantasy Freud complained in a letter to Lou Andreas-Salomé, on February 9, 1919: "I am afraid that the whole primeval history of the family is still suspended in the stretch of time beyond my grasp, although I know that only its allocation with reference to the other dates of evolution can bestow on it its full value" (1966, p. 100). In the following decades nothing changed in this respect: "No date has been assigned to this, nor has it been synchronized with the geological epochs known to us: it is probable that these human creatures had not advanced far in the development of speech" (1939, p. 81).

falteringly the two scandalous characteristics of the drive model in his phylogenetic fantasy: first, in that it depicts the psychic condition of each and every one of us by maintaining that at that time *all* those who were exposed to the hardships of the Ice Ages and the violence of the primal father were then what psychoneurotics are now;[22] and second, in that his construction of the evolutionary beginnings of neurosis and psychosis conceptualizes these as phylogenetically normal conditions arising during successive stages of anthropogenesis, the frontier between mental health and illness becomes blurred.

In passing I would like to draw attention to the fact that in Freud's phylogenetic fantasy the outline of yet another configuration becomes discernible—something like a mythological contraction for the unique anthropological position of man with his "dual relationship" (Lorenzer, 1986, p. 1165) to nature and society. Freud attempted to take this into account by emphasizing the radically new epistemological position that psychoanalysis holds, with its dual relationship to the natural and the social sciences, to biology and hermeneutics (Grubrich-Simitis, 1985, p. 99 and p. 105f.). Again and again he tried to conceptualize the complex interrelatedness of three realms of reality: first, the natural and social outer world; second, the inner-outer body reality; and third, the inner world which is, although drive-controlled, highly variable because of the capacity for symbolization. Lacking a more suitable theoretical framework for his intellectual endeavor, he made use of neo-Lamarckian ideas, even at that time thoroughly unpopular. His interest was not, however, merely theoretical; it was also therapeutic in view of the fact that psychoanalytic interpretation, when it succeeds, exerts its mutative and liberating influence on this interdependence.

If Freud had to content himself in his metapsychology from the '90s onward with many prescientific concepts and purely metaphorical descriptions, in 1915, in discussing the phylogenetic disposition in his twelfth metapsychological essay he moves, open-eyed, into the realm of myth.[23] But scarcely having permitted himself this liberty, having felt his way from the darkness of biology to the darkness of prehistory,[24] he confiscated his sketch and returned to the solid

22. "An essential part of the construction is the hypothesis that the events I am about to describe occurred to *all* primitive man—that is, to *all* our ancestors" (1939, p. 81; my italics).

23. One should, however, recall Freud's question to Albert Einstein: "It may perhaps seem to you as though our theories are a kind of mythology. . . . But does not every science come in the end to a kind of mythology like this? Cannot the same be said to-day of your own Physics?" (1933b, p. 211).

24. Significantly Freud remarks in a letter to Lou Andreas-Salomé on May 29, 1918,

ground of his daily scientific work. The last sentence of the draft reads, disenchanted: "In sum, we are not at the end, but rather at the beginning of an understanding of this phylogenetic factor" (p. 20). Three days after sending the manuscript to Ferenczi, he wrote him, as though once more calling himself to order: "I hold that one should not make theories—they should arrive unexpectedly like uninvited guests, while one is busy investigating details" (quoted in Grubrich-Simitis, 1985, p. 83).

IV

Nevertheless in the later works we can still find offshoots of the phylogenetic fantasy. Freud's failed attempt to link the trauma and drive models with the help of a phylogenetic construction in 1915 continued to make itself felt, especially in the *Introductory Lectures on Psychoanalysis* (1916–17), the case study of the "Wolf-Man" (1918), *Beyond the Pleasure Principle* (1920), and later, once again in a splendid climax in *Moses and Monotheism* (1939). I would like to follow up a few of these offshoots of the phylogenetic fantasy.

All the main themes of the twelfth metapsychological essay reappear in the *Introductory Lectures* written shortly afterward: among them the six points of view in the structural comparison of the neuroses and the classification of the etiological formula on the basis of a complemental series of internal and external factors (1916–17, p. 346ff.). The discussion of trauma, here retraced to the earliest pregenital stages, as in the example of weaning (p. 366), and again presented with ambivalence, occupies a prominent position. On the one hand, Freud deals with the traumatic neuroses, especially in the form of the then topical war neuroses, in a train of thought disconnected from psychoanalysis, admitting that he had not yet "succeeded in bringing them into harmony with our views" (p. 274).[25] On the

---

relating to a possible explanation of a small boy's plant phobia: "Here the witch prehistory or phylogenesis must be called to our help" (1966, p. 89)—a variation on that *Faust* quotation to which he later used to allude in connection with metapsychology (1937, p. 225).

25. Looked at superficially one might indeed gain the impression that Freud had used "the dark and dismal subject of the traumatic neurosis" (1920, p. 14) as a not wholly unwelcome opportunity obstinately to maintain the disjunctive opposition between trauma model and drive model and thus to preserve, as it were, the pure drive model. A closer inspection, however, reveals that immediately after World War I, he had already suspected, as with the psychoses, that the traumatic neuroses too would fit into the psychoanalytic scheme "as soon as a successful outcome has been reached of our investigations into the relations which undoubtedly exist between fright, anxiety and narcissistic libido." He then continues in a vein that anticipates our modern view

other hand, one is struck by the many formulations that link the drive and trauma models. As when Freud emphasizes that traumatic experiences also play a part in the pathogenesis of the psychoneuroses, that these patients too can remain caught in their traumas. However, the etiological formula developed together with Josef Breuer in his preanalytic period had proved, as Freud now states, to be "not sufficiently comprehensive" (p. 275), "a greater wealth of determinants for the onset of the illness" must be taken into account; and: "we may also suspect that there is no need to abandon the traumatic line of approach as being erroneous: it must be possible to fit it in and subsume it somewhere else" (p. 276).

If one studies the diagram of the etiological formula in the twenty-third lecture carefully, one can observe how Freud inserts precisely this traumatic factor at all ends of the causal network: in those events occurring from *without* and leading to the onset of the neurosis, the traumatic "accidental experience" of the adult falling ill; but equally in the *internal* factors which promote the illness in a particular individual, his or her "disposition due to fixation of libido" which, in turn, develops from traumatic childhood experience and the individual sexual constitution. And once again, as in the phylogenetic fantasy, it is the constitution, heredity, that Freud considers to be effective in transmitting the primaeval traumatic experiences of our ancestors transgenerationally in a neo-Lamarckian mode. When patients' accounts of childhood seductions and castration threats, etc., verifiably fail to correspond with real events in their early lives, these accounts are, nonetheless, not arbitrarily invented untruths but compelling *primal fantasies*. In Freud's opinion, these relatively few typical primal fantasies are anchored hereditarily in each and every one of us as "a phylogenetic endowment" and preserve the record of real events in the life history of primal man. "In them the individual reaches beyond his own experience into primeval experience. . . . It seems to me quite possible that all the things that are told to us to-day in analysis as phantasy—the seduction of children, the inflaming of sexual excitement by observing parental intercourse, the threat of castration (or rather castration itself)—were once real occurrences in the primaeval times of the human family" (1916–17, p. 371).

The primal fantasy theme also pervades the copious clinical mate-

which modifies the sharp boundary between traumatic neuroses and psychoneuroses: "The theoretical difficulties standing in the way of a unifying hypothesis of this kind do not seem insuperable: after all, we have a perfect right to describe repression, which lies at the basis of every neurosis, as a reaction to a trauma—as an elementary traumatic neurosis" (1919, p. 210).

rial from the treatment of the "Wolf-Man." As has already been mentioned, the renewed confrontation with a pathogenic *real* infantile seduction in the anamnesis of this patient had influenced Freud's thinking in the second part of the twelfth metapsychological essay. However, there is also evidence for an interaction in the opposite direction—from the phylogenetic fantasy to the case study published in 1918. To the version written in 1914 but withheld from publication, Freud added comments on the "prehistory of neuroses" (1918, especially p. 95ff.), which, as in the *Lectures,* suggest an integration of the drive and trauma models by way of the archaic heritage. Finally he speaks of "phylogenetically inherited schemata, which, like the categories of philosophy, are concerned with the business of 'placing' the impressions derived from actual experience" (p. 119) and draws an analogy from such "hardly definable knowledge" to the *"instinctive* knowledge of animals" (p. 120).

Freud made a further attempt to integrate the drive and trauma models in his speculative paper *Beyond the Pleasure Principle* (1920) published two years later—without, however, considering the phylogenetic dimension. Still under the impression of the war neuroses he tried to capture—in his concept of the *repetition compulsion*[26]—the typical rhythm of attempts to bind the excitation elicited by traumatic experiences. The necessity for such assimilation arises from the preceding traumatic breach in the otherwise effective "shield against stimuli" (1920, p. 31). In the idea of a somatically anchored stimulus barrier we again encounter the body's inner-outer reality. Stimulus-flooding can occur through external events at the body's perceptual end; it may, however, also be caused by excitation from within, especially through "the organism's 'drives'" (p. 34). On this occasion Freud goes so far in bringing the two models together as to state that a failure to master such endogenously produced stimulus-flooding "could provoke a disturbance analogous to a traumatic neurosis" (p. 35) induced by external stimulus-flooding. It seems that we can regard the complex notion of repetition compulsion as a linking concept well-suited to integrate the drive and trauma models; the same could be said of the notion of primal fantasies.

The *Lectures,* the case study of the "Wolf-Man," and *Beyond the Pleasure Principle* merely offer a few examples of the many passages in the

26. In the *Moses* book Freud, without further ado, associates the fixation to the trauma with the repetition compulsion and, significantly enough, mentions the following example: "A girl who was made the object of a sexual seduction in her early childhood may direct her later sexual life so as constantly to provoke similar attacks" (1939, p. 75f.).

work in which Freud, after giving up the phylogenetic fantasy, continued quietly and unceasingly, to try and include the traumatic causal factors into his etiological formula. A virtual revival of the phylogenetic fantasy, however, is to be found in his book of old age, *Moses and Monotheism* (1939), initially intended to be entitled *The Man Moses: A Historical Novel* (Freud and Zweig, 1968, p. 102)—that final variation on the great theme of the murder of the primal father, broached in *Totem and Taboo*. I refer especially to the third essay in the book that Freud published with misgivings in 1939 only after his emigration to London. The book was written in the shadow of Hitler's seizure of power and of "a relapse into almost prehistoric barbarism" (1939, p. 54), as Freud stated in a preliminary note drawn up while still in Vienna.

A clear presentiment of the approaching World War II and hitherto unknown excesses of anti-Semitism and persecution of the Jews, a collective trauma of extreme proportions, seems to have driven Freud to renew his reflections on trauma and its effects. Several passages in the third essay read—even in the use of language—as though a copy of his old, discarded manuscript of the twelfth metapsychological essay lay beside him on his desk.

Once again the origins of religion are set in analogy to the etiology of the neuroses. Anew, he raises questions about *real* traumatic events in the external world, about "historical truth" (p. 58), to which, in the last resort, the strength of conviction and the compulsive nature of both religious beliefs and pathogenic fantasies can be attributed. Once more, he reverts to the "audacity" of his neo-Lamarckian construction that "cannot be avoided" (p. 100) and retells the story of those archaic acts[27]—murder or castration or expulsion of the sons, killing and eating the father—that exist in each of us as hereditarily anchored contents, independently of our personal life experience. These can emerge from primal repression, as the return of the repressed, moving from the unconscious into our consciousness. In comparison with the phylogenetic fantasy of 1915, Freud expatiates more upon those events supposedly occurring after the murder and ingestion of the primal father which resulted in a kind of social contract, in the first institutions, in drive renunciation, incest taboo, and exogamy, i.e., in "the beginnings of morality and law" (p. 82).

Even more resolutely and openly than in the draft of the twelfth

27. The speculations about the effects of the Ice Ages on the evolution of the human psyche, as expressed in the first part of the phylogenetic fantasy, were, however, not taken up again in the *Moses* book.

metapsychological essay Freud connects his phylogenetic speculation in the Moses study with considerations of trauma and its effects within the context of his etiological formula. In a new attempt to link the drive and trauma models, he qualifies the differences between external and internal causation by stating:

> But the gap between the two groups [that is, neuroses, in the origins of which infantile traumas are clearly demonstrable, and those where this is not the case] appears not to be unbridgeable. It is quite possible to unite the two aetiological determinants under a single conception: it is merely a question of how one defines 'traumatic'. If we may assume that the experience acquires its traumatic character only as a result of a quantitative factor—that is to say, that in every case it is an excess in demand that is responsible for an experience evoking unusual pathological reactions—then we can easily arrive at the expedient of saying that something acts as a trauma in the case of one constitution but in the case of another would have no such effect. In this way we reach the concept of a sliding 'complemental series' as it is called, in which two factors converge in fulfilling an aetiological requirement. A less of one factor is balanced by a more of the other; as a rule both factors operate together and it is only at the two ends of the series that there can be any question of a simple motive being at work. After mentioning this, we can disregard the distinction between traumatic and nontraumatic aetiologies as irrelevant [p. 73].

Under traumas Freud now includes "impressions of a sexual and aggressive nature" as well as "early injuries to the ego (narcissistic mortifications)" (p. 74).[28] They were suffered early and as a rule sank into oblivion through repression. After a latency period of "apparently undisturbed development" (p. 77) it may happen in puberty or later that "experiences occur which resemble the repressed so closely that they are able to awaken it" (p. 95); thereby the "change" takes place "with which the definitive neurosis becomes manifest as a belated effect of the trauma" (p. 77). Notwithstanding the widened trauma concept, the reader may well be reminded of the preanalytic ver-

---

28. Here the trauma concept appears yet again in a further widened form, namely, to include those narcissistic injuries occurring during primary structuralization with their corresponding effects upon defense organization, ego alterations, and character formation; i.e., including a dimension that was later to be explored further by Sándor Ferenczi (e.g., in his concept of the "narcissistic split of the self," 1931, p. 135), René A. Spitz (in his studies reaching back into the '30s, of the damaging "cumulative" effects of a failure of coenaesthetic communication between mother and infant, 1967, p. 156f.), D. W. Winnicott (e.g., with his "false self" concept, 1960), M. Masud R. Khan (in the theory of "cumulative trauma," 1963, 1964), and by many others.

sion of the trauma model in the form of the seduction theory, at times word for word as when the temporal sequence of pathogenesis is delineated as follows: "Early trauma—defence—latency—outbreak of neurotic illness—partial return of the repressed. Such is the formula which we have laid down for the development of a neurosis" (p. 80). Thus the old Freud in his Moses essay; the young Freud could well have written similarly to Wilhelm Fliess 40 years earlier because, in the Moses study, in contrast to the draft of the twelfth metapsychological paper, trauma is once again explicitly included in ontogenesis. Traumatization lies at the heart of the etiology of an individual neurosis in the same way as it also characterizes the group psychological events operating in the origins of religion: "in both cases the operative and forgotten traumas relate to life in the human family" (p. 80).

One might really think, for a moment, that in his Moses study Freud himself had occasionally lost sight of his drive model. However, he again sets the etiological formula back in psychoanalytic order, when he declares unequivocally:

> When we study the reactions to early traumas, we are quite often surprised to find that they are not strictly limited to what the subject himself has really experienced but diverge from it in a way which fits in much better with the model of a phylogenetic event and, in general, can only be explained by such an influence. The behaviour of neurotic children towards their parents in the Oedipus and castration complex abounds in such reactions, which seem unjustified in the individual case and only become intelligible phylogenetically—by their connection with the experience of earlier generations. It would be well worth while to place this material, which I am able to appeal to here, before the public in a collected form. Its evidential value seems to me strong enough for me to venture on a further step and to posit the assertion that the archaic heritage of human beings comprises not only dispositions but also subject-matter—memory-traces of the experience of earlier generations [p. 99].

And with impressive obstinacy, Freud professes himself once again to his neo-Lamarckian convictions, against the "compact majority" (1925, p. 9) of the biologists of his time: "I must, however, in all modesty confess that nevertheless I cannot do without this factor in biological evolution" (1939, p. 100).[29]

29. In this passage Freud briefly considers yet another transgenerational mode of transmission, alongside the Lamarckian one, for the "universality of symbolism in language": "The symbolic representations of one object by another . . . is familiar to all

These extensive quotations show that Freud here, in a renewed intellectual effort and in a similar way, tried once more to achieve a main aim of his phylogenetic fantasy: the integration of the drive and trauma models. It is probably no coincidence that such thoughts are to be found in a work with which Freud was as dissatisfied as he had been with his twelfth metapsychological essay and about which he had also thought, when it was first written, that he would never publish it (1939, p. 55f., p. 103). When he, in exile in London, did finally release it for publication, he apologized more than once for its shortcomings. We are accustomed to link the undeniable imbalance in form and content of the third Moses essay, which in Freud's judgment "included what was really offensive and dangerous" (p. 103) in the entire book, with the theme of Moses' relationship to the people of Israel, reflected upon shortly before the Holocaust. However, Freud's ambivalence might well have been amplified by his attempt to integrate the drive and trauma models outlined in the same text.

In other passages of his writings where Freud also endeavors to do

---

our children and comes to them, as it were, as a matter of course. We cannot show in regard to them how they have learnt it and must admit that in many cases learning it is impossible. . . . Moreover, symbolism disregards differences of language; investigations would probably show that it is ubiquitous—the same for all peoples. Here, then, we seem to have an assured instance of an archaic heritage dating from the period at which language developed. But another explanation might still be attempted. It might be said that we are dealing with thought-connections between ideas—connections which have been established during the historical development of speech and which have to be repeated now every time the development of speech has to be gone through in an individual" (p. 98f.). Finally, a reminder of yet another mode of transgenerational transmission that Freud had considered in *Totem and Taboo:* "psycho-analysis has shown us that everyone possesses in his unconscious mental activity an apparatus which enables him to interpret other people's reactions, that is, to undo the distortions which other people have imposed on the expression of their feelings. An unconscious understanding such as this of all the customs, ceremonies and dogmas left behind by the original relation to the father may have made it possible for later generations to take over their heritage of emotion" (1913a, p. 159); see similar formulations a little later (1913b, p. 320). This genuinely psychoanalytic argument conforms more to our contemporary attempts to understand transgenerational transmission of trauma than the neo-Lamarckian concept. When the primary object has been so severely traumatized that the trauma cannot be assimilated by the psychic metabolism, it is then unconsciously passed on to the next generation in order to be mastered—implanted, as it were, like a foreign body. The transmission seems to occur along primitive paths of communication that are as yet little understood, from unconscious to unconscious, through archaic transferences and countertransferences—scarcely on the level of the mental ego but more on that of the body ego. This happens with such oppressive inevitability and so close to the soma, that the idea of hereditary transmission of acquired characters easily comes to mind. (See, e.g., Balint, 1985; Loch, 1985, p. 10; and Lebovici, 1986.)

this, one is struck by incongruities unusual in a writer of his rank—as when he somewhat abruptly breaks off his chain of thought[30] or makes mistakes in cross-referencing.[31] Pithy comments such as the following, banished in a footnote: "this is the most delicate question in the whole domain of psycho-analysis, . . . no doubt has troubled me more; no other uncertainty has been more decisive in holding me back from publishing my conclusion" (1918, p. 103, n.)—are connected with the problem of assessing the appropriate etiological value given to infantile fantasies, on the one hand, and to real traumatic childhood experiences, on the other.

Evidently throughout his life Freud retained the attitude which had arisen in the Fliess period during the creation of the psychoanalytic paradigm, not least because of a struggle against powerful personal resistance. He continued to suspect that the comparatively agreeable trauma model might endanger the radically new, permanently offensive "more difficult and more improbable" (1918, p. 103) drive model.[32] Therefore all his attempts to integrate both causal sequences are beset by conflict and handicapped by ambivalence as in the 1915 phylogenetic fantasy. Freud's concern could be summarized as follows: By drawing attention to external traumatic factors in the etiology of neuroses, one opens, wittingly or unwittingly, an escape hatch out of the uncanny, threatening inner world that dominates our thinking, feeling, and actions and whose tormented and proud systematic discoverer he had become in the '90s. With regard to the external causal factors, he therefore personally took up a position that,

30. For example, in 1916–17, p. 350 (second paragraph); 1918, p. 97, where he himself speaks of an "unsatisfactory conclusion"; 1920, p. 14.

31. As in 1918, p. 103, n. 1.

32. This becomes particularly evident in Freud's contradictory attitude toward Otto Rank's theory of the birth trauma (1924). He admits to Ferenczi, in an unpublished letter of March 26, 1924, that he has not yet recovered from "the first shock of dismay," "that our intricate aetiological structure should be replaced by the crude birth trauma." Although Rank "nowhere explicitly states that he wants to place the trauma where the Oedipus complex stands, everyone hears this implicitly. . . . Hence the strong opposition." To Rank personally Freud had already written, on November 20, 1923, in a letter containing somewhat ironical commentaries on the interpretation of one of his dreams: "you are the feared David, who will bring about the devaluation of my work with his birth trauma" (quoted from an unpublished transcript). In fact, according to a letter from Ferenczi (March 24, 1924), Freud, when he first heard of it, had celebrated Rank's theory almost headlong as the most important step since the discovery of psychoanalysis. This can be taken as evidence for the attraction that trauma theories on the etiology of neurosis could still exert on him spontaneously—with the result that he had to distance himself from them all the more vehemently, in a second step, as he had done with regard to his own seduction theory, in the '90s.

because he naturally never lost sight of the helplessness and vulnerability of the human infant and child,[33] could be summed up in the sentence: *The traumatic is always self-evident.*[34] By contrast, Freud's typical manner of continually emphasizing the internal etiological factors seems appropriately expressed in a sentence from the third Moses essay: *"There are things which should be said more than once and which cannot be said often enough"* (1939, p. 104; my italics).

V

This attitude has been handed down to later generations of psychoanalysts up to the present day, perhaps more unconsciously than consciously. This may well have contributed to the superficial and erroneous impression that psychoanalysts refuse to be aware of and take seriously the significance of the external world and the damaging effects of real traumas. In fact, psychoanalysts since Freud have in no sense merely been concerned with pathogenic fantasies, dreams, and drive vicissitudes, but also always with the immediate as well as the long-term effects of traumatic breaches in the stimulus barrier[35] through flooding by excessive external stimuli.

This is the case, for example, when we investigate the effects on children's development of parental loss, physical and/or mental handicap in siblings, personal illness, surgical procedures and hospitalization, severe accidents, social and cultural displacement as the aftermath of war and persecution. It is also the case when, in the investigation of earliest ontogenesis, we pose questions with regard to the influence of pathological inner states and disturbed behavior in the primary object on psychophysical structuralization in the infant and toddler. As is well known, such studies may proceed as participant observation of the mother-child dyad, but equally as reconstructive understanding of transference and countertransference phenomena in the treatment of narcissistically disturbed adult patients, or as care-

33. "A small living organism is a truly miserable, powerless thing, . . . compared with the immensely powerful external world, full as it is of destructive influences. A primitive organism, which has not developed any adequate ego-organisation, is at the mercy of all these 'traumas'" (1926, p. 202).

34. In analogy to a sentence that Freud liked to quote, from the tragicomical novel *Auch Einer* by Friedrich Theodor Vischer: "The ethical is always self-evident" (1879, e.g., p. 21, p. 57).

35. More recent investigations, especially of the first year of life, have meanwhile cast doubts on the usefulness of Freud's concept of the stimulus barrier and have led to further differentiations; see Esman (1983) for a summary account.

ful attempts to influence therapeutically a pathogenic "fantasmatic interaction" (Lebovici, 1986) between mother and baby. Finally our attempts to reach a psychoanalytic understanding of the severe transgenerational inner damage resulting from the Holocaust—even though these began only after a long period of withholding of empathy—are also an example of the psychoanalysts' readiness not to deny permanently the effects of extreme traumatization caused by a real crime of unique proportions.

Was Freud correct in his assumption that we might be seduced into escaping from psychoanalysis with its unabatedly disturbing and narcissistically mortifying insights at the trauma end, so to speak?

As Sándor Ferenczi's clinical diary of the year 1932, published in 1985, shows, even this brilliant friend who had stimulated Freud to his phylogenetic fantasy, at times, toward the end of his life, abandoned the drive model, along the path of an exclusive emphasis on infantile traumatization. With regard to technique, this return to preanalytic concepts corresponded to an emphasis on the *real relationship* at the cost of the *transference relationship*. In the utopian wish to compensate for—or even undo—those infantile traumatizations through a tender and devoted "mutual" analyst-analysand relationship, Ferenczi at times revived cathartic and suggestive measures.[36]

36. This correspondence between trauma model/drive model, on the one hand, and real relationship/transference relationship, on the other—whereby drive model and transference relationship, i.e., the truly new and genuinely psychoanalytic concepts, represent "the more difficult and more improbable view" (1918, p. 103, n.)—can also be found, with inverted emphasis, in Freud. In his explicitly technical papers (the most important of which originated almost simultaneously with the twelve metapsychological essays), he especially stressed the transference relationship, presumably for the same reasons that led him again and again to place the drive model in the foreground in the etiology of the neuroses. From his analysands' many recorded accounts we know that he allowed the real relationship plenty of scope. This was for him no doubt as self-evident as the traumatic factor, and he therefore paid little attention to it in his theory of technique. On January 4, 1928, in a letter to Ferenczi, he complains that he had frequently been misunderstood because he had elucidated only certain aspects of the therapeutic process in his technical papers: "my recommendations on technique of that time were essentially negative. I thought it most important to stress what one should not do, to point out the temptations that run counter to analysis.... What I achieved thereby was that the Obedient submitted to these admonitions as if they were taboos and did not notice their elasticity" (quoted in Grubrich-Simitis, 1986, p. 271). When the Freud-Ferenczi letters are published, the reader will be in the position to follow Freud, step by step, as he accompanied Ferenczi's technical experiments and the corresponding etiological reflections with a mixture of initial benevolence and increasing uneasiness—benevolence with regard to Ferenczi's ingenuousness in following paths from which he had distanced himself with such great inner effort in his psychoanalytic beginnings ("activity" of the analyst, positive regard for acting out, emphasis on the

We can take it for granted that the resistance to Freud's burdensome anthropological formula will be revived again and again, although—or more precisely, because—in view of our experience in this century it proves to be very realistic indeed. The need to throw it off once and for all, even at the cost of a crude abrogation of logical reasoning, appears to have increased in recent times. In such an atmosphere it turns out that precisely those authors (e.g., Masson, 1984) who acknowledge solely the traumatic factors in pathogenesis, in fact, who wish to declare Freud's paradigm null and void, are able to arouse a certain interest in the media and in the general reader who is unacquainted with the subtleties of psychoanalytic theory and technique. Such attacks might have been facilitated by the fact that psychoanalysts, in the tradition described above, do not make a great ado about their researches into the pathogenic effects of real traumas—or even by the fact that some, in a mistaken excess of zeal, seemed for a while to ignore these altogether in their exclusive emphasis on internal causal factors, in sharp contrast to the founder of psychoanalysis.

To conclude I want to return to the phylogenetic fantasy of 1915. As psychoanalysts, we can extract three lessons from the newly discovered text:

The first lesson reads: We should continue explicitly, and henceforth relieved of ambivalence, to try and integrate the traumatic factors in pathogenesis into the genuinely psychoanalytic etiological formula, that is, into the drive model. If we get no further on the ontogenetic level, we should not hesitate to consider the phylogenetic dimension.[37]

The second lesson follows from the first: We should definitely take the phylogenetic part of Freud's legacy more seriously than we do at present. This would at the same time imply support for the undiminished theoretical claims of metapsychology. This, in turn, would mean that those of us who have a command of the appropriate knowledge or who could acquire it in dialogue with representatives of related disciplines must be ready to revise in Freud's metapsychological writ-

---

experiential factor in the analytic process); dismay, because he soon suspected that the paths opened up here could indeed "lead away from psychoanalysis" (p. 267).

37. See the attempts made by Krause (1983, 1987) to formulate a new and psychoanalytically relevant theory of affects in which he takes the phylogenetic point of view into account and presupposes culturally invariant primary affects which are "verifiably biologically programmed" (1983, p. 1030).

ings not only the obsolescent physicalism but also the equally outdated conceptions of evolutionary biology. In 1920 Freud had already clear-sightedly predicted that biology would prove to be "a land of un-limited possibilities": "We may expect it to give us the most surprising information and we cannot guess what answers it will return in a few dozen years to the questions we have put to it. They may be of a kind which will blow away the whole of our artificial structure of hypoth-eses" (p. 60). Even more succinctly, in some as yet unpublished work-ing notes, he wrote: "Science humbles the individual, greatness shrinks before the difficulties of acquiring real knowledge; each indi-vidual can conquer only a small area, each must go astray after a cer-tain point, only the succeeding generations can do it properly." Al-though the anti-Lamarckian furor of Freud's time has abated (Mayr, 1972), this has not changed the fact that the neo-Lamarckian con-struction drafted in the phylogenetic fantasy is apparently not tenable in this form. Nevertheless, we should not, as if embarrassed, set it aside too quickly as a conceit before we have taken pains to under-stand the conceptual sketch, which Freud also draws with it, on man's intricate dual relationship to nature and society. It is conceivable that the contribution to a possible solution of the body-mind problem[38] might one day be counted among the undying Freudian achieve-ments—along with the discovery of the unconscious and of infantile sexuality and the invention of the psychoanalytic method—and that in this "in-between area" the modernity and viability of Freud's think-ing would again be borne out.

And finally the brief third lesson: At the frontiers of our knowledge we should, with a gay naturalness, dare to indulge in creative fantasy, which also means, we should have the courage and the capacity to play.

BIBLIOGRAPHY

BALINT, E. (1985). Unconscious communication. Unpublished.
ESMAN, A. H. (1983). The "stimulus barrier." *Psychoanal. Study Child*, 38:193–207.
FERENCZI, S. (1913). Stages in the development of the sense of reality. In *Sex in Psychoanalysis*. New York: Basic Books, 1950, pp. 213–239.
———— (1924). *Thalassa: A Theory of Genitality*. New York: Psychoanal. Quar-terly.

38. For an account of the present interdisciplinary discussion of the body-mind problem, see Vollmer (1980); certainly as yet without consideration of the psycho-analytic contribution and the unconscious dimension of the "internal aspect."

_____ (1931). Child-analysis in the analysis of adults. In *Final Contributions to the Problems and Methods of Psycho-Analysis*. London: Hogarth Press, 1955, pp. 126–142.

_____ (1985). *Journal clinique*. Paris: Payot.

FLIESS, W. (1906). *Der Ablauf des Lebens*. Leipzig & Wien: Deuticke.

FREUD, S. (1896a). Further remarks on the neuro-psychoses of defence. *S.E.*, 3:162–185.

_____ (1896b). The aetiology of hysteria. *S.E.*, 3:191–221.

_____ (1900). The interpretation of dreams. *S.E.*, 4 & 5.

_____ (1906). My views on the part played by sexuality in the aetiology of the neuroses. *S.E.*, 7:271–279.

_____ (1913a). Totem and taboo. *S.E.*, 13:xiii–161.

_____ (1913b). The disposition to obsessional neurosis. *S.E.*, 12:317–326.

_____ (1914). On the history of the psycho-analytic movement. *S.E.*, 14:7–66.

_____ (1915a). Instincts and their vicissitudes. *S.E.*, 14:117–140.

_____ (1915b). Repression. *S.E.*, 14:146–158.

_____ (1915c). The unconscious. *S.E.*, 14:166–215.

_____ (1915d). Thoughts for the times on war and death. *S.E.*, 14:275–300.

_____ (1916). On transience. *S.E.*, 14:305–307.

_____ (1916–17). Introductory lectures on psycho-analysis. *S.E.*, 15 & 16.

_____ (1917a). A metapsychological supplement to the theory of dreams. *S.E.*, 14:222–235.

_____ (1917b). Mourning and melancholia. *S.E.*, 14:243–258.

_____ (1918). From the history of an infantile neurosis. *S.E.*, 17:7–122.

_____ (1919). Introduction to *Psycho-Analysis and the War Neuroses*. *S.E.*, 17:207–210.

_____ (1920). Beyond the pleasure principle. *S.E.*, 18:7–64.

_____ (1925). An autobiographical study. *S.E.*, 20:7–70.

_____ (1926). The question of lay analysis. *S.E.*, 20:183–250.

_____ (1933a). New introductory lectures on psycho-analysis. *S.E.*, 22:5–182.

_____ (1933b). Why war? *S.E.*, 22:199–215.

_____ (1936). A disturbance of memory on the Acropolis. *S.E.*, 22:239–248.

_____ (1937). Analysis terminable and interminable. *S.E.*, 23:216–253.

_____ (1939). Moses and monotheism. *S.E.*, 23:7–137.

_____ (1950). *The Origins of Psycho-Analysis*. New York: Basic Books, 1954.

_____ (1971). *James Jackson Putnam and Psychoanalysis*, ed. N. G. Hale. Cambridge: Harvard Univ. Press.

_____ (1985a). *A Phylogenetic Fantasy*, ed. I. Grubrich-Simitis. Cambridge: Harvard Univ. Press, 1987.

_____ (1985b). *The Complete Letters of Sigmund Freud to Wilhelm Fliess 1887–1904*, ed. J. M. Masson. Cambridge: Harvard Univ. Press.

_____ & ANDREAS-SALOMÉ, L. (1966). *Briefwechsel*, ed. E. Pfeiffer. Frankfurt: S. Fischer.

———— & ZWEIG, A. (1968). *Briefwechsel*, ed. E. L. Freud. Frankfurt: S. Fischer.

GRUBRICH-SIMITIS, I. (1985). Metapsychology and metabiology. In S. Freud (1985a), pp. 75–107.

———— (1986). Six letters of Sigmund Freud and Sándor Ferenczi on the interrelationship of psychoanalytic theory and technique. *Int. Rev. Psycho-Anal.*, 13:259–277.

GUTTMAN, S. A. (1980). *The Concordance of the Standard Edition of the Complete Psychological Works of Sigmund Freud.* New York: Int. Univ. Press.

JONES, E. (1957). *The Life and Work of Sigmund Freud,* vol. 3. New York: Basic Books.

KHAN, M. M. R. (1963). The concept of cumulative trauma. In Khan (1974), pp. 42–58.

———— (1964). Ego-distortion, cumulative trauma and the role of reconstruction in the analytic situation. In Khan (1974), pp. 59–68.

———— (1974). *The Privacy of the Self.* London: Hogarth Press.

KRAUSE, R. (1983). Zur Onto- und Phylogenese des Affektsystems und ihrer Beziehungen zu psychischen Störungen. *Psyche,* 37:1016–1043.

———— (1987). Psychodynamik der Emotionsstörungen. In *Enzyklopädie der Psychologie,* ed. K. R. Scherer. Göttingen: Hogrefe (in preparation).

LEBOVICI, S. (1986). Interaction fantasmatique et transmission intergenerationelle. In *Communications du laboratoire de recherches au 3ème Congrès Mondial de Psychiatrie du Nourrison de Stockholm.* Université Paris Nord, pp. 8–27.

LOCH, W. (1985). *Perspektiven der Psychoanalyse.* Stuttgart: Hirzel.

LORENZER, A. (1986). Review of S. Freud, *Übersicht der Übertragungsneurosen. Psyche,* 40:1163–1166.

MASSON, J. M. (1984). *The Assault on Truth.* New York: Farrar, Straus, & Giroux.

MAYR, E. (1972). Lamarck revisited. In Mayr (1976), pp. 222–250.

———— (1974). Behavior programs and evolutionary strategies. In Mayr (1976), pp. 694–711.

———— (1976). *Evolution and the Diversity of Life.* Cambridge: Harvard Univ. Press.

RANK, O. (1924). *Das Trauma der Geburt und seine Bedeutung für die Psychoanalyse.* Leipzig & Wien & Zürich: Int. Psychoanalytischer Verlag.

ROSTEN, L. (1971). *The Joys of Yiddish.* Harmondsworth: Penguin.

SPITZ, R. A. (1967). *Vom Säugling zum Kleinkind.* Stuttgart: Klett.

STRACHEY, J. (1957). Editor's introduction. In *S.E.,* 14:105–107.

VISCHER, F. T. (1879). *Auch Einer.* Stuttgart & Berlin: Deutsche Verlagsanstalt, 1917.

VOLLMER, G. (1980). Evolutionäre Erkenntnistheorie und Leib-Seele-Problem. In *Wie entsteht der Geist?* ed. W. Böhme. Karlsruhe: Evangelische Akademie Baden, Selbstverlag, pp. 11–40.

WINNICOTT, D. W. (1960). Ego distortion in terms of true and false self. In *The Maturational Processes and the Facilitating Environment.* London: Hogarth Press, 1972, pp. 140–152.

Early Reviews of
The Interpretation of Dreams

MARK KANZER, M.D.

IT IS TRADITIONAL THAT FREUD'S *THE INTERPRETATION OF DREAMS* (1900)
was predominantly ignored or condemned by the reviewers, both
laymen and scientists, at the time (Freud, 1950, 1985; Jones, 1953).
Latter-day biographers (Bry and Rifkin, 1962; Decker, 1975, 1978;
Ellenberger, 1970; et al.) seem to lean to the view that a one-sided and
inaccurate viewpoint was established. There can be no doubt that
Freud himself was greatly disappointed and chagrined when years of
effort which meant so much for his future, his family, and his work
received less acclaim than he had hoped. In our current approach
examining some of the earliest reviews, we have the special advantage
that Freud (1950, 1985) himself commented on them in his letters to
Wilhelm Fliess. We also have the opportunity to examine the original
critiques in full where Freud disposed of them in a few words, predominantly disparaging. Thus gaps between his reactions and impressions of later commentators can more readily be compared. Moreover,
we are able to examine the unabridged reviews in their original language, German, drawn from journals at the turn of the century, which
are not readily available for consideration in this country.

It would not be sufficient to show that Freud and his followers may
have formed a one-sided impression of these reviews. We favor rather
the recommendation of Bry and Rifkin (1962) that the exchanges be
viewed in terms of the history of ideas as interactions were formed
between Freud and typical cultural representatives of the period. In so
doing, we shall be fulfilling what Heinz Kohut (1976) has called the

Clinical professor of psychiatry (ret.); director, Division of Psychoanalytic Education
(ret.), State University of New York (Downstate); faculty, Psychoanalytic Institute, department of psychiatry, New York University Medical Center.
Freud lecture at Yale University, April 2, 1987.

ongoing task of each generation of analysts—namely, to continue the self-analysis of Freud from which their science was differentiated. At the same time, they continue their own self-analyses from which contemporary analytic science is being differentiated (Kanzer and Glenn, 1979).

I shall approach this task from the standpoint of Freud's mental state as the volume approached publication. To learn about this, we turn to the invaluable letters he wrote to Wilhelm Fliess, which he never expected to reach the public and which have not entirely done so even yet. Doubtless, he was much troubled by the intimate revelations that the dream book would bring to light about his personal life and relationships. This fearful anticipation has disturbed many a budding author of a first novel which reveals, allegedly in fiction, so much of his actual experiences to the family and friends who have been a part of them. The theme, "You can't go home again," is not always part of the fiction, but Freud with a wife and six children as well as a close circle of friends and patients did not have likely alternatives. Actually, he considered moving into the suburbs and building a new practice. In his case, the personal revelations that he had to make extended into areas that few novelists would undertake to follow. His daring could be justified only by its acceptance as a valuable contribution to science, but it was precisely among his fellow scientists, as he knew, that this was least likely, which indeed proved to be the case.

Moreover, it was not merely personal revelations that he had to fear but an approach to the scientific study of the mind itself which was to prove unprecedented and invited a shocked rebuff. Dreams were considered scarcely worthy of scientific notice. For ages, they had been the preoccupations of the superstitious, the seers into the future, and at the best of the philosophers and the imaginative creators of literature and drama. Shakespeare could effectively conjure up the ghost of Julius Caesar warning Brutus that the time of retribution was at hand—a hallucination that provided a very effective dramatic device—but Caesar could not be persuaded to enter the neuropathologist's laboratory for explanations and measurements!

Our exploration of Freud's troubled mental state as the date of publication, November 4, 1899, approached, begins a week earlier with a letter to Fliess on October 27, wherein he declares that he is awaiting the results with "resigned suspense" (1985, p. 380). The next letter, on November 5 and following the event, begins on a dismal note. In the book, he has given the name of Hannibal's father as Hasdrubal, who was a brother, instead of Hamilcar. He lamented that of course he knew better. His own identification with Hannibal, the Semitic general who could not reach Rome, perhaps for psychological reasons, is expounded in the dream book itself, while in a later work he discussed the oedipal determinants of his choice of the brother over the father (1901). We learn that it was his guilt at surpassing the father that entered into his own travel phobia about reaching Rome, and similar conflicts almost certainly entered into thoughts of surpassing him by writing a book.

The belated recollection of similar mistakes as well as early unfavorable reactions from others to whom he had mailed copies continued to dishearten him. On November 7, he reported that a reference to a close friend who had died offended the widow, another distressing casualty. Possible internalization of his woes followed—he referred to a migraine and writer's cramp which had befallen him. Next, two of his children were stricken with illness, and his wife and her sister commented on the resemblance of one of them to a relative who had died of tuberculosis. Apparently the atmosphere in the house had turned morbid. Friends who probably had not had time to read the book, or had little qualification for passing judgments on it, made only brief remarks which he regarded as condescending. Others found further errors. Apparently not a good word was said about it, and even Fliess stopped writing at this juncture. By November 19, Freud was complaining to him of cardiac symptoms for which his friend in Berlin had treated him in the past and which now were obviously an invitation for renewed care and sympathy. Impatiently he wrote on the same day, "It is a thankless task to enlighten mankind a little. No one has yet told me that he feels indebted to me . . . for having been introduced to a world of new problems" (1985, p. 387). (His own dream theories explained why people did not want a world of new problems!)

The first review actually appeared before the end of 1899 and should probably entitle the writer, Carl Metzentin, to a certain lasting recognition, but it cannot be said that Freud offered him much. His article appeared in a local Viennese journal, *Die Gegenwart* (The Present), and we take cognizance of it from Freud's own "counterreview" in a letter to Fliess on December 21 (1985, p. 392). It was not exactly a letter of thanks for a long-awaited Christmas present: "as a critical evaluation it is empty," he declared, "as a review it is inadequate. It is just a bad patchwork of my own fragments." "However," he conceded, "I am willing to forgive everything because of the one word 'path-breaking'" with which Metzentin characterized it. One might have supposed that this was some sort of critical evaluation. What sort of evaluation could Freud have possibly expected from an ordinary newspaper columnist confronted with such an extraordinary work by an almost unknown author? Even the title, accorded by the reviewer, "On the Scientific Interpretation of Dreams," conveys its own respectful message, and it is likely that Metzentin was too overawed in the presence of science to do more than use the author's own words as far as possible. In any event, the Christmas present was sent back except for the one word "path-breaking."

Freud added on reflection: "We are, after all, terribly far ahead of our own time" (p. 392). Since he was aware of this, we must wonder all the more at his severity with an admiring reviewer cognizant apparently that he was entrusted with a special book and a special responsibility in bringing it to public attention. Presumably Metzentin was practiced in gaining access to the language and minds of his readers. The fact is that he devoted no less than four columns to instructing them as to the details and significance of the dream book, all respectfully and instructively phrased. He pointed out such important aspects as that Freud placed the dream within the psychological context of everyday life and "astutely" traced it to childhood memories. The division between manifest and latent contents emerges as he admires the "thoughtful evidence" with which Freud justifies his conclusions. In historical perspective, he places him with Aristotle and Plato and above such contemporary authorities as Wundt and Eduard von Hartmann! The conclusion that the dream book is "path-breaking" provides a summary, not an addition. What indeed could Freud have been expecting?

Yet he was certainly not to be identified alone with the tensions that beset these critical moments and from beneath the surface of his personality; as I have been describing it, there emerged signs of the deeper core that had launched psychoanalysis. On December 29, as the new century was dawning, he dispatched another letter to Fliess—apparently a poem, even a hymn, which was not explained and has no apparent connections either with what came before or after, but is undoubtedly related to his reactions at this time. I shall quote the essentials of these few lines:

Hail
To the valiant son who at the behest of his father appeared at
the right time,
To be his assistant and fellow worker in fathoming the divine
order.
But hail to the father, too, who just prior to the event found
in his calculations
The key to restraining the power of the female sex

And to shouldering his burden of lawful succession;
No longer relying on sensory appearances, as does the
mother,
He calls upon the higher powers to claim his right,
conclusion, belief, and doubt;
. . . May . . . the legacy of labor be transferred from father to
son and beyond the parting of the centuries
Unite in the mind what the vicissitudes of life tear apart [p.
393f.].

As I have said, there is nothing that comes before or after to explain
this prayer or vision except the impact of the coming century and the
stake that Freud had now invested in the dream book. Perhaps that is
why his executors assigned it to the archives from which it emerges into
Masson's newly published version of the letters to Fliess. I myself can
recall only one really analogous thought in Freud's writings, and that is
in *Moses and Monotheism* (1939) in which his long latent identification
with Moses comes to the surface. There he suggests, with that touch of
mysticism which alternated and sometimes coexisted with his science,
that Judaism is an intellectual religion based on the affinity between
God and the older son, while Christianity is a more sensuous outlook
arising from the bond between the mother and the younger son (pp.
88–91).

Actually, this strikes me as reproducing in reverse the transition
from the oedipal phase in the boy to the formation of the superego.
Freud would have had experiences as a younger son in respect to
siblings from his father's first marriage and as older son in connection
with the marriage between his own parents. There is also an intermediate formulation in which he envisions the mother as protecting and
favoring the youngest son from whom the epic poet evolves (1921, p.
136). Elsewhere I have sought to explain these concepts in terms of his
own life history (Kanzer and Glenn, 1979, pp. 285–296). Relevant also
to the unexplained greeting to the new century is the wording by his
father of a dedication which accompanied the gift of the family Bible to
him on his thirty-fifth birthday in 1891 (Jones, 1953, p. 19).

Returning to the more everyday sequences in the correspondence
with Fliess, we find another possible allusion to the father. The next
century is now upon them and Freud's view of it remains gloomy. He
feels that the most predictable part of the twentieth century is that it
contains the date of their deaths. Then he concludes this thought with
the news, in an unbroken sentence, that it has brought him so far
nothing but another "stupid review." This is by Max Burckhard in *Die*

Zeit. The writer, former director of the Burgtheater, is not to be confused with "our old Jacob" who happens to bear the name of Freud's father and is one of his favorite authors. His counterreview is terse and succinct (contrasting greatly in these respects with Burckhard!). "It is hardly flattering, uncommonly devoid of understanding, and—worst of all—to be continued in the next issue" (1985, p. 394).

This conclusion is echoed in the opinion of Ernst Kris as editor of the 1950 correspondence with Fliess that the Burckhard review presented "an ironic and malicious distortion of Freud's ideas" (p. 307). This was of course a very brief opinion without further details, but even so we are not prepared for the comment of Henri F. Ellenberger (1970) that it was in fact an "extensive and learned, though somewhat glib review. Actually, it was by no means negative" (p. 784). Other recent critics have been in accord with Ellenberger, and we are reminded of the traditionally different measurements of an elephant depending on which part of his anatomy is being studied. It is incumbent to give Burckhard's own measurements not only to help form our own judgments but also to obtaining a glimpse into the reception given the dream book by a considerable segment of the Viennese population. I must remark that when Freud referred to this reviewer as the former director of the Burgtheater, I get the impression of a trace of a sneer, as though he must put up with even such an opinion. Yet as he was well aware, the cultured circles were more favorably disposed to accept his teachings than the scientists with their demands for exactness and proof, which are still used to reject psychoanalysis. Writers and artists have always been disposed to give weight to the imagination, and decades of experience with Dostoyevsky, Ibsen, Strindberg, and others had given acceptance to the meaningfulness of dreams, symbols, and even free association, which was being used as an established technique by writers long before it became the basis of psychoanalysis.

The theatrical background of Max Burckhard should prepare us nevertheless for the somewhat dramatic and authoritative way in which he conducted his review of Freud's book as he gave it a tryout. Where Metzentin had been impressed by Freud's scientific credentials, gave the title of his review as "The Scientific Interpretation of Dreams," and set himself the task of explaining it to the general public, Burckhard was not going to be put at a disadvantage so easily and simply used the title, "A Modern Dreambook." Though he began by conceding that the book was very interesting, he at once found fault with Freud's careful introduction in which he stated that he would not go beyond the bounds of neuropathology. To be sure, there was some conflict here with his obvious wish to win over the general public.

This elicited only sarcasm from Burckhard, who remarked that the book seemed intended only for the narrow circle of the author's colleagues, while others were being warned to keep their "hands off," a phrase he used in the original English, perhaps to show how wide his own background was. Next, he made the point that his public was accustomed to forming opinions about books on mathematics, philology, astronomy, etc. (under his tutelage, of course!), and will do the same about a dream book without the leave of a faculty of neuropathologists. After all, they may have common sense to offer in return—all this in the days of the absolute Hapsburg monarchy!

After this temper tantrum and the establishment of his own turf, Burckhard finally turns to the book itself and praises its introduction as comprehensive and instructive. However, he does become deflected at one point and that is where Freud quotes Aristotle as declaring that the best interpreter of dreams is the one who best grasps similarities—such as the poet. Unfortunately, it turns out that he is familiar with Greek as well as English, Latin, and medieval German and does not quite agree with Freud as to his understanding of Greek. This goes on for line after line of quotations in the original Greek from Aristotle without translation and I am unable to venture any opinion about this. However, this must have hurt Freud deeply as his mastery of Greek won him a special award when he was graduated from the gymnasium. In fact, he had been reading *Oedipus Rex* in Greek at the time simply for his own enjoyment and not as a classroom assignment—an eventful predilection!

Then, after delineating the mechanisms of dream formation as postulated by Freud, Burckhard actually announces that he himself can subscribe to them without reservation—certainly a great concession from this argumentative ex-theater director and scarcely in the realm of "malicious distortions." However, he does find an area in which he can be self-assertive and thus permit his ego to become dominant again. He disagrees with Freud more or less strongly on the subject of wish fulfillment, as did many of the reviewers at the time. It is not so much that Freud is wrong as that he is not always right in this matter. In refutation, he cites his own dreams which, remarkably, match Freud's experiences over and over again—dreams of the dead father, examination dreams, typical dreams, etc. It is the detailed presentation of his own dreams that makes his review so long.

Sometimes his dreams show wish fulfillment, sometimes they do not, and one may gain the impression that he is now offering the first revised edition of the dream book. Yet there is another aspect which was not remarked upon by Freud or his followers in their angry rejections of such reviews. The critics, like Burckhard, repeatedly cited their own dreams in weighing Freud's and automatically confirmed his viewpoint by taking dreams seriously and attaching rational meanings to them, correlating them with day residues, more or less accepting concepts of the manifest and latent contents, censorships, childhood memories, etc. There is no reason to doubt that many readers were being impelled to do the same, even as Freud was lamenting that his book was making no impression. Readers of the reviews did not have to buy the dream book to register their interest, but by 1902 when followers began to seek Freud out and he established the Wednesday night groups which were the nuclei of the psychoanalytic movement, they were largely laymen from cultural circles drawn by the dream book and associated writings, sometimes spread by word of mouth (Kanzer, 1971).

In seeking to understand Freud's failure to grasp at first the possibility and significance of such trends, we find references in his letters to untalented would-be students of the dream who sought him out and soon would be demanding to be analyzed rather than prove serious and detached investigators of dreams. We get another relevant glimpse into Freud's outlook when he informs Fliess, "I have given up my lectures this year in spite of very sizable enrollments and do not plan to resume them in the near future. I have the same horror of the uncritical adulation of the very young that I used to have of the enmity of their elders. Besides, the whole thing is not ripe" and he quotes from Horace in Latin, "Let it be kept quiet till the ninth year" (1985, p. 347). It is difficult to say under what terms Freud would have considered such relationships acceptable. Periodically he threw old notes into a scrap basket, not exactly a contribution to an understanding of the history of psychoanalytic ideas or their relationships to his personality. His technique of analysis combined both his fondness for resolving the riddle of the Sphinx in others and remaining himself a Sphinx in relation to them (Kanzer, 1984).

Although he dismissed it tersely, Burckhard's review continued to rankle in Freud's mind and later he hazarded the opinion that the former had found writing it odious and therefore had written an odious review (1985, p. 408). One can only wonder if he realized that the versatile Burckhard was also editor-in-chief of *Die Zeit* and had no need to publish an odious paper, much less write the review himself, especially in such a brief time and with an undeniable degree of self-involvement. While analysts often assumed that the external world came by degrees to accept Freud, it would also seem that there was a distinct reciprocity here. We can consider this aspect more clearly after reading the review to which Freud looked forward for so long—that of an academic scientist.

This took a while longer and materialized in 1901 with an article by a psychologist, Wilhelm Stern of the University of Breslau, in an unimpeachably academic Journal for the Psychology and Psychophysiology of the Sensory Organs (pp. 130–133). Freud's counterreview was limited to nine words. Not only did he not mention Stern by name, but he economically used these words to include another scientific review by Hugo Liepmann (1901) which appeared at about the same time. "Naturally," he said in detachment, "both are shocked by the intrusion into science" (1985, p. 454). Masson, as editor, adds in a footnote that Stern's commentary "is particularly disagreeable in tone" and includes the remark that "A special tendency, namely, to see sexual meaning in all possible and impossible dream contents, is made so much of in the book that it would serve no purpose to cite a single example: the fact that the material comes primarily from hysterics probably is responsible. The unacceptability of this kind of dream interpretation as a scientific method must be emphatically stressed, for the danger is great that uncritical minds might take pleasure in this interesting fantasy game and thereby drag us into complete mysticism and chaotic arbitrariness" (p. 455). A third voice, that of Ernest Jones (1953), establishes a consensus when he declares that Stern's review was "almost as annihilating as complete silence would have been" (p. 361).

Thus there seems to be an open and shut case for the rejection of the dream book by the first scientific commentary until Bry and Rifkin (1962) came along and actually found the same review "laudatory"! This is startling and, since we have learned that these authors are careful, competent, and well disposed toward Freud, we are bound to reflect that so far we have been given only two brief statements by Stern to consider and that in all scientific fairness we should grant his work a more detailed hearing.

Stern begins with the comment to his presumably confused readers, who have subscribed to a journal oriented to the sensory organs as the gateways to the mind, that *The Interpretation of Dreams* is not to be approached on that basis but rather through the inner meaning of dreams. Then he hastens to assure them that the author is a neurologist and not a mystic—a consideration that presumably will keep them from turning the pages and getting on with the next review! The title of his own, incidentally, is quite noncommittal, "The Interpretation of Dreams."

Stern then elaborates further on the meaning that Freud attaches to dreams. This is of something subjective derived from underlying important psychic processes which are disguised by the apparently absurd, confused, and disconnected façade of the dream and are related to the essential features of the dreamer's personality as anchored in childhood memories that are registered in the unconscious. These are translated into current experiences by the dream work which, however, rarely represents them directly among the manifest contents. The latter express wishes that may not be recognized as such but appear rather as undesirable. Their apparent subjects may be day residues. The divisions of the mind into unconscious, preconscious, and conscious components, and the roles of the censorship as delineated by Freud, are outlined. As with most other commentators, no challenge is offered to these unprecedented distinctions.

Stern next points to the background of Freud's view in his work with hysteria and apparently grants them an empirical scientific basis. In correct scientific fashion, Stern presents all this material before offering his own critique. "We must confess," he begins with a significant choice of words, "that this new way of looking at dream life and forming analogies with pathological conditions opens many interesting perspectives, but [we] must reject the theory on which it is based." The apparently reluctant confession as to the useful perspectives receives amplification along the lines which Bry and Rifkin have presumably been measuring when calling the review laudatory.

What seemed most valuable to him, Stern declared, were the many threads of thought, so little known, that reach into the nuclear world of the affects and in so doing make the choice of ideas intelligible. (Here he has obviously absorbed Freud's distinctions between the manifest and latent contents and the censorships between sleeping and waking life.) "In addition," he continues, "the book offers many details that are most stimulating, fine observations and theoretical outlooks as well as extraordinarily rich material with very exactly recorded dreams which will be very welcome to every worker in this field" (p. 131). This evaluation certainly bears the earmarks of admiring recognition and incentives to become better acquainted with this book. The tone leaves nothing to be desired.

Then there is the caveat about which he has warned us—certain aspects of theory that were taken up alone by Freud and indignant followers. First he finds that free association permits the interpreter to make arbitrary interpretations that are not convincing. Secondly, as pointed out, he argues that Freud finds sex everywhere (which his theories indeed called for) and could not be followed here either. Indeed, Freud alone at the time had formed these theories, which rested on clinical work not available to others and are largely excluded from the dream book. His theories about sex were sketchy and would undergo many modifications in later years.

If Freud wanted the reactions of the scientists of the day, he was getting them through Stern, which he must have expected. Yet, basically the tone was not ugly, nor were the commentaries, as we have seen, "annihilating." On the contrary, Stern seems to be finding extenuating circumstances by suggesting that Freud's sexual ideas were derived from his studies on hysteria, which to a considerable extent they were (tactfully omitting to observe the frequent references to self-observation).

This is a first recorded impact of the dream book on the world of science, and the reservations mingled with more approval than one might expect from an academic psychologist completely unprepared for such an outlook should have been far from discouraging. It must also be said that from the standpoint of the development of ideas, the need for academic psychology to become accommodated to psychoanalysis was only one part of the equation. Psychoanalysis was only gradually to free itself from the dangers of elaboration into wild analysis that troubled Stern. Interpretations became increasingly restricted to trained individuals in an analytic setting, accompanied by careful testing of resistances and transferences in gradual approaches from the surface. Actually dreams became only a portion of the analytic procedure instead of the mainstay, as one can also say of sexuality and its relation to the total personality. In 1938, when Freud wrote *An Outline of Psychoanalysis,* he announced at the beginning that he would present his material concisely and dogmatically since he did not believe it could be understood except with long experience in the analysis of individual cases. Fortunately, he published the dream book with greater confidence in the public than that.

With these reflections, I shall turn to a dream that Stern selected to bear witness to his difficulties with Freud's interpretations. It was the dream about R. being his uncle (1900, pp. 137–141), which has become a classic of psychoanalysis, but then all of Freud's dreams, unlike Burckhard's, have become classics of psychoanalysis. Oddly enough, it has almost nothing to do with sex and belongs, as do many of Freud's reported dreams, largely in the realm of preconscious memories and ideas. Briefly, and I am sure no extended presentation is necessary here, and I shall bring out later why I am dwelling on it at all, R. is a colleague who, like Freud, had not been able to attain the coveted status of a professor. Freud decided that the uncle in question was named Joseph, who committed illegal acts and was imprisoned. Jacob, Freud's father, was so grieved at this mishap that his hair soon turned gray. The dream interpretation offered is that R., who had committed some small offense, had been rejected for a professorship because of this minor "crime," not because of religion, which seemed much more likely. This gave Freud an opportunity to develop the fantasy that his own chances of obtaining a professorship were enhanced, since his own record was blameless.

Certainly the validity of such an interpretation depends to a considerable extent on the convictions of the dreamer and may well seem unlikely to others, as it did in this case to Stern. In actual analytic dream interpretation as it has evolved, immediate interpretations have largely given way to partial solutions which only with gradual penetration of the dreamer's mind reveal their full meaning. Even so, a gradual interpretation of the above, and other dreams, can be worked out if one becomes aware of Freud's canny techniques of apparently unrelated syntheses which led some commentators to refer to his "cunning."

It is noteworthy that the "Uncle Joseph dream" does not refer to childhood elements which Freud says must be there for a full understanding of the dream. At a later and apparently disconnected point, Freud tells us that the name Joseph in a dream often screens his own ego, for both of them were dream interpreters. Even so, he does not tell us that both were the younger and favored sons of a patriarch named Jacob. Applying this to the "Uncle Joseph" dream, we must wonder if the faultless Freud could have committed some crime which greatly grieved his father.

The dream book for the most part indicates great affection and respect between them. But there is a "minor" incident recorded which on closer examination may not be so minor after all. It deals with an episode in childhood, which itself evokes thoughts about the missing and indispensable portion of the "Uncle Joseph" dream that we require for its full understanding. Sigmund was disposed in childhood to bed wetting, which he later came to associate with the character trait of ambition—which, to the child, is to equal and excel the father. On one occasion it was not uncontrollable bed wetting but a deliberate action in which urination was used as a challenge and affront to the father.

> When I was seven or eight years old there was another domestic scene, which I can remember very clearly. One evening before going to sleep I disregarded the rules which modesty lays down and obeyed the calls of nature in my parents' bedroom while they were present. In the course of his reprimand, my father let fall the words: 'This boy will come to nothing.' This must have been a frightful blow to my ambition, for references to this scene are still constantly recurring in my dreams and are always linked with an enumeration of my achievements and suc-

cesses, as though I wanted to say: 'You see, I *have* come to something' [1900, p. 216].

The recurrence of this dream points to an unsolved problem in his self-analysis, and I believe that we can go further than he did in explaining it and relating this to the immediate problem he had in confronting his reviewers. There is certainly more involved in the case of this 7- or 8-year old boy, otherwise so well behaved and the darling of both father and mother, in his violation of "the rules of modesty" in choosing quite consciously to urinate before his parents, who were presumably in bed. It may well be assumed that the background was a primal scene and younger siblings were constantly putting in their appearance. It would seem that this was no ordinary "lapse in courtesy" but a genuine and heroic challenge in the oedipal tradition directed at parents who were abandoning him. Pathetic and megalomanic competitive exhibitionism at the root of "the character trait of ambition" obviously upset the usually fond and understanding father who responded with the contemptuous superego sentence, "This boy has nothing and never will"—e.g., castration threats.

This rejection by the father had the force of a constant countercathexis, for it became the subject of repetitive dreams which found no peace except for confrontations when, armed with new resources and achievements as he grew older, he dared to assert: "You see, I have come to something." At this particular time when Freud's neurosis was sufficiently severe to keep him in the throes of a travel inhibition which kept him from reaching Rome, it makes much sense to see him appearing before the critics with his great contributions on the dream and to expect unconsciously that they would disparage his accomplishments.

In the "Uncle Joseph" dream there are allusions to Freud's own resemblances to the disgraced uncle who so grieved father Jacob. There is no reference to the actual transgressions of the law which put an end to the former's career. As we now know, it was the passing of counterfeit money, and we are in no position to confirm the "wild" analytic interpretation that Freud, so long a member of the organically minded neuropathological community, shared with them in part the misgivings about the authenticity of his newer findings which even Breuer and Fliess, his closest associates in his researches, regarded dubiously.

Very relevant to these considerations is a passage in the introduction to the second edition of the dream book, which did not appear until 1909: "this book has a further subjective significance to me personally—a significance which I only grasped after I had completed it. It

was, I found, a portion of my own self-analysis, my reaction to my
father's death—that is to say, to the most important event, the most
poignant loss, of a man's life. Having discovered that this was so, I felt
unable to obliterate the traces of the experience" (1900, p. xxvi). Self-
analysis had found its limits in the bedrock of the father-son relationship.

This passage, which has so often produced wonder and criticism by
others who have not written dream books, bears testimony to the fact
that his major volume has claim to being a none too successful effort at
working through guilt after the father's death and carried over in
relation to critics the recurrent dream problem as to whether his father
was dead or still alive. Jacob Freud died on October 23, 1896. At that
time, Freud's views of neuroses were shaped by his conviction that
these illnesses were occasioned by seduction of the child by the father—an event that befell boys as well as girls. We find unmistakable
allusions to his own father in this connection. He interpreted one of his
own dreams in a letter of May 31, 1897 as occasioned by the wish to
"pin down" his father as a seducer (1985, p. 249).

In September 1897, as the first anniversary of his father's death
drew near—a very important event in the Jewish religion—significant
changes in Freud's outlook and life took place. He announced to Fliess
that he had given up the theory of seduction by the father as the cause
of neurosis and, while this left him at a loss to find a substitute, he was
glad to have done so. Then an inner remedy showed the way. He began
to dream almost every night; and with the dreams childhood memories
returned and the beginnings of recognition of the oedipus complex as
the cause of neurosis set in. It was not the sin of the father, it was the
inborn disposition of the child that was responsible.

Freud's incessant dreams launched his self-analysis. He recorded
them in much the same order as he dreamed them, and they became
the vehicle for his inner reconciliation with the father, in part mediated
by his constant letters to Wilhelm Fliess as father-substitute. This inner
Odyssey is certainly one of the most intriguing in the history of the
mind, one of the most productive. I believe that the history of Freud's
relations to the reviewers of the dream book and later of his other
works has much to teach us in rounding out our understanding of this
aspect of his development which stands intermediate between the collapse of his dependency on Wilhelm Fliess in 1901 and the beginnings
of a new substitutive force in 1902, the acceptance of a father's role to
his disciples, who discussed his work with him. The latter may be
regarded as the effective reviewers of the dream book and their de-

mands for analysis for themselves were pragmatic steps, like Freud's own earlier history, in achieving this end.

Summary

The analytic tradition holds that Freud's basic volume, *The Interpretation of Dreams,* was ignored or rejected by the earliest reviewers. Later commentators found, on the contrary, that the reception was remarkably favorable. My own research into the subject, drawing upon these reviewers at greater length than is generally available, tends to substantiate more recent historians.

The question is raised as to why Freud was so prone to feel himself ignored and rejected. Perhaps the most fundamental was his realization some years later, as his own self-analysis continued, that the dream book represented a working through of guilt feelings that followed the death of his father. I have explored the relevance here of an angry reaction by the older man, Jacob Freud, to his son, the future dream interpreter (Joseph) declaring that he would never amount to anything, which constituted a superego injunction, probably instigated by an interrupted primal scene. The dream book, as a supreme manifestation of the undying ambition to excel the father, drew rebukes from expectations of rejection by the reviewers.

BIBLIOGRAPHY

Bry, I. & Rifkin, A. (1962). Freud and the history of ideas. *Sci. & Psychoanal.,* 5:6–36.
Burckhard, M. (1900). Die Traumdeutung. *Die Zeit,* Jan. 6, 22:9–11; Jan. 13, 22:25–27.
Decker, H. S. (1975). Book review: *The Interpretation of Dreams* by Sigmund Freud. *J. Hist. Behav. Sci.,* 11:129–141.
———— (1978). Psychoanalysis and the Europeans. In *American Psychoanalysis,* ed. J. M. Quen & E. T. Carlson. New York: Brunner-Mazel, pp. 1–19.
Ellenberger, H. F. (1970). *The Discovery of the Unconscious.* New York: Basic Books.
Freud, S. (1900). The interpretation of dreams. *S.E.,* 4 & 5.
———— (1901). The psychopathology of everyday life. *S.E.,* 6.
———— (1921). Group psychology and the analysis of the ego. *S.E.,* 18:67–143.
———— (1938). An outline of psycho-analysis. *S.E.,* 23:141–207.
———— (1939). Moses and monotheism. *S.E.,* 23:3–137.
———— (1950). *The Origins of Psychoanalysis.* New York: Basic Books, 1954.

———— (1985). *The Complete Letters of Sigmund Freud to Wilhelm Fliess,* ed. J. M. Masson. Cambridge, Mass.: Harvard Univ. Press.

JONES, E. (1953). *The Life and Work of Sigmund Freud,* vol. 1. New York: Basic Books.

KANZER, M. (1971). Freud, the first psychoanalytic group leader. In *Comprehensive Group Psychotherapy,* ed. H. I. Kaplan & B. J. Sadock. Baltimore: William & Wilkins.

———— (1984). Freud: The Greek family romance. Freud lecture, New York Psychoanalytic Institute.

———— & GLENN, J. (1979). *Freud and His Self-Analysis.* New York: Aronson.

KOHUT, H. (1976). Creativeness, charisma, group psychology. In *The Search for the Self,* ed. P. W. Ornstein. New York: Int. Univ. Press, 1978, pp. 793–844.

LIEPMANN, H. (1901). Über den Traum, S. Freud. *Mschr. Psychiat. & Neurol.,* 10:273–279.

METZENTIN, C. (1899). Über wissenschaftliche Traumdeutung. *Die Gegenwart,* Dez. 16, 30:386–389.

STERN, W. (1901). S. Freud, Die Traumdeutung. *Z. Psychol. & Physiol. Sinnesorgane,* 26:130–133.

PSYCHOANALYTIC
THEORY

The Transference Neurosis in Child Analysis

JUDITH FINGERT CHUSED, M.D.

THE DEVELOPMENT OF A TRANSFERENCE NEUROSIS, MANIFESTED BY SYMP-
toms or the intensification of characteristic, pathological modes of perception and interaction in relation to the analyst, is, I believe, the *sine
qua non* of psychoanalysis. Although every attempt at analysis does not
result in a transference neurosis (or an analysis), when a full analytic
process occurs, analysis of the transference neurosis is a central element. Many analysts believe it to be the pivotal mutative experience in
adult analysis; this, however, is not the general opinion for child analysis. Until recently, most child analysts in the United States (other than
the followers of Melanie Klein) saw the child as having a limited capacity to form and sustain a transference neurosis. Although this perception of analysis with children is changing, and a growing number of
analysts today practice "adult-type" child analysis, there remain many
who believe children do not develop transference manifestations and
transference neuroses as adults do, in either frequency, endurance, or
depth. The determinants of this belief lie both in the preconceptions
and political struggles that mark the history of child analysis and in
certain characteristics of child analysis itself.

I have not found intense transference manifestations developing
around the person of the analyst unusual in children; quite the contrary, without it I find there is no analysis (though there may be very
good psychotherapy). However, if the term "transference neurosis" is
limited to the development within the analytic situation of a new neurosis, complete with a new set of symptoms, then I have to agree that
this is not a regular occurrence in the analysis of children (or adults).

Training and supervising analyst at the Washington Psychoanalytic Institute, Washington, D.C., and an associate clinical professor of psychiatry at George Washington
University School of Medicine.

This is the definition recommended by Marjorie Harley (1971). But if "transference neurosis" is broadened to include the intensification of pathological character traits and modes of relating within the analytic setting, with the gradual emergence of regressive, incestuous fantasies, conflicts, and impulses experienced in relation to and centered on the analyst, and with the intensity of affect and sense of reality described by Bird (1972), then an analyzable transference neurosis can develop almost as frequently with children as with adults. This definition of transference neurosis is similar to that advanced by Sandler et al. (1975): "By transference neurosis we mean the concentration of the child's conflicts, repressed infantile wishes, fantasies, etc., on the person of the therapist, *with the relative diminution of their manifestations elsewhere*" (p. 427).

If the development and utilization of a transference neurosis can be an integral part of child analysis, then when children *fail* to develop an analyzable transference neurosis, we need to question why this is. After a child has developed sufficient capacity to retain a memory of human interactions and to form an internal mental representation of an object, he has the capacity for transference, to "misperceive" an interaction with one person so that it "feels" the same as with another. And when he has sufficient structural development to sustain intersystemic conflicts (Panel, 1966), and the ego capacity to tolerate (even minimally and only transiently) conflictual feelings, impulses, and fantasies, he can develop a transference neurosis. But whether the child develops a transference neurosis, and if he does, how it is utilized for the work of analysis, will depend not only on his level of development and his individual psychopathology, but also on the theoretical position of the analyst. The analyst's theory and his expectations, regardless of his neutrality, always influence his perceptions and his technique.

One consequence of the skepticism about transference neurosis in children is that it has led to a discrediting of conflict resolution as the major mutative element in work with children. Although theoretical discussions support conflict resolution as the core therapeutic agent in child analysis, clinical presentations often emphasize other elements, such as the relationship with the analyst as a "real object," as important for the therapeutic efficacy of the work. On occasion this has obfuscated the distinction between child analysis and child psychotherapy, leading analysts of adults to declare that "child analysis isn't really analysis."

Historically, child analysis began with Freud's analysis of Little Hans (1909) conducted through the child's father. The report of this case opened up a world of possibilities to analysts, who hoped that because children were in close temporal proximity to the origin of their neurotic conflicts, the conflicts would be available for rapid resolution through the analytic method. However, analysts trained in working with adults quickly found the work with children extremely frustrating; Ferenczi (1913) decided that "direct psycho-analytic investigation was therefore impossible" (p. 244) when his attempts with a 5-year-old boy failed because the child was bored and wanted to get back to his toys. Analytic work with children soon became the province of educators and pediatricians. From the start, therapists such as the teacher Hug-Hellmuth (1921, 1924), Anna Freud (1927), and Dorothy Burlingham (1932), whose work Hug-Hellmuth influenced, were sensitive to the unique characteristics of the child and felt that the techniques and tools of child analysis would have to be modified; specifically, that the relative abstinence and neutrality utilized in adult analyses should be set aside as intolerable to children who would neither participate in nor benefit from analysis under nongratifying conditions. They also believed that since the child was still very attached to and quite dependent on his original objects, his parents, there would be no transference or transference neurosis formed around the person of the analyst. At this time the difference between the psychic representation of the child's earlier relationship with his parents and the external reality of his present relationship with them was not yet elucidated; the relationship of the past and present were seen as the same, and being currently active, as nontransferable. In addition, the awareness of the developmental need for a positive attachment between mother and child led to a belief among these early child analysts that if analytic work was to enable the child to resume progressive development, a similar type of positive attachment to the analyst was essential.

The work of Melanie Klein and her colleagues, presented in a panel in 1926 and reported in the *International Journal of Psychoanalysis* in 1927, reveals a very different perception of child analysis. But until recently, their work has had little influence on the majority of child analysts in the United States.

It was Anna Freud who had the dominant influence on child analysis in the United States. Her beliefs, including that it was important for the child *to want* to come to analysis, led child analysts to present themselves as benevolent providers, with gifts, skills, or powers (even omnipotence) the child would value (A. Freud, 1927; Bornstein, 1949). It gradually became apparent that exuberant benevolence was not needed to ensure the child's participation in the analysis. But though the seductions and gratifications that occurred in the early years of child analysis are now no longer sanctioned, many analysts still believe it is important for them to be perceived as a "benevolent object." This has led to a self-perpetuating problem in child analysis: an analyst who believes the child cannot tolerate significant deprivation in analysis can justify the very gratification that interferes with the full development of transference and a transference neurosis. Thus it is not surprising that in a recent Panel (1983) on the reanalysis of child patients, those contributors who held this belief found that "A transference neurosis, which requires the ability to contain an internal conflict, does not develop before the end of latency" (p. 684), and that "the transference had not been analyzed" (p. 686).

By the 1950s and 1960s most analysts (Harley, 1986, p. 133) recognized that children had transference reactions to the analyst and that these could be utilized for interpretations and clarifications much as in work with adults. Yet there was still a general feeling that because of the immaturity of the child's psychic structure and the continuing dependence on the parents, transference neurosis as such did not occur with children; that since transference manifestations were so fluid and of such relatively short duration, they did not occupy the same central role in the child's analysis as in the adult's. Only when case reports of fully developed transference neuroses in children began to appear in the analytic literature (Kut, 1953; Fraiberg, 1966; Harley, 1967) did the concept gain more acceptance.

Anna Freud (1965) later modified her position, and her observation that a transference neurosis can develop in children but does not equal the adult variety in every respect (p. 36) is currently quoted or referred to in almost every article on transference neurosis in children. The accuracy of her observations of children's behavior in analysis (their inability to free associate, the preponderance of aggressive transference reactions, the use of the analyst as a real object, and their tendency to externalization of psychic structures onto the analyst) lends credence to her conclusion that the transference neurosis is less significant in child analysis than in adult analysis. However, the factors which she described as limiting the development of a transference neurosis in child analysis are also found in adult analyses, and some analysts (Bird, 1972) believe these are the very factors that constitu the transference neurosis. I sense, instead, that the specific limitin factor to the development of a transference neurosis in child analys arises from the analyst and the child patient automatically respondin to each other as *adult* and *child,* falling into customary roles of adu.. who educates and/or directs, child who learns, complies, or rebels. This is similar to the problem Bird (1972) alludes to in adult analyses when he said, "One of the most serious problems of analysis is the very substantial help which the patient receives directly from the analyst and the analytic situation" (p. 285).

For example, with an intensification of transference, not infrequently a child will create bigger and bigger messes in the office, regressively trying to engage the analyst in a reenactment of anal-phase struggles (P. Tyson, 1978, p. 227). It is extraordinarily difficult for the analyst to time his interventions so that the child experiences the impulse but does not become so overwhelmed by the associated affects that he loses the capacity to hear verbal interventions. Children move very fast—objects are broken, guilt escalates, and behavior gets out of control as the attempt to elicit punishment intensifies. A conflict is repeated rather than remembered and verbalized. At this point there is a temptation for the analyst to control the child's behavior and instruct (which often contains superego injunctions). However, if the analyst can provide (and the child receive) the structure necessary to halt regression and support self-observing ego capacities, if he analyzes rather than educates, a new solution based on experience can be forged. Enactment of a conflict, a common occurrence in child analysis, does not always require the interruption of an analytic attitude in the analyst. Abstinence is important not only in its effect on the patient; its effect on the analyst is to permit him to become more an "analyzing" and less a "modifying" force.

Unintentionally Anna Freud's words (1965) have contributed to a premature closure of the issue of transference neurosis in child analysis. Analysts have yet to explore adequately: (1) What inhibits the full development of transference and a transference neurosis in child patients? (2) In which ways does this inhibition alter the treatment? (3) How, if the development of a transference neurosis with child patients is useful, might it be facilitated? Excellent papers have been written (Sandler et al., 1975; Harley, 1986; R. L. and P. Tyson, 1986) in which transference and the transference neurosis in children are discussed. Unfortunately, they offer little new understanding as to its infrequent appearance, with Harley's doing just the opposite: looking for something out of the ordinary in the child who does develop a transference neurosis.

In my experience, transference and transference neuroses are not uncommon in the analysis of children, although they do differ in some respects from their adult counterparts. In children, as in adults, oedipal conflicts are a significant feature of the transference neurosis, with these conflicts reflecting not only pathogenic experiences during the oedipal period but also organizing pathology derived from earlier preoedipal phases. When the developmental level of the child's ego functions, including cognitive development, affect tolerance, narcissistic vulnerability, and maturity of defenses are taken into account, as well as the nature of the child's attachment to his current objects (R. L. and P. Tyson, 1986), a thoughtful analytic procedure, with strict attention to the analysis of resistance and to countertransference interferences, can lead to a full-blown transference neurosis in the child patient.

I reached this conclusion several years ago when I was analyzing, concurrently, two girls, Sarah (11 years old) and Molly (10 years old), both of whom had an intensely negative transference to me. During the many months when exploration of the determinants of their negative feelings did little to alter their behavior, I had ample time to examine our interactions. Three observations stand out: (1) The negative transference from these children was much more unpleasant than negative transference from adults—they were hypersensitive to and openly critical of my failings, and I, in turn, was sensitive to their comments. (2) Even though there was no evidence of any positive feeling from either child and both spoke of wanting to quit the analysis, material continued to emerge that could be beneficially utilized. (3) My initial response to their negative feelings was less abstinent than with adults. Specifically, my attempts to educate them about transference as a phenomenon were clearly defensive, as were some of my interpretations, which in retrospect were intended to dissipate the transference rather than understand it. In both cases, the patients picked up on my defensiveness: one became frightened she had hurt me and went through a brief period of "goodness" with some hypochondriacal obsessing during the sessions; the other became more sullen and withdrawn, as if she experienced my defensiveness as coercive, which, I fear, it was unconsciously intended to be.

With adults one expects negative transference reactions; their absence raises concern about defensive compliance, the possibility of a "good" patient who "loves" analysis but derives no lasting benefit from it. Yet during training, most child analysts are taught to maintain a positive therapeutic alliance with the child patient. They learn that though they should not gratify with the aim of suppressing the child's hostile feelings, they must prevent deprivations which would arouse so much negative affect that active participation in the analytic work ceases (Sandler et al., 1980).

I was powerless to alter, through any change in my demeanor, Molly's and Sarah's dislike and distrust of me, their perception of me as potentially hurtful, instead of helpful. And, with an abstinence dictated as much by the patient as by theory, what began as negative transference went on to become a transference neurosis, similar in that both girls concentrated their rage and feelings of deprivation and injury on me (with an increasingly positive interaction with the outside world), but different in the specific content and course of development. However, in both children the transference neurosis was relatively uncontaminated by any attempt on my part to maintain a therapeutic alliance or be a benevolent "good object."

The analytic process with these two children was interesting. Molly, who had recreated with me the horror of her fourth through sixth years, when she had spent many hours alone in a hospital waiting room while her already depressed and unavailable mother attended to her baby brother who had leukemia, continued to feel negative about me until termination. However, during the last year she continued in the analysis voluntarily (that is, she no longer begged her parents to let her quit), because she thought it was doing her some good. During the earlier "months of hate," the ideational content of her negative attitude changed several times. Her perception of me as nonempathic and "not too smart" (which developed in the sixth month in response to what had been intended as neutral questions about her drawings and description of a future world) shifted gradually to a quite competitive and aggressively taunting battle over when and what she would talk about, followed by a long period in which I was seen as intrusive and controlling. The associations in this period were to her father, and were both provocative of and defensive against the gratification she had experienced when he (in part in response to his wife's preoccupation with their ill son) had begun to spend large amounts of time with Molly, instructing her about intellectual matters in a domineering, impatient manner.

After the termination date was set, Molly's attitude toward me changed dramatically. As we examined the change during our final months together, she was able to talk about her longing to be nurtured and loved by me, her disappointment in me, and her awareness that she could not see me as anything but disappointing—anything more would have been too scary (and too stimulating) and would have made thoughts of the past too painful.

Sarah, on the other hand, had a more abbreviated period of negative feeling about me, though hers was the more intense, with a definite paranoid flavor. In addition to imagining that I was taping the sessions with the aim of blackmailing her, she also feared, for a one-week period, that there was poison gas in the office room and during several other isolated sessions was frightened that I was trying to hypnotize her. What emerged during the course of her analysis was an erotic attachment to her mother, which played itself out in the transference neurosis, complete with perverse sexual fantasies and intense rivalry with the male patient whose hour followed hers.

The analysis of these two girls added to my appreciation of the therapeutic value of analytic abstinence with children. Let me make it clear, however, that by abstinence I do not mean withdrawal or withholding. For along with being abstinent, the child analyst needs to be available, speaking and behaving in a manner that is understandable to the child, and that, as nearly as possible, conveys what the analyst intends to convey. Thus I will tie the shoe (when asked) of a child who has not yet learned to perform this task. On the other hand, I will not offer to tie a child's shoe unsolicited, no matter how often the child trips—and will both interpret the value of "tripping" when that seems appropriate (which may include pointing out the wish to have me offer to help) and try to avoid making interpretations that are really covert suggestions. Similarly, depending on the age of the child, I often answer direct questions—my first name, my age, my dog's name, etc.— because with the very young child not to do so seems strange, and I can think of no explanation that would make sense at the beginning of an analysis to a child under 5 or 6. As time goes on, and the child has a sense of me, I say that I prefer to hear what the child imagines the answer to be, and though this often seems "silly," my refusal to answer becomes another aspect of the analytic situation, like the way I talk, the color of my hair, my clothing, the decor of the office, the toys and the limits. All these things—physical and behavioral—may become recipients of transference, to be perceived as the child's internal conflicts, wishes, fantasies, past and present experiences dictate.

With an older child who I feel can better understand, I usually make some statement, in response to questions at the beginning of the analysis, about my not answering; that my interest is, instead, to figure out what led to the question. This not infrequently leads to a "drying up" of the questions, a retaliative refusal to respond to *my* questions, provocative questions, or battles over why I don't answer—but all this is subject for analysis.

My office provides considerable structure, which helps me and the patient understand the meaning behind the process of our interactions. Each child has a drawer to which no one else is permitted access. Drawings, favorite toys, Lego constructions, whatever, can be kept private in the drawer, but I request that nothing be taken home during the course of treatment. If the child is insistent about taking home his drawings, we analyze it. I do not struggle with him about it, nor say,

"It's okay." Instead, if he takes something home, his "breaking a rule," feeling of guilt, concern about my anger (and, not infrequently, his wish to stimulate it) are analyzed. If the child is worried that another patient or one of my children will go into his drawer and take his stuff, we analyze it. And if the child thinks I am mean, we analyze it. One 4-year-old child, Robert, was so frightened of his rage (which he projected onto me), that he refused to come into my office for three weeks. We had his sessions outside on the street with Robert inside his car and me talking to him through the window. Later, when he returned to my office (after spending the hours outside repetitively telling me that the car was his and I could not get into it), we spent many months sitting with our legs drawn up, in chairs across from one another, pretending that the floor was an ocean filled with sharks, the chairs our boats, and the back of the chairs control panels for our defense against the sharks. The sharks had one end in mind—eating us, eating our penises, getting into us—and in this displaced way we explored Robert's fantasies, both feared and wished for. The earlier experience and resolution of Robert's tremendous fear of me had increased his capacity to distinguish reality from fantasy and gave him a sense of control over his fantasies. This, in turn, made possible the full flowering of the shark fantasies and their connection with his own wishes.

Robert's difficulties (insomnia, stool retention, marked separation anxiety, temper tantrums, and rage reactions directed at his younger sister) had begun after the birth of this sister, his only sibling. Robert was the product of his father's second marriage, and was much adored by this loud, large, and forceful man, who had lost contact with the children of his first marriage. Robert was terrified that he would lose his father after his sister was born, and he was jealous of his mother having the father's baby. He also wanted to have his adored mommy for himself and to get rid of the baby that his daddy had made. In essence, his fear of the consequences of both his negative and positive oedipal rivalry, of his wish to be pregnant and what that would do to him, had disrupted the course of his development. Some of his wishes and fears about his family members were conscious at the onset of the analysis and others became conscious later—but it was his fear of me, his later identification with me in the shark play, and the connection of the two in the interpretation of the transference that led to Robert's recovery.

During Robert's analysis I often wondered about the therapeutic importance of the reconstructions we made, for example, of his feeling jealous when his mother became pregnant. In general, I am uncertain about the value of reconstruction in child analysis, particularly since a child analyst's investment in the reconstruction of past events can interfere with the development of a transference neurosis in his patients. If an analyst wants verbalized content, ideas, information—and wants it from the child, not the parents—then he needs a patient who is willing not just to talk but also to "tell" things, and not just things he feels an urgency to tell but things he feels the analyst wants to hear. Such a patient needs both to understand what is expected of him and to be willing to provide that. This means that the analyst has conveyed his desire for information *and* created a relationship with the patient (albeit covertly or even unconsciously) in which the latter performs as is expected. In so doing the analyst deviates from neutrality and abstinence (Hoffer, 1985) with respect to the direction of the analysis and the use of his power to direct it.

I also have some reservation about the value for conflict resolution of "knowing" the reconstructed distant past. The ego that reconstructs has changed markedly since the events reconstructed (Kennedy, 1971); past experience has been overlaid with other experiences which alter the impact and meaning of earlier events—as with the Wolf-Man's primal scene experience (Freud, 1918). In child analysis (but also in work with adults), genetic reconstructions often seem to be for the analyst's benefit, to achieve closure (for example, understanding all the determinants of a particular compromise formation) when closure is impossible, or to reaffirm, for the analyst, the truth of his theories.

The process of reconstruction does increase the child's appreciation of the influence of past events on current thinking, feeling, and functioning, which adds to his understanding of the phenomenon of transference (E. Furman, 1971). Reconstructions can also lead to reorganization of memories with a beneficial change in both object and self representations. In addition, when a reconstruction leads to the recovery of the associated affect, in particular, affect associated with a recent experience (such as five minutes earlier during the analytic hour), it can significantly enhance a child's ability to self-observe. Useful are the reconstructions/constructions/remembering of immediate past events as, for example, when a child has a specific thought or feeling (like Robert's fear of me) during the course of analysis and the determinants, in terms of unconscious fantasies or affects (like Robert's wish to cut open my stomach), are constructed from the conscious associations (the shark's wish to eat my insides). In the work with Robert, we eventually articulated his early wish to cut the baby out of his mother and eat it—thus destroying it, turning it into stool, and having this gift from the father for himself. However, I believe it was his experiencing how his wishes in the transference and the associated aggression turned to fear of me, not the knowledge of past fantasies, that was most therapeutic for Robert.

The perception of the analyst as a benevolent object may lead, through identification and/or a wish to please him, to development in many areas, including a cognitive precocity that can enhance intellectual understanding. It may even help the child tolerate his internal conflicts and modify his behavioral and affective response to these conflicts. However, the wish to please neither resolves conflicts nor increases ego autonomy. Nonetheless, the "basic transference" continues to be cited as a useful if not essential ingredient of child analysis (Ritvo, 1978, p. 300f.), with the child turning to the analyst for help as toward a benevolent parental figure. Certainly a perception of the analyst as exclusively aggressive, destructive, or overstimulating will interfere with any analysis, particularly that of a child with immature observing ego functions. But the opposite is also true; a perception of the analyst as exclusively benevolent can contaminate the transference template and dilute the mutative force of anxiety-producing impulses.

Those analysts who believe in the importance of *experiencing* during the analytic process tend to emphasize the development of as full an analytic transference as possible; *shared cognitive understanding* seems to be the goal of those who stress the need for a therapeutic alliance strongly rooted in a positive relationship. I sense that without the first (experiential) phase of Strachey's (1934) mutative interpretation, the therapeutic value of the second (interpretive) phase lies largely in strengthening defenses for more adaptive functioning—which, of course, can enhance development. In contrast, the experience of the transference, with an elucidation of defensive behavior and the inadequate and inappropriate compromise formations that wish and fear engender, can lead to therapeutic change even without complete genetic understanding.

When Geleerd (1967, p. 10) speaks of the development, after a period of time in analysis, of verbal ability and self-observation that is far beyond the child's maturation, I feel concern lest the precocious ego development reflects a tendency to intellectualization based on a partial identification with the analyst. Such intellectualization either diminishes the force of the internal conflicts so they can be more successfully repressed or shifts the economic balance by providing more successful defenses (augmented by the auxiliary ego strength of the analyst) without really resolving the conflict. As Abrams (1980) observed, "cognitive growth is stimulated in the analysis of children. . . . Generally, this serves the treatment process, but it may backfire and prove disruptive if a proper balance is not maintained between the freeing of the unconscious, on the one hand, and the stimulation of cognition, on the other . . . there may be a fixing of earlier organizational modes if the therapist fosters submission to an omnipotent id-wisdom; or there may be a further encapsulation of the entrapped unconscious if analysis builds a wall composed of a precocious cognitive system" (p. 306).

A relationship with a benevolent object can have enormous therapeutic power. Analysis is not the only form of child psychotherapy; criteria of analyzability and whether one can or should analyze children with major ego deviations remain important issues for child analysts. I am reminded of Susan, a 5-year-old girl I saw in psychotherapy four times a week for two years. Her mother had been severely depressed after Susan's birth, and aside from times of feeding and diaper changes, she had left Susan alone in her crib for the first six months. (The mother was already on lithium when I began treating Susan; and although no longer clinically depressed, she was always anxious and emotionally distant.) Susan's two older siblings occasionally played with her, but basically she had no consistent human contact during early infancy. When I first saw Susan, she had no language. The most striking thing about her, aside from her markedly retarded cognitive development, was the juxtaposition of a warm, seemingly responsive smile and complete unavailability.

Work with Susan was exhausting, frustrating, and ultimately exhilarating. I began treatment by imitating Susan's movements and speech as closely as possible, rolling on the floor, drawing, or bouncing a ball when she did; essentially, I tried to enter her world. With excruciating slowness she began to take notice of me and to express anger when she felt I was "doing it wrong." Perhaps the most dramatic achievement over those two years was her becoming aware of the difference between "you" and "me." Susan went on to many years of treatment with other therapists, including a long stay in a residential treatment center. She is now a young adult and functioning quite well with a job, an apartment of her own, and a boyfriend—able to communicate not only in English but also in German.

The most successful treatment I have participated in was Susan's, but it was not analysis. I was a very specific person for Susan—an intrusive, benevolent force, whose job was to convince her she got more from being with me (even though it made her very mad at times) than from not being with me (even though that meant she was sometimes very sad when I wasn't there). Her therapy clearly contributed to her development—I could see that in the two years we were together—but it was not analysis. Analysis is a quite specific treatment for individuals whose development and function are handicapped primarily by unconscious internal conflicts, not by environmental interferences or by structural deficits, except when the latter are the results of fixations secondary to retreat from conflict. Neurotic individuals also can be helped by learning new ways to deal with conflicts. However, if therapy is aimed at the resolution of conflict (with an underlying assumption that with conflict resolution, development will resume of its own accord), then, to that end, there is nothing so effective as the development of a transference neurosis within the analytic setting. And if an analyst believes that intense transference (or a transference neurosis) is essential for a successful analysis, he needs to learn what interferes with its emergence and what promotes its development.

Many of the techniques of child analysis are based on the same principles as those used in the analysis of adults. Nonetheless. there are some significant differences in how they are employed, differences dictated by (1) the maturity of the child's ego apparatus (including his cognitive skills, his reality testing, his capacity for self-observation, and his system of defenses); (2) the appearance and pressure of drive derivatives; (3) the phase of superego development; and (4) the intensity of current developmental demands. Although the "use of the analyst as a new object" in a current phase of development can require technical adaptations in child analysis, it should not be cited as a justification for deviations from an abstinent analytic position. The child (and adult) will use the analyst concurrently as a transference object, a "new type" of object to rework preceding phases of development, and an object to fulfill current developmental needs (Chused, 1982). But in all instances the patient's use of the analyst must be dictated by the patient's needs and perceptions—not by the analyst's preconceptions of the patient's needs. The use of the analyst should be determined by the patient's psychic reality, not by the analyst's "real" behavior.

I shall use the analysis of 11-year-old Sarah as illustration. During the course of her treatment, she made many references to the deprivation she suffered at her mother's hands. She was highly critical of her mother—not only for being self-indulgent and infantile, but also for being ugly, silly, flirtatious, poorly dressed, and overly made up. It was clear there was nothing the mother could do that was acceptable to Sarah. Yet it was only after her complaints turned on me, in the transference, that we were able to explore her hunger for her mother's attention, her rage at feeling rejected after her brother was born, as well as the tremendous competitiveness with her mother. During the course of her analysis, Sarah entered adolescence. This, as a phenomenon, was fascinating to watch and hear about—in particular the progression from disgust over boys first, to a fear, embarrassment, and displacement of her impulses (lots of criticism of "boy-crazy" class-mates); then, to a relentless pursuit of boys, a combination of coun-terphobic behavior and active defense against passive vulnerability; subsequently, to a feeling of terror when one young man began to pursue her; and finally, at the time of termination, to real pleasure in early sexual exploration. Throughout this struggle to establish a femi-nine identity, her scrutiny of me was intense. She carefully noted my dress, my makeup, my laugh—in a way that is typical of adolescent girls' scrutiny of their mothers. But interposed with this ceaseless yet relatively objective nonmalevolent scrutiny were repeated hostile at-tacks, with negative, fantasy-filled observations. All was in the sub-tleties: her comment, "That's an interesting color [pointing to a mauve skirt]; I never thought of wearing it with purple; I wonder, did you try to match your lipstick to your blouse?" had a different feel (and differ-ent determinants) than "Yuk, one of my teachers still wears bell-bot-toms; that's probably from the '60s; that's when you were young, isn't it? I don't mean to say that you look funny—but quite honestly, it's hard to trust you when you look so, I don't know, weird; I wonder if you're still married or divorced; I heard that women really begin to live in the past when they can't get a man; I don't mean to make you mad, but. . . ." The first seemed an attempt to use me as a new object for identification; the second a transference perception of me as a de-valued oedipal rival. At other periods of the analysis, when Sarah became able to mourn the loss of the nurturing mother, she fantasized having me be her mother. This was a hard phase of the analysis; it was difficult to distinguish what was an expression of loss from what was a regressive defense against oedipal feelings. One of the clues I used was how the transference affected her participation in the analytic process: when her words became whining and endlessly repetitive, when she misheard my comments as critical and behaved as if she were too injured to analyze, her complaints of deprivation were understood as a defensive transference resistance against the emergence of oedipal rivalry.

It was clear that many of Sarah's observations about her mother's self-preoccupation and unavailability were correct. However, Sarah needed me as an analyst, not a substitute mother; it was the resolution of conflict which enabled her to use me as a current object for identifi-cation (without my ever altering my analytic stance); and it was the resolution of conflict that allowed her to mourn not having a "warm mommy for the little Sarah" and to find two teachers at school for whom she could excel and who treated her as a favorite. That it was two teachers instead of one defended against any impulse to act out her strong erotic attachment to women. This had entered the transference at age 12 when she talked about wanting to touch and kiss me and her fear of being homosexual. Her anxiety was intense during the analysis of these wishes; but before the determinants had been fully explored, her homoerotic concerns disappeared. As she was comfortable with her relationship with these two teachers, I decided not to "push" an exploration of the unconflicted compromise (two objects) she had made in the outside world. Similar decisions are made in the analysis of adults, but usually after a longer period of working through. With children in whom development is still in flux, the analyst may wonder whether to "push" harder to create conflict over what appears to be a potentially pathological solution that might affect future development. Child analysts differ in their belief in the importance of neutrality (and other issues), and their belief affects their analytic stance. I decided it was appropriate to remain abstinent in regard to influencing the direction of the analysis, and not to push Sarah to examine issues that troubled primarily me. I hoped this would allow Sarah to feel that the analysis was really hers; that she would return for further work if and when difficulty with intimacy became a problem for her.

My decision was influenced, in part, by an awareness that adolescents are frequently conflicted over assuming responsibility for their actions; they both wish for and fear external influence—and are very sensitive to it. I believe an important developmental goal in adolescence is the achievement of comfort with self-determined action (even if it is only relatively autonomous with respect to unconscious determinants). Others differ; for example, Harley (1970) recommended that masculine, phallic behavior be reinforced during the analysis of passive adolescent males.

Adaptations of technique dictated by the specific needs and developmental stage of the child are to be distinguished from modifications which can distort or even disrupt the analytic process, such as interventions aimed at changing the patient's environment or explanations given to correct the child's sexual misconceptions without first analyzing the underlying fantasies (Harley, 1986, p. 130). However, justifications for "adaptations" must not blind the analyst to any potential interference with the development and understanding of the transference.

The child's relationship with his parents cannot be ignored, and frequently it necessitates behavior in the child analyst that differs from his behavior with families of adult patients. The child's attachment to his analyst may lead to jealousy and guilt in the parents and loyalty conflicts in the child, which can distort the expression of the transference or lead parents to withdraw the child from treatment prematurely. Parental support of the analysis is essential. Thus, after an initial evaluation, even if I feel the child will need analysis, I often meet with the parents alone for several months (not seeing the child at all during this period so as not to contaminate the eventual analytic relationship) and try to alleviate their guilt (to prevent a defensive denial of the need for treatment) and help them understand what it means for a child to have internal conflicts. During this time I support their wishes to do what they can to make the child less troubled, but I try to help them understand why environmental changes are often not effective.

The experience of the analyst as available and nonjudgmental can diminish the tendency to undermine treatment that develops in some parents. In addition, even if a child is consciously antagonistic toward analysis, therapist, or parents, he is much more accepting of treatment if he believes parents and analyst are allied in supporting it. Five-year-old Annie quite proudly told me that thinking sometimes gave her a headache, like her father had from work, but that her mother said I was probably trying to get her to think so I could discover things about her. With that she handed me the picture she had colored and said, "You discover this!"

To repeat: the major goal with parents is to get them to support the analysis. Once sufficient data are obtained for a complete diagnostic evaluation, there is usually little need for information from the parents concerning the child's behavior or daily life—the analytic work is enough. Although parents may need to be seen at regular intervals to insure their continuing support, one should not yield to parental requests for advice or information in a way that could undermine the child's trust or contaminate the transference. But even when the analyst is abstinent with the parents, just the fact of their knowing each other will influence the child's productions; however, I have yet to see this create unanalyzable difficulties, even with adolescents.

The external reality of the child's relationship with his parents and the analyst's psychic response (including but not limited to countertransference) to this relationship can interfere with the analysis. For example, many child analysts (Geleerd, 1967, pp. 43–44, 201, 304) move their interpretative focus too rapidly to the parents, deflecting the child's attention from the transference with interventions that sound like defensive displacements or premature genetic interpretations (and which would certainly be so labeled if the patient were an adult). This tendency may be a reaction formation against unconscious competition with the parents. Parents can be rivalrous with the analyst, while, at the same time, wanting him to take over. Single parents, or those that are self-preoccupied or insecure in their parenting, may want the analyst to parent. When the analyst feels drawn into that role, he may defend against it by referring back to the parents whenever strong affective responses become manifest in the transference. This deflection of affect can be disruptive to the development of a transference neurosis.

The relationship with the parents of the past—both real and fantasized versions—*are* "transferred" to the parents of the present; when they contribute to pathological interactions, the presence of a transference neurosis may be obscured (P. Tyson, 1978, p. 215). Once an analytic relationship is established, however, this extra-analytic transference can be recognized as such and pathological interactions, stemming from the child's behavior, can often be aborted by appropriate interpretations. Unfortunately, parental behavior may continue to be pathogenic even after a child enters analysis. Child analysts have tried a number of therapeutic interventions aimed at decreasing disturbing experiences with parents. One is parent guidance, with direct manipulation of parental behavior, concurrent with analysis of the child. Sometimes the guidance is part of a well-thought-out plan; other times it spontaneously emerges, as when I felt an irresistible urge to tell the mother of a 10-year-old girl to stop checking her daughter's body for pubic hair development. Parent guidance concurrent with a child analysis can be beneficial; however, it can also be hazardous, with the modification of the parent's behavior only temporary or with only the form of the pathogenic relationship changing.

When interactions detrimental to the child's development are fueled by both the child's and the parents' pathology, simultaneous treatment of the parent(s) by another therapist, including psychoanalysis, can prove of enormous value to the work with the child. This leaves the child's analyst free to deal with the inevitable displacements and transference split between himself and the parents within the child's analysis—intervening as indicated by the work with the child, attending both to the purpose of the split and to the way the displacement is moving (from parent to analyst or vice versa), without fearing the effect of such phenomena on the parents' support of the analysis.

Although it is helpful to be able to distinguish transference of past relationships from habitual modes of relating (Sandler et al., 1975) or displacement onto the analyst of current conflicts with the parents, such distinctions are often not clear-cut. Current conflicts with the parents may be a repetition of aspects of an earlier relationship with them, or may be precipitated by a displacement of the analytic transference or a split in the transference between the analyst and the parents. In addition, habitual modes of relating may eventually evolve into transference, as the component elements which resulted in their formation are experienced in relation to the analyst (Harley, 1971). In general, the most effective verbal interventions in these situations are those in which there is an accurate understanding of the immediate experience; in which a distinction is made, for example, between the externalization of a superego attitude and the transference repetition of the original introjections which made up the superego.

An example of a conflicted response which first began as a displacement from a current relationship with a parent but later became part of the transference neurosis comes from the analysis of Annie, the 5-year-old compliant, "good" girl mentioned above. Annie came for treatment with marked separation anxiety and tremendous fear of robbers, kidnappers, and being poisoned. During an early session, she expressed some fear about touching either the split or intact geodes I had in my office. (Geodes are rocks with a rough, unattractive exterior and an exquisite crystal interior that is exposed when they are cut.) Initially she feared that the rocks were poison and would kill her if she touched them. She spoke of her mother's injunctions not to touch things that didn't belong to her, not to take food from strangers, not to put nonedible items into her mouth. Intermittently, for many months, the geodes were the focus of her attention. Eventually they were seen as something precious, and she feared I would hurt her if she touched, played with, or damaged them. At this time she continued to talk of her mother—moving to mother's instructions not to suck her thumb nor touch herself (her genitals). Later, as she began to want to take the geodes home and to entertain fantasies of how she would get them from me, the focus was almost exclusively on me, with the geodes seen as a gift from my husband. The geodes had become, by the end of the analysis, a metaphor for my womb-baby-penis, through which Annie's envy, narcissistic injury, fear of retaliation, fear and feeling of loss of her mother's love were all explored. Although some reconstructions were made about the birth of her younger sister and the fears stimulated by her oedipal rivalries, the bulk of the work was done in the transference, with an analysis of her defensive behavior, her wishes, and her fears of my retaliation.

With Annie, as with other young children, the immaturity of ego functioning required adaptations of analytic technique. To do analysis as we know it, with a consolidation of transference manifestations around the person of the analyst, the child must have the capacity for reproducible internal self and object representations (which implies fairly intact functions of perception and memory), for symbolization and verbalization, for repression, and at least a minimum tolerance for unpleasant affect. This tolerance is often only minimal, however, and as a child's defense mechanisms tend to be more primitive and less dependable than an adult's, even interventions which address conscious material can lead to outbreaks of anxiety, aggression, or poorly modulated erotic impulses. Thus the analyst of children *must* pay particular attention to the patient's level of arousal. In addition, with children under 7 (Shapiro and Perry, 1976), for whom speaking or thinking often seems the same as doing, the analyst may need to spend considerable time addressing the very process of affects being stimulated by words; as in my telling Annie, "When my words talk of worries, it seems like the words hurt just like the worries do. Then you don't want me to talk." When the child can hear that, an important step has been taken; the action of verbalizing, of interpreting, is objectified, can be talked about, and is less likely to create feelings of helplessness in the child. To counteract the sense of helplessness, the analyst can elicit the child's help with timing, saying something like, "I'm thinking of what you just said; let me know when you want me to tell you my thoughts." Such a statement with an adult would be heard as condescending; with a child, being "in control" of the flow of the analyst's words, being active rather than passive, adds to his tolerance of the words. Often a child can tell me when my tact or timing is off; not in those words, of course, but as Annie did when she said, "Those words are like needles, put it in a picture first." Of course, both the content and the intent of interpreting are still subject to transference misperceptions, and these misperceptions need to be interpreted.

To my surprise, I have found that even for very young children, it is often more comfortable to talk about feelings and impulses directly in the transference than in displacement to outside objects or even toys (which can be endowed with a magical quality to retaliate). Annie, in an expression of rage, stimulated by the story she was telling me about her mother's favoritism toward a younger sister, began to go on an "ant hunt" in my office, using long, pointed pick-up sticks as weapons. She took pleasure in collecting the ants, torturing and then killing them, but as she asked me if ants could talk, fear of retaliation disrupted her play. However, when she later began to blame me for not giving her powerful enough weapons, she was able to stick with her rage and to elaborate on her fantasy about the equipment I could provide my patients, if only I wanted to.

Young children do not have the capacity to abstract that is required to simultaneously experience the transference and perceive it "as if." The analytic structure with its curtailment of gratification (of both patient's and analyst's aggressive and libidinal impulses) protects the child from excessive anxiety over the consequences of his wishes and makes the expression of drive derivatives tolerable. Without analytic abstinence Annie might not have risked the full expression of her ire. Had I behaved as a benevolent object, upon whom Annie had come to depend for emotional supplies (and who could withhold as well as give), this would have both distorted the transference perception *and* interfered with her comfort in "enacting the past" in the therapeutic setting.

Children and adults differ in the level of their superego and ego development; this is reflected in their differing capacity and desire to control urgent impulses and restrict discharge to verbalization. Both adult and child patients, in the throes of strong affects generated by a transference neurosis, find it difficult to remain within an analytic mode of exchange. With the regression in ego and superego function that accompanies the development of the transference neurosis, there is a strong tendency to "act out" or "enact" via a transference resistance. Depending on the complexity of the symbolization, these "actualizations" of the transference are often responsive to interpretation; for example, the child who reports she won't be returning because I want her to play "dirty" may be dealing with an externalization of her own drive derivatives and/or the beginning repetition in the transference of an early or fantasized seduction or primal scene experience. Whichever it is, as she struggles to find a more comfortable compromise formation for her affects, wishes, and fears, analysis with her, beginning with an exploration of her fantasies of my intent in wanting her to play "dirty," is not unlike analysis with an adult.

However, the child who throws a pillow or glass vase at the analyst, the child who tries to pinch or who repeatedly climbs into the analyst's lap or grabs at his genitalia, presents another type of problem. It matters little whether this behavior is a complex compromise formation or the primitive expression of a drive derivative via an ego that is so overwhelmed it has little ability to "force a compromise." This behavior is destructive; it destroys the analyst's and the patient's comfort with their interaction, and it makes clear that at least one member of the dyad is in no position to analyze. In addition, the very experience of beng "out of control" is exciting, painful, and potentially shameful and is not conducive to the child's future participation in the analytic work.

Behavioral limits, particularly limits to the physical contact between analyst and child, are extremely important in child analysis, for immature ego functions are often weakened by the regression induced by transference. When a child wants to play doctor with me as the patient, I offer a doll as a substitute—and analyze rather than gratify or evade the issue when the doll substitution is unacceptable. Analysts often feel some awkwardness in speaking directly about the genital arousal stimulated in their patients by the analysis. This is a particularly difficult task with a child, as the initial clarification of behavior may be heard as a seduction, increasing the press of the impulse, the associated anxiety, and the push to action. Hence there is sometimes a tendency to leave transferential sexual material unanalyzed. Although hugs or blows are rarely useful, an avoidance of physical gratification *without commentary* is liable to be received by the child as a condemnatory prohibition and may lead to a maladaptive identification. Verbalization of thwarted impulses is extraordinarily important in child analysis, for both the analysis of conflicts and to protect the ongoing superego development of the child.

For example, when Annie wanted to measure me, my initial response was simply to decline. It was only when she retreated to a distant point in the room that I became aware of how hurtful my refusal without clarification had been. Overcoming my own resistance, I said I understood that she had wanted to touch me, and that she had heard my "no" as saying it was wrong to want that. We needed to talk about it, because I thought her "wants" were part of her "worries." This "speech," to some extent, was heard within the transference as a challenge and led to an increase in action as well as to repeated questions about "What will you do if I do something you don't want me to do?" However, the questions and behavior led to further analysis of her conflict over impulses, analysis that would have been aborted if the erotic impulses of the transference had not been addressed directly.

Just as internal controls or the wish for controls are less well developed in the child than in the adult (even the obsessional child's rigid superego is usually more brittle than an adult's), so drive derivatives tend to be more primitive, less sublimated or well modulated in their expression, and more urgent in their push for gratification. In addition, the child has fewer resources available to deal with the frustration, feeling of rejection, and narcissistic injury that follows non-gratification. This has been used as an argument for being more gratifying to the child, as if the strength of his demands or the pain of frustration would be lessened by partial or substitute gratification. Actually, I have often found the opposite to be true; partial gratification of most wishes just intensifies the push for full gratification. The child feels more comfortable knowing when and which impulses will *not* be gratified. Of course, limits should not be so confining that the analysis is unremittingly frustrating. Nonetheless, in child as in adult psychoanalysis, frustration is the key to understanding the unconscious wishes and fantasies (and corresponding dangers) that underlie pathology. As with other aspects of the analytic structure, the limits set by a child analyst should take into account the amount of frustration the child can tolerate, the importance of abstinence and neutrality for the emergence of the transference, and the analyst's own psychic requirements for the maintenance of an analyzing stance.

Depending on the developmental level of the child, a degree of responsiveness to requests (such as providing tissues, playing games, helping with constructions) is appropriate in child analysis. However, these "gratifications" should be part of the regular procedure of the analysis of that particular child and not increase, or suddenly become available, at times of stress or increased anxiety. As Sandler et al. (1980) pointed out, "therapists who express fear of adversely affecting the transference really mean that they are afraid of disturbing the positive transference, and their fears of refusing certain gratifications may be rationalizations they use in order to avoid the child's hostile feelings. This is a countertransference problem" (p. 197).

Abstinence neither means nor leads to the absence of all gratification; it does require the frustration of escalating demands for transference gratification. However, a child can leave an office filled with rage at the analyst, even convinced, on one level, of the analyst's malevolent intent and return the next day and the next to continue the work of analysis.

Children do not like being overwhelmed by their impulses anymore than adults do; they are simply more vulnerable to being overwhelmed because of the immaturity of their ego functions. In addition, they have less ego resources to aid in recovery of their equilibrium. When abstinence is perceived as deprivation, it can be analyzed within the transference; exciting gratification confuses the issue and renders the analyzing equipment inoperative. To repeat: consistent limits are more conducive to establishing an analytic situation than partial gratification. The only gratification which *must* be available to the child is the analyst's interest and his continual attempt to understand. Of course, patients can perceive gratification even from potentially nongratifying situations. An example is Robert, who said to me, after a very difficult (for both of us) analysis in which, from his perspective, I had been quite withholding, "I know you cared because you didn't have to prove it." In spite of my abstinence, Robert had perceived me as nurturing and, like Phyllis Tyson's (1978) patient, Colin, first openly demonstrated his positive oedipal longings with me as the object.

This brings me to the issue of the analyst's role as new object during an ongoing phase of development. Although development is continual in both child and adult, the intensity of the developmental thrust and the associated process of identification with important objects are much greater in the child than the adult. Consequently, the child patient makes more frequent use of the analyst as a "new object." The question is not whether this use is "analysis," but what the analyst's active participation in ongoing development should be.

Often when a child comes for analysis, he is unable to use any object in his world for successful navigation of developmental pathways; it is analysis, with the exposure and resolution of instinctual conflicts within the transference, that permits object relations to be more tolerable and development to resume.

Phyllis Tyson has suggested that when a child is "trying to cope with the upsurging drives accompanying a new developmental phase" (1978, p. 229), the energy required for the elaboration of a transference neurosis is unlikely to be available. I disagree with this. When an analysand begins to take a new developmental step utilizing the analyst as a "real" object, his perception of the analyst will be distorted by his current needs as well as by his past conflicts—the analyst is no more "real" in this mixed utilization than he would be in the expression of transference alone. In essence, transference reactions and a transference neurosis will continue to exist even during a period of active development. Their manifestations may be different, as the balance of drives and defenses change and the relative contribution of impulses from different libidinal zones shifts. Yet the object relationship in which the drives are expressed will continue to be distorted as before—reflecting pathological interactions of the past, longed-for idealized objects of the past and present, and perceptions of the original objects that are distorted by projection of the child's own libidinal and aggressive impulses and fantasies.

A child frequently resumes or reworks (Chused, 1982) development around his relationship with the analyst. But the analyst does not need to depart from a neutral, abstinent analytic position for this to occur—the child will make of the analyst what he needs him to be. Special kindness or reassurance reflect the "benevolent object fallacy," so-called because what is intended as kindness may be understood as condescending; what was meant to be reassuring, experienced as controlling or intrusive. It is much better for the analytic process, and for the development that proceeds from it, if the child's perceptions of the analyst are (relatively) autonomous, both in the transference and in the transformations of transference which constitute the analyst as "new object." This does not require new technique, only a tolerance for being a passive participant rather than the active initiator of the analytic process—a tolerance for being neutral as to how the child uses analysis. Child analysis offers multiple therapeutic opportunities (A. Freud, 1965); optimally, a child in treatment will make use of those elements he needs.

When the child uses the analyst as both transference object and new object, perceptions which are not caught up in conflict need not be subject to interpretation, even though they may reflect a distortion of reality (such as Robert's perception of me as nurturing). This fits in with Ritvo's point (Panel, 1980) that the analyst need work only on the identifications that are used defensively or for resistance—not the identifications and object relations that are part of the silent process of development of psychic structure and growth. On the other hand, behavior of the analyst which is misperceived within a transference framework (or just misunderstood because of lack of experience) and is liable to be used for maladaptive identifications in the development of superego and ego structure (such as my declining to be measured by Annie) needs to be addressed and interpreted.

Child analytic training does not provide a theoretical basis for responding to ongoing developmental demands with the same degree of clarity that it does for the demands dictated by unconscious conflicts. When a 5-year-old repeatedly trips over untied shoes, one can wonder with him about his tendency to fall and hurt himself without taking the obvious precautions. But when a 5-year-old asks you to tie his shoes so he won't trip, to interpret that his failure to tie them himself was either self-destructive or indicative of a regression to a dependent position is ridiculous if the child has not yet learned to tie. One may wonder with him why he can't tie; a missing skill may represent a neurotically determined inhibition or developmental interference, as well as reflect a constitutional delay in development. The analyst may also tie the shoe if a refusal to do so would be a senseless withholding to the child, but having done so, the analyst must monitor himself carefully for a countertransference reaction to what the child does with the tied shoe. Does it stay tied, or does it get undone as a way to damage what the analyst (and whom he represents in the transference) has to offer? This is where the work of the analysis lies; this is the point where the transference, and later the transference neurosis, manifests itself; and this is where child psychoanalysis often fails to become analysis and remains psychotherapy.

There is another characteristic of the analytic process with children that makes work with the transference neurosis difficult. Children often do not have the interest or the psychic structure that is required for a lengthy working through. Once a conflictual issue has been resolved sufficiently so that a new piece of behavior is possible (for example, learning to read), a symptom is no longer obligatory (like a hand-washing ritual or psychogenic limp); or anxiety is diminished enough for an inhibition to be overcome (such as social isolation); action takes over, the economic balance shifts, and the conflict disappears. The conflict may reappear later in a new context, but often not with the multiple repetitions that seem to be required to make transference interpretations believable to adult patients. It is not just a lack of interest or ability that keeps the child from working through. In my experience, children seem to require less repetition of conflictual situations within the transference in order to have insight result in change, perhaps because their psychic structure is less fixed and more flexible.

Some of the child analysts who question whether a child is capable of repeating with the analyst, through restricted reenactment, enough of his conflictual past experience to benefit from an analysis of transference similar to that in adult analyses, continue to believe that the child has less tendency or need to make transferences to the analyst because his primary love objects are available in his daily life for instinctual drive gratification (reported by Ritvo, 1978). However, there is abundant clinical material (Harley, 1971; P. Tyson, 1978) which demonstrates that independence from the original objects is not a determining factor in the development of a transference neurosis in children; the degree to which processes of internalization have taken place is far more important. In addition, as with adults, it is not the need or wish for gratifying objects that brings children to analysis, but rather the unconscious conflicts over gratification, conflicts rooted not in current relationships but derived from past experiences and their incorporation into psychic structure. Potentially gratifying objects are frequently available in our patients' lives; the problem is a patient's inability to be gratified.

Another factor contributing to a disbelief in transference neurosis in children, the educational background of many early child analysts, was alluded to earlier. Educators had observed that children learned best in a positive teacher-student relationship. The combination of wishes to please and to emulate a teacher leads students to work harder and be more intellectually productive. And pediatricians were aware that a positive, nurturing mother-infant relationship was essential for optimal development of the young child. Their combined knowledge, together with the observations that, in general, a child's frustration tolerance is small and his negative responses intense, led the early child analysts to assume that a positive relationship, with some degree of "real" gratification (emotional or material), was essential for the child to be an active participant in the analysis. As Kramer and Settlage (1962) stated, "The entire technique [of child analysis] presupposes the willingness and ability of the child to communicate with the analyst verbally and symbolically, giving material which lends itself to verbal interpretations, which in turn can be understood and accepted by the child" (p. 515). They continued, "it is necessary that the child develop a good relationship with the analyst, because he can bear the tension associated with analysis only if he likes the analyst . . . negative feelings toward the analyst, regardless of whether they are caused by events in treatment or are manifestations of transference or resistance, are not well tolerated by the child. They usually are dealt with immediately in order to keep them from becoming a wedge between child and analyst. On the other hand, positive feelings are encouraged to grow gradually" (p. 524). ". . . strong negative transference for any length of time does not augur well for child analysis" (p. 527). Harley (1986) sums it up: "we had felt it indispensable to maintain only a positive transference" (p. 133f.). In this way, I believe, analysts prevented transference neuroses from developing in their child patients.

Child analysts who have had no adult analytic experience (true of many trained in England) seem to have an idealized or distorted conception of the analytic process with adults. In articles contrasting child and adult analysis (A. Freud, 1965), the adult is often presented as an active, cooperative participant in the process. I believe a more accurate description of adult analysis can be found in Bird's (1972) discussion of transference resistance; how, in the heat of the transference, the patient expresses his wish to destroy the analyst by attempting to destroy the analytic process. At this point in the analysis, regardless of the patient's original motivation, the last thing he wants is for the analysis to work. No matter how good the therapeutic alliance seemed, it has disappeared under the force of transference resistance.

As Freud (1912) observed, "Over and over again, when we come near to a pathogenic complex, the portion of that complex which is capable of transference is first pushed forward into consciousness and defended with the greatest obstinacy" (p. 104).

Without intense transference resistance, reflective of a consuming transference neurosis, the analysis may remain a didactic exercise, a comforting experience—which may be therapeutic, but isn't analytic. This, unfortunately, is what child analysis often becomes. It is hard to resist trying to calm an enraged or frightened child. "Poor Susie, you're so unhappy; I have all these toys and you feel you have nothing," said in response to Susie's provocative, "Shut up! . . . Pretend I'm all chained up and you're beating me" (R. L. and P. Tyson, 1986, p. 36) may be accurate, but it fails to help the child understand the connection between her manifest behavior and its determinants. In addition, it presents the analyst as omnipotently knowing what the child is feeling. Even when an analyst is trying to prevent the overwhelming of an immature ego, it is counterproductive (and potentially infuriating) for a child to be told what he is thinking or feeling— it strips him of autonomy and deprives him of the opportunity to learn both to observe himself and to observe his effect on others.

Some of my observations on the development of a transference neurosis in children have also been made by others: Selma Fraiberg (1967) suggested one could see a transference neurosis in children if the analysis was conducted along the lines of the adult model "conceding only to the use of play, free movement, and the substitution of another therapeutic contract for the analytic rule" (p. 101). She also said, "increased appreciation of transference by child analysts . . . may lead to changes in technique toward minimizing supportive measures and encouraging autonomy. The very change in technique may create an atmosphere which facilitates the development of transference manifestations. The result will be a decrease in the tendency to manipulate the transference and an opportunity to encourage the full development of the transference" (p. 102f.). On the other hand, Anna Freud, in one of her last contributions, indicated that she felt it was often appropriate to provide a child with sweets, a toy kit, or Christmas or birthday presents (Sandler et al., 1980, p. 194).

Melanie Klein, early in her work, recognized the child's capacity for transference and the development of a transference neurosis. However, the tendency of many Kleinian analysts to make early interpretations about the unconscious determinants of behavior, interpretations which seem to bypass defenses and create great anxiety in the child, may have kept other child analysts from appreciating the value of

Klein's contributions and led to a discrediting of her idea that children do have the potential to develop a transference neurosis. Kleinians often seem to interpret as if the child speaks and behaves in universal symbols; his individual history and level of ego development appear to have little influence on their interventions. This, plus a seeming lack of sensitivity to the importance of the child's affective arousal remaining within tolerable limits (some Kleinian interventions sound almost like verbal rape), has led many non-Kleinian analysts in the United States to disregard the work and ideas of Melanie Klein. Although I disagree with her timetable of libidinal development and her understanding of early ego functioning, I am impressed by her realization that the pedagogical and benevolent position advocated by Hug-Hellmuth and initially by Anna Freud interfered with the development of a transference neurosis and the ultimate therapeutic benefits of analysis (Klein, 1927).

All of the above factors contribute to the failure of child analysts to see the development of a transference neurosis in their own work with children. But also contributing is their response to the child's behavior, to his frequent progressive and regressive shifts in ego functioning, and to his rapid move to action when stressed. It is much easier for an analyst to maintain an analytic stance behind a couch than when face to face with a child. This more direct interaction continually taxes the child analyst's capacity to be neutral and abstinent.

Deviations from abstinence and neutrality occur in all analyses. Every analyst has certain preconceived notions of what is therapeutically effective; each tries to create an atmosphere in which what he believes will work has a chance to do so. An analyst who believes that the regressive transferences (most fully developed in the transference neurosis) are the major therapeutic tools of child, adolescent, and adult psychoanalysis establishes a structure in which thinking and talking are encouraged by example and, perhaps, initial education, but then accepts the "actualizations" (Boesky, 1982) of the transference that inevitably occur and, where appropriate, analyzes them. On the other hand, the analyst who believes that for treatment to be effective the patient needs to be a willing, contributing participant in the attempt to understand must make a continuing effort to maintain a therapeutic alliance.

The therapeutic alliance, dependent as it is on the "basic transference," can function as a resistance (Greenacre, 1968; Novick, 1970; Brenner, 1979; Stein, 1981); when it contains an unanalyzed desire to please or is actively supported by the analyst's behavior, it may obscure the transference. Even more than with an adult this is a danger during the treatment of a child, who, being genuinely dependent on adults, is less likely to question the roles of kind doctor and good patient. For the child, who is in the process of developing autonomous functioning with respect to both the drives and the external world, conflicts over autonomy and control, expressed through rebellion and compliance, are part of what led to a need for analysis in the first place. To the extent that the analyst contributes to the perpetuation of compliance in his patient, the compliance (or a rebellious reaction against it) is unavailable for analysis.

The "teasing out" of when and what to interpret with a child (Blos, 1979) is a difficult process—it often requires the analyst to be a silent participant in a drama which can make him quite uncomfortable. The most difficult part of child analysis is being this silent participant, eventually interpreting misperceptions, yet remaining abstinent long enough for them to be fully understood by both analyst and child. When I err with a child, it is on the side of talking too much, too soon. The "real" dependency needs of all children (but particularly those children who have suffered emotional deprivation), their potential for growth, their tremendous vulnerability to external forces, and the wish to have them grow successfully with minimum suffering, are all powerfully seductive forces which lead to countertransference interferences with the development of a transference neurosis.

There will be many crises throughout development for both the child and the adult. In the process of growth many wishes, fantasies, and ideals must be given up, and even children must mourn. Analysis can assist with the mourning process by making it a shared experience. But only through the transference neurosis can we learn *what* is being mourned.

In summary, there is a historical precedent for the child analyst to behave primarily as a benevolent object. Unfortunately, too much benevolence can interfere with the development of a transference neurosis. Psychoanalysis as a therapy based on a theory of conflict-determined psychopathology relies on the emergence of derivatives of conflict within the transference for its efficacy. When analysts begin to practice the same abstinence and neutrality with children as with adults, I believe they will see much more intense transference and full-fledged transference neuroses, have more opportunity to make experience-based interpretations, and be able to keep hypothetical genetic reconstructions to a minimum. The child patient differs from the adult—this demands changes in technique. But the analytic stance with both should be the same.

BIBLIOGRAPHY

ABRAMS, S. (1980). Therapeutic action and ways of knowing. *J. Amer. Psychoanal. Assn.*, 28:291–308.

BIRD, B. (1972). Notes on transference. *J. Amer. Psychoanal. Assn.*, 20:267–301.

BLOS, P. (1979). Gender and its relationship to transference and countertransference in the analysis of the preoedipal and oedipal child. Panel discussion of the Association for Child Psychoanalysis (unpublished).

BOESKY, D. (1982). Acting out. *Int. J. Psychoanal.*, 63:39–55.

BORNSTEIN, B. (1949). The analysis of a phobic child. *Psychoanal. Study Child*, 3/4:181–226.

BRENNER, C. (1979). Working alliance, therapeutic alliance, and transference. *J. Amer. Psychoanal. Assn.*, 27:137–157.

BURLINGHAM, D. (1932). Child analysis and the mother. *Psychoanal. Q.*, 4:69–92, 1935.

CHUSED, J. (1982). The role of analytic neutrality in the use of the child analyst as a new object. *J. Amer. Psychoanal. Assn.*, 30:3–28.

FERENCZI, S. (1913). A little chanticleer. In *Sex and Psychoanalysis*. New York: Basic Books, 1950, pp. 240–252.

FRAIBERG, S. (1966). Further considerations of the role of transference in latency. *Psychoanal. Study Child*, 21:213–236.

———— (1967). Repression and repetition in child analysis. *Bull. Phila. Assn. Psychoanal.*, 17:99–106.

FREUD, A. (1927). Four lectures on child analysis. *W.*, 1:3–69.

———— (1965). Normality and pathology in childhood. *W.*, 6.

FREUD, S. (1909). Analysis of a phobia in a five-year-old boy. *S.E.*, 10:5–149.

———— (1912). The dynamics of transference. *S.E.*, 12:99–108.

———— (1918). From the history of an infantile neurosis. *S.E.*, 17:3–122.

FURMAN, E. (1971). Some thoughts on reconstruction in child analysis. *Psychoanal. Study Child*, 26:372–385.

GELEERD, E. R., ed. (1967). *The Child Analyst at Work*. New York: Int. Univ. Press.

GREENACRE, P. (1968). The psychoanalytic process, transference, and acting out. *Int. J. Psychoanal.*, 49:211–228.

HARLEY, M. (1967). Fragments from the analysis of a dog phobia in a latency child. *Bull. Phila. Assn. Child Psychoanal.*, 17:127–129.

———— (1970). On some problems of technique in the analysis of early adolescents. *Psychoanal. Study Child*, 25:99–121.

———— (1971). The current status of transference neurosis in children. *J. Amer. Psychoanal. Assn.*, 19:26–40.

———— (1986). Child analysis, 1947–1984. *Psychoanal. Study Child*, 41:129–153.

HOFFER, A. (1985). Toward a definition of psychoanalytic neutrality. *J. Amer. Psychoanal. Assn.*, 33:771–795.

HUG-HELLMUTH, H. (1921). On the technique of child-analysis. *Int. J. Psychoanal.*, 2:287–305.

_____ (1924). *New Paths to the Understanding of Youth.* Leipzig-Wien: Franz Deuticke.

KENNEDY, H. (1971). Problems in reconstruction in child analysis. *Psychoanal. Study Child,* 26:386–402.

KLEIN, M. (1927). Symposium on child analysis. *Int. J. Psychoanal.,* 8:339–370 (and papers by J. Riviere, M. N. Searl, E. F. Sharpe, E. Glover, and E. Jones; *ibid.,* pp. 370–391).

KRAMER, S. & SETTLAGE, C. F. (1962). On the concepts and technique of child analysis. *J. Amer. Acad. Child Psychiat.,* 1:509–535.

KUT, S. (1953). The changing pattern of transference in the analysis of an eleven-year-old girl. *Psychoanal. Study Child,* 8:355–378.

NOVICK, J. (1970). Vicissitudes of the working alliance in the analysis of a latency girl. *Psychoanal. Study Child,* 25:231–256.

PANEL (1966). Problems of transference in child analysis. H. Van Dam, reporter. *J. Amer. Psychoanal. Assn.,* 14:528–537.

_____ (1980). Conceptualizing the nature of the therapeutic action of child analysis. L. Shabot, reporter. *J. Amer. Psychoanal. Assn.,* 28:161–179.

_____ (1983). Reanalysis of child analytic patients. A. L. Rosenbaum, reporter. *J. Amer. Psychoanal. Assn.,* 31:677–688.

RITVO, S. (1978). The psychoanalytic process in childhood. *Psychoanal. Study Child,* 33:295–305.

SANDLER, J., KENNEDY, H., & TYSON, R. L. (1975). Discussions on transference. *Psychoanal. Study Child,* 30:409–441.

_____ _____ _____ (1980). *The Technique of Child Analysis.* Cambridge: Harvard Univ. Press.

SHAPIRO, T. & PERRY, R. (1976). Latency revisited. *Psychoanal. Study Child,* 31:79–105.

STEIN, M. H. (1981). The unobjectionable part of the transference. *J. Amer. Psychoanal. Assn.,* 29:869–892.

STRACHEY, J. (1934). The nature of therapeutic action. *Int. J. Psychoanal.,* 15:127–159.

TYSON, P. (1978). Transference and developmental issues in the analysis of a prelatency child. *Psychoanal. Study Child,* 33:213–235.

TYSON, R. L. & TYSON, P. (1986). The concept of transference in child psychoanalysis. *J. Amer. Acad. Child Psychiat.,* 25:30–39.

A Current View of the Psychoanalytic Theory of Depression

With Notes on the Role of Identification, Orality, and Anxiety

DAVID MILROD, M.D.

BEFORE DISCUSSING THE SUBJECT OF DEPRESSION WE MUST BE CLEAR about the differences between sadness, grief, mourning, and depression. Sadness is the emotional response of the ego to suffering, brought on by an experience or fantasy of loss or deprivation (Jacobson, 1957). Grief or mourning, which I will use here synonymously, are special types of sadness caused by a specific form of loss, namely, the permanent loss of a love object in reality. However, experiences of loss do not always evoke sadness. They may also trigger rage and hostile responses. If that rage is turned on the self representation and then transformed to a mood state, we are dealing with a depression. The essential elements in a depression are the self-directed aggression and the mood state to which it leads.

Because depressions are mood disorders, a brief digression about the nature of moods seems appropriate. A mood is an ego state which colors all ego functions, substructures, and modes of discharge with a uniform quality. It comes about by the spreading of a focal affective discharge process over the entire ego, whether the spreading is caused by the high intensity of the stimulus, or a low capacity on the part of the ego to relieve tension by focalized discharge. This redistribution of

Training and supervising analyst at the New York Psychoanalytic Institute.

An earlier version of this paper was presented at a panel on depression held at the New York Psychoanalytic Society as part of a scientific meeting on April 24, 1984.

drive energy in the ego always affects the self representation and the representation of the object world alike. In fact, unless both self and object representations are affected, there would be no mood state. Moods are maintained by a temporary denial of opposite qualities. In a high mood when the world seems wonderful and rewarding, it is important to deny all contradictory evidence in order to sustain that mood. In a depressed or low mood, all evidence of worthiness and self value must be denied or the mood will be brought to an end. Moods have the economic function of facilitating the discharge of high levels of psychic tension which the ego cannot handle by focal discharge, whether aimed at an object, interest, or activity. When I say, therefore, that depressions are mood states, I mean that the affect accompanying the self-directed aggression has spread over the entire ego, coloring all its manifestations and contents, affecting all discharges and transferences. Of special significance is the fact that both self and object representations are thus affected. Moods are therefore quite different from focalized, object-directed affect states such as love or hate (Jacobson, 1957).

Returning to our main theme, we can see that experiences of loss may lead to sadness or to depression. In sadness it is the libidinal drive which is involved; in depression it is the aggressive drive.[1] The sad person may feel diminished, but he does not feel, "I am bad; a failure; deserving of punishment." There is no hostile cathexis of the self representation and therefore no significant narcissistic disturbance. In depression the opposite is the case. The self representation is cathected with aggression and there is therefore a significant narcissistic disturbance. In sadness the value which is lost is pleasure or gratification. In depression what is lost is the sense of one's own worth, which attests to the fact that in depression the self representation is the focus of the psychopathology.

Narcissistic blows of this type, so intimately connected with depression, account for the fact that depression is a universal phenomenon. No one can escape insults to his or her narcissism as maturation and development unfold, and some of these insults will lead to self-criticism or self-condemnation. Of these a certain number will evolve to a mood state, whereupon we are dealing with a depression.[2] Self-directed con-

1. Freud's original distinction between mourning and melancholia in his classic 1917 paper already pointed to this difference, although he was dealing with a complex and specific form of sadness, namely, mourning, and a very specific form of depression, namely, melancholia.

2. Mahler (1966) also pointed to the universality of depression in ascribing the development of a basic depressive affect to the vicissitudes of the rapprochement subphase.

demnation that remains focused and does not spread to a mood state will not produce a depression. In fact, it may be a specific self-criticism that leads to constructive change, without a loss in the sense of self-worth. But more important than its universality is the question of diagnosis. Does the depression belong to the normal, neurotic, borderline, or psychotic variety? Here, in addition to our regular diagnostic criteria, we have a special tool to help—the nature of the denial maintaining the depressive mood. All moods, because of the denial, distort reality. They are normal if they yield when reality asserts itself in the area being denied. To the degree that unconscious infantile conflicts participate in a mood, reality testing is precluded and the mood is repetitive until the unconscious sources are made conscious. Moods stemming from narcissistic sources are even less influenced by reality testing. Those stemming from psychotic sources are beyond the influence of reality.

Depressions belong to the group of moods stemming from narcissistic sources. The sense of loss which always accompanies depression underscores its narcissistic basis because it is brought about by a significant fall in the level of libidinal investment in the self representation below that necessary for the maintenance of its integrity and well-being. It is this loss of libidinal cathexis that produces the loss of self-esteem which most contributors since Freud have noted in all depressions. The libidinal cathexis is then replaced by a hostile one and the flow of narcissistic supplies to the self representation is shut down, whether that flow originated from the love object, from the ego, or from the superego. These are the three sources of libidinal supplies for investment in the self representation. We will see that the different structural configurations a depression may take are related to one or the other of these sources of supply. It is not the affect that distinguishes one type of depression from another; it is its structure which does.

The simplest structural form of a depression is one in which the narcissistic injury, whatever its stimulus, is caused by the self representation falling too far short of the goals and standards in the individual's wished-for self image (Milrod, 1982). In everyday terms this means that a wide gap develops between the individual's view of himself in worldly terms and the image of what he aspires to be. When that happens, the individual will condemn himself for not being equal to his ambitions. Included here are such familiar examples as depressions triggered by career or financial disappointments as well as the large group of depressions related to the aging process. Once the self representation falls to a critical level below that of the wished-for self image, narcissistic supplies from the ego are cut off and the libidinal cathexis of the self representation is replaced by a hostile cathexis instigated by the self-critical function of the ego. It then spreads to a mood state. This form of depression involves an *intrasystemic* process without superego participation. Thus the self-condemnation carries no moral flavor and can be translated as the feeling, "I am a failure."

A second type of depression, structured differently, occurs when the narcissistic injury is caused by the self representation falling too far short of the moral and ethical values built into the ego ideal. Here the individual condemns himself for some moral or ethical failure. Guilt feelings and superego punishment are the regular outcome whenever a person fails to live up to his ego ideal. In depression, which is only one of a variety of possible superego punishments, libidinal supplies to the self representation from the superego (Schafer, 1960) are cut off and replaced by a hostile cathexis. Depression results if it becomes a mood state. In this type of depression an *intersystemic* process is involved in which the superego participates via its punitive function, producing a hostile cathexis of the self representation. Here the self-condemnation will carry a definite moral flavor and so can be translated to carry the meaning, "I am bad!" or "I deserve punishment."

A third form of depression with yet a different structure occurs when an ambivalent love object continues to be the essential source of libidinal supplies for the self representation. In this case a loss of the object or of the object's love produces the narcissistic blow responsible for the loss of libidinal investment in the self representation and its replacement by a hostile cathexis, all experienced as a loss of self-esteem. Such a situation implies that there is an insufficient degree of differentiation between self and object representations or, put somewhat differently, object relations still retain a significant degree of symbiosis. Because the object plays such a vital role in the psychic economy of these people, derogation of the object is intolerable. When it happens, as it inevitably will, it produces a reactive defensive shift of libido from the self representation to the object representation. The result is an exaggeration of the subject's flaws in order to reinstate the virtues of the ambivalent object. But if the process goes too far or lasts too long, the narcissistic libido (libido invested in the self representation) may become depleted and the person may be unable to restore the object representation to its former lofty image, leading to a hostile devaluation of both object and self representations. Both then participate in a sense of worthlessness. This represents the primary disturbance of the melancholic, and depressions can and do occur at this stage. The external world has failed him; and as the process goes on, his last line of defense is retreat from the external world by a total decathexis of the object representation. But these are people who cannot do without their love objects and in a last attempt to recover the lost position, the lost decathected object is restored in the form of an introject in the self representation. Now the structure of the full melancholic syndrome is set in place. In fact, as Abraham (1924) and Rado (1928) pointed out, there are two introjects formed. The good aspect of the decathected ambivalent object forms an introject in the superego; the bad aspect becomes an introject in the ego (self representation) and hostility is directed at the latter by the former. The role of the superego in this third structural form of depression is quite different from that in the second where it does not depend on an introject.

Freud's seminal paper on "Mourning and Melancholia" (1917) was carefully limited to a detailed analysis of a form of depression which is related only to the third structural type described above. Many authors have made the mistaken assumption that the same structure and the same dynamics apply to all depressions. Some have even confused the dynamics of mourning with those of depression.

In order for a depression to result following any of the three kinds of narcissistic injury described above, a mounting tide of aggression must develop which will have two characteristics as it is deployed. First, it always cathects the self representation producing the subjective experience of "I am bad," or "I am a failure." Second, it always leads to a mood state. The entire process is complex, and it can produce a variety of clinical pictures, depending on a number of factors. Prominent among them I would include the nature of the narcissistic blow, and the degree of maturation, structuralization, and stability of ego and superego. The conscious and unconscious significance of the narcissistic blow would lead us to expect that less severe narcissistic insults will, in general, cause less severe depressions. But we must always be aware that what seems a relatively light narcissistic injury on the surface may touch on a long-standing, repressed injury of more profound proportions than would ordinarily be expected, resulting in a more severe depression.

By far the most important variable in determining the clinical picture is the degree of maturation and structuralization of ego and superego, and particularly this includes the ego's capacity to neutralize the drives. In depressions the ability to neutralize the aggressive drive is of special importance. I would also include under the ego and superego structure the nature of the person's object relations. Where more mature object relations prevail, depressions will tend to be milder, and ties to the object world will be maintained. This is so even if disappointment in, and hostility toward, the object are part of the dynamic picture. Sometimes the defenses of denial and idealization of the object may prove effective in dissipating the depression. Similarly, reality testing may dispel the denial of positive attributes in the self, and with it the depressive mood and the sense of being bad. In these situations the ego is sturdy, object ties sound, ambivalence not intense, and the propensity to regression much less. The object world remains intact.

By contrast, with greater degrees of ego disturbance, deneutralization, and disorders of object relations, a narcissistic insult may lead to total decathexis of the object representation, and with this some break with reality. If we are dealing with a manic-depressive psychosis, the loss of the object cannot be tolerated, and in a desperate attempt at restoration, an introject is formed, leading to the picture of melancholia which Freud so carefully delineated. If we are dealing with a depression in a schizophrenic, further regression occurs even to the point of fragmentation of ego and superego and disruption of the self representation. Restitutive efforts to recathect the object world then produce bizarre recombined forms of fragmented elements of a grossly disorganized ego and superego, producing a clinical picture we recognize as schizophrenic.

As we move from neurotic to psychotic depression, we find that the spectrum of increasing pathology of object relations and of ego and superego structure runs parallel to, and is the result of, an increasing degree of deneutralization of aggressive drive energy (Hartmann, 1953). Total decathexis of the object representation in melancholia, for example, is an economic description of the destruction of the object representation and is related to a fantasy of killing. Abraham (1924) linked it to an unconscious fantasy of destroying the object by anal expulsion. Also, the shallow nature of object ties, shown by the ease with which the object representation is given up, something Freud described as early as 1917, is due to the predominance of aggression over libido during the period of development when object and self representations are being formed. But even the mildest and most transient depressions in the relatively healthy are dynamically linked with aggression. The affectively charged thought, "I am bad!" is an indication that aggression is directed at the self representation. It follows, therefore, that in order to understand depression we must take into account the role of aggression and ambivalence.

The above considerations can help us understand a number of perplexing questions that have always been associated with the subject of depression. For example, does identification with the ambivalent love object always occur in depression? To answer we must first understand that there are different kinds of identification. Freud (1917) described a process in melancholia which he called identification. But he took the trouble to explain that it was different from the identification which occurred in hysteria. In melancholia, the object representation was totally decathected only to have "the shadow of the object" fall on the self representation in a restitutive effort. He was very clear on this point, using strong terms of emphasis. Given his mastery of language, he must have wanted especially to underscore it. Several times in the course of his paper he said that the object cathexis was "abandoned," or "brought to an end," or "shattered." By contrast, in hysterical identification the object cathexis, he said, was sustained in an ongoing way.

But Freud was not finished with the subject of identification. He returned to it repeatedly for many years, adding an insight here and there which enlarged our understanding, but not without a degree of lack of clarity. The early stage of his theory building and the changing models with which he was working were partly responsible for the confusion. Also, it was to be 33 years before the concept of the self representation as distinct from the ego would be clearly enunciated by Hartmann and Jacobson. As a result terms like narcissism and identification were impossible to define precisely. In retrospect it is remarkable how much Freud made clear without having more recent concepts at his disposal. In retracing his steps we can discern that he was struggling to clarify distinctions between ego and superego identifications; the nature of libidinal object ties and their relationship to identification of the ego and superego type; when object ties develop and whether they are necessary for early identification; or, on the contrary, whether identifications precede object ties; and the question of how identification processes relate to superego formation. And in the midst of these ideas he kept returning to the concept of the total decathexis of the object, which he first described in "Mourning and Melancholia" (1917). There he wrote about "an *identification* of the ego with the abandoned object" (p. 249), "the shadow of the object fell upon the ego" (p. 249), and an object cathexis being replaced by an identification (pp. 249–252). In *Group Psychology* (1921) he spoke of identification being the original form of emotional tie to an object, so that it could represent a regression from an object tie. In addition, it could express a wish to put oneself in the same situation as another, even when there had been no previous libidinal tie. He differentiated two kinds of identification, one of which he called simply identification, while he referred to the other as "putting the object in the place of the ego ideal" (p. 130). This was his first hint that ego identification was different from superego identification.

By 1923 Freud had decided that the identification he described in

1917 for melancholia was very common. In fact, the process by which the ego and its character are built up is the same process, he said, namely, an object cathexis is *replaced* by an identification. Today we would raise questions about identification *replacing* the object cathexis in ego building, since the object cathexis is generally ongoing and sustained in these situations. Foreshadowing future theoretical developments Freud said in the same work that the first, most important identifications with parents are *not* the outcome of an object cathexis but are direct immediate identifications earlier than an object cathexis (p. 31). This could only refer to a period of development before complete self-object differentation, when boundaries between self and object representations are blurred, and when there are experiences or fantasies of merging. Later, writing on the formation of the superego, he contrasted the identification in melancholia with that in superego formation. He said that in both, the object cathexis is given up, which was the reason he grouped them together for purposes of comparison. In superego formation this happens at the height of the oedipus complex. But unlike melancholia, these latter identifications form a precipitate in the ego which is able to confront the other contents of the ego as a new psychic structure, the superego. Although he said that with the demolition of the oedipus complex, the child must give up the *object cathexis* of the parent of the opposite sex, a little later he made it clear that it is the *incestuous erotic cathexis* that must be given up. It is not therefore a total object decathexis. The object cathexis continues and is even strengthened by the formation of the superego.

These insightful, penetrating ideas about identification form a group of seemingly unrelated observations, difficult to integrate into a coherent whole. But they fall into place more easily when we take a leap in time to view the problem from the point of view of modern ego psychology. Now we would define identification as a complex process by which the individual becomes more like the object in reality terms. Qualities of the object representation become part of the self representation in a more or less stable ongoing way. The self representation is, in other words, altered so that we can say identification is a process that builds structure. Although the focus is on the change in the self representation, this always involves changes in ego functions, ego interests, and ego activities as well. Hartmann and Loewenstein (1962) said that identification was complex because it referred to the process as well as the end result. It is also complicated by the fact that the process goes through a developmental evolution, only the final, mature form of which is represented by the above definition. To follow Jacobson's ideas on identification (1964), the process goes through a developmental line (A. Freud, 1965) consisting of three major steps.

1.The first step is the early stage of merging self and object images prior to clear self-object differentiation. This is the stage Freud alluded to in *The Ego and the Id* (p. 31). As we saw, Freud had at one time speculated that identification was the first form of tie to a love object, and that an object cathexis developed only later. It was not an idea he held to for long. Today we would say that identification and object relations begin at the same time and are motivated by the identical maturational event, namely, the beginning of differentiation, self from nonself, inner from outer, self from object images. At first the differentiation is rudimentary and temporary. But from this single stimulus, two developmental lines begin. One aims at regaining the lost undifferentiated or merged state (a return to the familiar) and is the developmental line of identification which unfolds in increasingly mature forms with time. The second developmental line has the aim of adapting to the new state of the ego with self and object representations separating and differentiating from one another. This is the developmental line of object relations, which also follows a course of increasingly mature forms with developmental growth.

2. The next step is a more differentiated stage, called imitation, in which there is a wishful *fantasy* of merging with the object that is idolized, at a time when maturation and differentiation preclude actual merging. Imitation is total, magical, and temporary. It does not alter the structure of the self representation. One need only observe a child playing at being Superman or some other idol to see all this in operation.

3. The final stage in the developmental line is selective mature identification based on realistic change of the self representation to conform with admired, selected qualities of idolized love objects.[3] This stage occurs after the formation of the wished-for self image (Milrod, 1982).

These complications do not exhaust the difficulties we face in defining identification. All that has been said so far deals with ego identifications. There is, in addition, the area of superego identification, where the major identifications occur at the time of the resolution of the oedipus complex, and the focus of influence is not the self representation but the newly formed superego. Where ego identifications are

3. The struggle to become more like an idolized object is an aspect of the complex identification process which can achieve consciousness.

highly personified, superego identifications are depersonified. Ego identifications deal with values concerned with gratification, power, speed, possessions, and phallic qualities. Superego identifications deal only with moral and ethical values. On an economic level, ego identifications bind aggression; superego identifications release aggression for the use of the superego. It should be clear that the focus of influence or the end product of identification may vary and may include the self representation, the wished-for self image, or the superego. In addition, identifications may be active or passive, conscious or unconscious. The whole subject is quite complex. Freud was very impressed by the kind of identification he described so carefully in melancholia. Although he did not mention it in 1917, after mourning there is also an identification with the deceased. It may be as circumscribed as taking over a mannerism, or it may involve a more profound identification. However, this is a very different form of identification from that in melancholia because the object cathexis is retained.

It would be helpful at this point to draw a distinction between introjection and the formation of an introject. We generally sense that they are different, and yet the distinctions have not been noted clearly enough. Most analysts accept that in melancholia an introject of the lost object is formed in the ego. With that the case, Freud defined the process for us in 1917. That is to say, the formation of an introject must be preceded by a total decathexis of the object representation. And to be consistent all introjects should be thus defined. It follows that introjection, a universal mental mechanism, does not always lead to introject formation, and that the normal identifications made by a growing child, which utilize the mechanism of introjection, are not introjects. It is true that in discussing melancholia, Freud spoke of the formation of an introject as an "identification." But he clearly knew this was a special form of "identification" because he took pains to contrast it with the identification in hysteria where the object cathexis is retained. Today we would add that in melancholia the self representation is not altered by the process in any way and does not become in reality like the ambivalent and degraded object representation. It is merely judged by the superego *as if* it were the degraded object. Freud said (p. 249), "judged . . . *as though* it were . . . the forsaken object." Strictly speaking, the melancholic type of "identification" is not a mature identification at all. Rather the introject has been kept separate and not assimilated or made part of the self representation. When the melancholic episode passes, we can see this very clearly because the old self reemerges. It is remarkable, indeed, to see how felicitous Freud's phrase

(1917) fits with all this: "the shadow of the object fell upon the ego" (self representation) (p. 249). It is the shadow, not the substance.

There is one exception to this definition of an introject and that concerns the formation of the superego. There we also speak of the new structure as an introject of depersonified moral and ethical qualities of the parents. In that special instance, it is the erotic and hostile cathexes of the oedipal objects which must be renounced, given up, or decathected prior to the formation of the introject, i.e., prior to the formation of the superego. But the object ties are retained. In fact, the formation of the superego protects and strengthens those object ties. So here, too, there is a renunciation or decathexis, but only of the forbidden wishes and impulses, not of the basic object cathexis.

Now we are in a position to be more specific about the role of identification in depressions. In melancholia or psychotic depression of a cyclothymic type the formation of an introject of the decathected object is universal. But we would not consider it an identification in the usual sense. It is only in this condition that Freud's comments about narcissistic identification (the formation of an introject) and regression from object cathexis to narcissism apply. By contrast, in neurotic depressions identification with the ambivalent love object may or may not occur. If it does, cathexis of the object representation is constantly maintained. An obsessive-compulsive mourner, for example, may develop a depression and in the process identify with the hated aspect of the ambivalent lost object in his self-condemnation. But the cathexis of that object representation is constantly sustained, so there is neither an introject nor a break with reality. Narcissistic identification with the object does *not* occur, and the obsessional ego rebels against superego punishment, unlike the melancholic ego which readily submits. On the other hand, when a person defies the moral standards in his ego ideal, or fails to live up to the values in his wished-for self image, there will follow some form of self-directed hostility from the superego or ego respectively, and this may develop to a mood state producing a depression. Yet identification with the object will play no significant part in the process. It follows that identification may or may not occur in neurotic depressions.

The role of orality poses another puzzling question associated with depression. Bibring (1953) and Brenner (1974, 1975, 1976, 1979) are correct, I believe, when they say that a narcissistic blow from any level of libidinal development (oral, anal, phallic, or oedipal) may trigger a depression. Both authors reason from this position that the classical view of depression is in need of revision because it emphasizes the universality of the depressive's fixation on orality. Brenner (1974, 1975) even suggests that phallic oedipal conflicts are more significant in depression. Yet the empirical findings of generations of analysts testify to the prominence of orality in these patient's dreams, fantasies, and character structure (Stone, 1986). But we can reconcile these views if we distinguish the dynamics of the precipitating event from those of the syndrome itself. It is not the precipitating event but the self-directed hostility spreading to a mood state which is essential to depression; and it is always accompanied by efforts to restore self-esteem. Some of the authors' clinical examples offered in support of the new theoretical approach do indeed demonstrate depressed patients who have phallic oedipal conflicts (e.g., Brenner, 1974, p. 27). But they fail to deal with the patient's depression per se, i.e., the self-directed hostility and mood state. We must ask why the pathology is focused on the self representation, and why a depression developed rather than some other neurosis based on oedipal conflicts. If we do not follow the problem to its basic elements including the preoedipal roots, neither the exaggerated self-denigration nor the efforts to restore lost self-esteem are dealt with. I would suggest that it is these restorative efforts which are basically oral in nature and which add to the clinical picture the quality of insistent neediness and demandingness. Even the oral incorporative fantasies which accompany the setting up of an introject in melancholia are one form of these restorative efforts. The infant's earliest sense of worth is instilled in the setting of the mother-child dyad by a proud and loving mother showering her affection on her newborn. The entire array of mothering activities is largely organized by the infant around the experience of feeding and is registered as mnemic images and affects related to the breast.[4]

Depressed patients have lost their sense of worth and are engaged in efforts to regain it. If easily regained, the depression is short-lived and will hardly become a clinical problem. Where restorative efforts are unsuccessful or blocked, regression to early oral modes or gaining self-esteem are brought into play. Since depressions are mood states, and the devaluation of the self representation is generalized, the feeling of being totally without worth or value calls for powerful measures to restore self-esteem. It is for this reason that the regression is deep and carries to early oral and restitutive devices. It also strongly suggests that an early trauma and fixation play a role in the predisposition to depression. Although orality plays a universal role in the depressive's efforts

4. Gaining a sense of worth should not be confused with gratification. It is quite possible to have experiences of gratification without gaining a sense of worth.

to restore self-directed libidinal supplies, it is more obvious in the more severe depressions. It should be clear from these considerations that orality, dealing as it does with efforts at restoring self-esteem, has nothing to do with the structure of depressions. When we say, therefore, that orality plays a role in all depressions, it does not mean that all depressions are alike, as some critics of classical theory have asserted.

Lewin (1961) addressed the same issue from a different vantage point. He held the conviction that all psychoanalytic theories about neuroses could be enriched if tested against sleep and dream psychology and to this end he drew comparisons between the two areas in a number of his papers. Assuming that the narcissistic regression in melancholia has the same meaning as that in sleep, he believed it implied a dreamless sleep state. Thus in Lewin's view, the manifest picture of melancholia becomes an analogue of the manifest dream, the result of intruding impulses from id and superego, properly disguised, which threaten to waken the sleeper. From this viewpoint melancholia is an unpleasant dream in which the wish to sleep at the breast is disturbed by what Lewin called the "weaners and wakeners," i.e., the well-known superego injunctions. They are disguised demands that the depressed patient give up the breast or waken. But like the manifest dream, the injunctions take a form that protects the narcissistic regression (sleep). Thus the depressed patient, hearing a constant voice from within saying, "Get away from your mother's breast! Wake up!" does not obey. The pathological element in melancholia is the refusal to be aroused and the insistence on holding on to the breast, a position driven by hostility. While on this subject we should note the parallel between the denial of external reality in sleep and the denial present in any mood state. In depression what is denied is one's sense of worth.

A further area of confusion arose when some recent contributors (Bibring, 1953; Brenner, 1974, 1975, 1976, 1979) equated depression with anxiety as parallel, basic, irreducible affects. Jacobson's (1971) reasons for disagreement with this position seem very sound. Her view is that anxiety is the motivation for defense, whereas depression is one of the symptoms resulting from defensive operations. Mahler (1966) supported this from another vantage point; she described the onset of ambivalence (ambitendency) during the rapprochement subphase when the mother's lack of emotional understanding lowers the child's self-esteem and leads to aggressive coercion of the parent. What follows is the turning of aggression against the self in a "feeling of helplessness" which produces the basic depressive affect. From this account it is clear that the basic depressive affect emerges out of conflict and is not the basic irreducible affect state these authors suggest. I would add that it is difficult to place depression parallel to anxiety when it is a mood disorder and thus an affective ego state with the defensive purpose of discharging ego excitations too strong for the ego to handle via focal discharge. Beyond this, anxiety is an affect based on a singular physiological model, namely, the birth trauma. Anxiety responses can be powerful but are always similar and in time are tamed by a developing ego, so that they can be utilized actively by the ego as a signal. By contrast, from the psychoanalytic point of view, depression, because it deals with feelings about oneself, is subjective in origin rather than physiological. It arises in relation to a variety of narcissistic injuries and never functions as a signal. In addition, anxiety is present from birth, and there must be a degree of ego structure with some form of delineated self representation before a person is able to develop a depression.[5] It is true that a depression can be warded off and defended against. But in that case it is the threat of an emerging depression which leads the ego to give the signal of *anxiety* which then triggers defensive efforts.

Yet another area of confusion has arisen with a recent theory of Brenner's which proposes to replace the classical theory of depression with one that places "depressive affects" alongside anxiety as two parallel forms of unpleasure, each of which can trigger defense. According to this theory, anxiety is the affect associated with a calamity about to happen; depressive affect is associated with a calamity after it has happened. Each triggers defenses to ward off unpleasure in accordance with the pleasure principle. There is a contradiction in replacing a theory about a clinical entity with a theory about signal affects. They do not deal with the same data. So it is no surprise to find that the term "depressive affects" is used in two different ways in this theory. When arguments are offered to change the classical psychoanalytic view of depression (the role of orality, aggression, identification, the basic level of conflict, etc.), it is implicitly used as a clinical entity. When the theory offers reasons to place "depressive affects" alongside anxiety as the two triggers of defensive operations, it is used as a signal affect. This suggests an important internal inconsistency in the theory.

Secondly, the theory is open to question on the basis that in a depression, what we see following the narcissistic injury which precipitates it is not so much defenses to ward off unpleasure, but the development of

5. Spitz (1946) was helpful in differentiating the group of anaclitic depressions he described from the general group of adult depressions. In his group there is a loss of the *real*, external love object, and not the object representation, which has not yet formed at the time of the trauma. Moreover, the self representation has not yet formed and cannot be the target of hostile discharge.

exaggerated unpleasure as self-directed condemnation is unleashed. In other words, because depressions are conditions in which there is a hostile discharge on the self representation, they do not follow the pleasure principle at all. The ego in depressions functions beyond the pleasure principle. The pursuit of pleasure is no longer the prime concern as the pleasure principle becomes subordinated to the economic necessity of restoring psychic equilibrium and preserving the psychic apparatus by the discharge of excessive hostile excitation accumulated in the ego. There is a pressing urgency to the discharge, and it occurs without regard for pleasure or pain. In some severe depressions even this process fails to lower the level of excitation sufficiently, and the individual may resort to the elimination of all psychic excitation in an act of self-destruction.

A further reason to raise questions about this theory is that it does away with so much that Freud carefully delineated for us in contrasting mourning and melancholia. With the new theory the differences are lost and become insignificant as both rest equally on calamities which have already occurred. The important distinctions of libido as the drive predominant in one and aggression in the other;[6] the differences in the work of mourning and the work of melancholia;[7] the retention as opposed to the loss of object cathexis; the difference in the role of reality in each; the formation of an introject in one and not the other; the role of narcissistic object choice in one and not the other—all these important distinctions carefully worked out largely by Freud are done away with as this theory shifts the focus to the question whether the calamity has already occurred or not. Freud taught us how mourning and depression are different. This theory tells us they are the same.

There is a wide variation in the degree to which a person may be aware of his own depression. There can be outright denial or projection or reaction formation brought to bear on depressions. A clinical elation may replace it, or the hostility may be bound in obsessional

6. Freud's clear-cut distinction made mourning emerge as a purely libidinal process, and melancholia as an ambivalent phenomenon with the emphasis on aggression. But most analysts today would agree that this is a puristic delineation, helpful for clarification, but almost unknown in reality. It is a rare mourner who has no ambivalence toward the lost object and who is not therefore depressed to some degree. In practice we deal with clinical phenomena that are mixed, the manifestations of which are determined by the proportions of libidinal and aggressive cathexis of the lost object. It nevertheless remains true that the grief component is related to the libidinal cathexis of the object, and the depressive component, to the aggressive cathexis.

7. In contrast to the work of mourning, which aims at freeing libido for new attachments by *decathecting* the representation of the lost object, a tactic which succeeds with the help of reality, the work of melancholia aims at *maintaining* a failing cathexis of the object, a task at which it does not succeed and in which reality plays no part.

character formation or entrenched in self-pity (Milrod, 1972). In more regressively organized ego structures, more primitive defenses may be used, such as the veering of aggression away from the self representation to the object representation or vice versa. This can happen without projection or introjection mechanisms. The former will ward off depression and produce a reaction of hostility to the world with a paranoid flavor. It constitutes a primitive defense to preserve the self representation. The latter turns hostility on the self representation, giving rise to depression in order to protect the object representation from psychic destruction.

CONCLUSIONS

The above information allows us to account for the fact that:

1. All depressions are painful, but not all painful states produce depression.

2. All depressions involve the loss of self-esteem; but, contrary to Bibring's view (1953), not all experiences of loss of self-esteem give rise to depression.

3. All depressions show a degree of helplessness, but not all experiences of helplessness produce depression.

4. All depressed people are self-condemning, but not all experiences of self-condemnation are connected with depression.

An effective theory of depression must account for all forms of depression, transient or persistent, neurotic or psychotic. In addition, there are three characteristics universally present in depression that an effective theory must explain:

1. In depression the self representation is always cathected with aggressive drive energy. The loss of self-esteem, universally present in depression, is related to this phenomenon.

2. Depression is always a mood state. That is, it is an ego state with generalized discharges and transferences.

3. In depression there is always a disorder in the area of narcissism. This is not surprising in a condition where the central subjective experience is, "I am bad," or "I am a failure."

A psychoanalytic theory of depression must include an explanation of *all* three of these characteristics before it can be considered complete.

BIBLIOGRAPHY

ABRAHAM, K. (1911). Notes on the psycho-analytical investigation and treatment of manic-depressive insanity and allied conditions. In *Selected Papers on Psycho-analysis*. London: Hogarth Press, 1927, pp. 137–156.

_____ (1916). The first pre-genital stage of the libido. *Ibid.*, pp. 248–279.

_____ (1924). A short study of the development of the libido, viewed in the light of mental disorders. *Ibid.*, pp. 418–501.

BIBRING, E. (1953). The mechanism of depression. In *Affective Disorders*, ed. P. Greenacre. New York: Int. Univ. Press, pp. 13–48.

BRENNER, C. (1974). Depression, anxiety and affect theory. *Int. J. Psychoanal.*, 55:25–32.

_____ (1975). Affects and psychic conflict. *Psychoanal. Q.*, 44:5–28.

_____ (1976). *Psychoanalytic Technique and Psychic Conflict*. New York: Int. Univ. Press, pp. 79–107.

_____ (1979). Depressive affect, anxiety and psychic conflict in the phallic-oedipal phase. *Psychoanal. Q.*, 48:177–197.

FREUD, A. (1965). *Normality and Pathology in Childhood*. New York: Int. Univ. Press.

FREUD, S. (1917). Mourning and melancholia. *S.E.*, 14:237–260.

_____ (1921). Group psychology and the analysis of the ego. *S.E.*, 18:67–143.

_____ (1923). The ego and the id. *S.E.*, 19:3–66.

HARTMANN, H. (1953). Contribution to the metapsychology of schizophrenia. *Psychoanal. Study Child*, 8:177–198.

_____ & LOEWENSTEIN, R. M. (1962). Notes on the superego. *Psychoanal. Study Child*, 17:42–81.

JACOBSON, E. (1957). Normal and pathological moods. *Psychoanal. Study Child*, 12:73–113.

_____ (1964). *The Self and the Object World*. New York: Int. Univ. Press.

_____ (1971). *Depression*. New York: Int. Univ. Press.

LEWIN, B. D. (1950). *The Psychoanalysis of Elation*. New York: Norton.

_____ (1961). Reflections on depression. *Psychoanal. Study Child*, 16:321–331.

MAHLER, M. S. (1966). Notes on the development of basic mood. In *Psychoanalysis—A General Psychology*, ed. R. M. Loewenstein, L. M. Newman, M. Schur, & A. J. Solnit. New York: Int. Univ. Press, pp. 152–168.

MILROD, D. (1972). Self-pity, self-comforting, and the superego. *Psychoanal. Study Child*, 27:505–528.

_____ (1982). The wished-for self image. *Psychoanal. Study Child*, 37:95–120.

RADO, S. (1928). The problem of melancholia. *Int. J. Psychoanal.*, 9:420–438.

SANDLER, J. & JOFFE, W. (1965). Notes on childhood depression. *Int. J. Psychoanal.*, 46:88–96.

SCHAFER, R. (1960). The loving and beloved superego. *Psychoanal. Study Child*, 15:163–188.

SPITZ, R. A. (1946). Anaclitic depression. *Psychoanal. Study Child*, 2:313–342.

STONE, L. (1986). Psychoanalytic observations on the pathology of depressive illness. *J. Amer. Psychoanal. Assn.*, 34:329–362.

On the Early Formation of the Mind

II. From Differentiation to Self and Object Constancy

VEIKKO TÄHKÄ, M.D.

IN THIS STUDY THE HUMAN MIND IS SEEN AS AN ENTIRELY SUBJECTIVE AND experiential entity which can be studied and understood only as such. Consequently, the only useful and operable psychoanalytic concepts are considered to be those that refer directly to the mental experience. As I discussed in part I of this presentation (Tähkä, 1987), mental experience is not to be equated with the experiences of a differentiated self; it includes the preceding experiences of an undifferentiated subject as well. Since this preself experience cannot be revived as conscious memories or reached by empathy, it can be approached only by inference and more or less likely speculations. However, to be at all useful and explanatory these inferences and speculations can only seek to say something about the emergence, primary dynamics, and development of the earliest constituents of the mental world of experience. The concept of mind is here considered to include everything that is experienced mentally and to exclude everything that is not (Tähkä, 1987).

From this standpoint it seems that such concepts as the primarily autonomous ego (Hartmann, 1939) or the "inborn structures" (Rapaport, 1960) are not useful. No doubt, a multitude of species-specific programmings and individual potentials can be postulated to exist in a newborn human infant, but these programmings and potentials are

Erik H. Erikson Scholar, Austen Riggs Center, Stockbridge, Mass.; professor emeritus of psychiatry, University of Kuopio; training and supervising psychoanalyst, Finnish Psychoanalytical Society.

not *mind* in any empirical sense; they are abstract constructions which do not contribute to a dynamic and experiential understanding of the early formation and functioning of the mind.

It seems probable that the earliest processes of sensory reception do not represent mental perception before they become connected with the first experiences of organismic tension reduction. It seems to me dynamically and phenomenologically more appropriate to assume that this experiential connection between primitive processes of sensory reception and the vitally necessary tension reduction *motivates* the emergence and cathexis of the baby's species-specific readiness of perceiving and storing engrams.

There exists no experiential justification to regard these readinesses as aspects of an a priori existing mind with cathexes and motivational status of their own. Although they can be inferred from the average course of human mental development, these specifically human potentials can start contributing to the emergence of mental phenomena only on condition that specific interactions take place between the child and his environment. The nursing activities of the mother bring about tension reduction and an experience of organismic relief in the baby with certain accompanying processes of sensory reception. Owing to this connection the sensory experiences involved become equated with the experience of tension reduction, which probably makes their repeated experience to become the first cathected aim of the child and thus simultaneously constitutes the most powerful motive for the emergence of perception and memory as the first representatives of mental activity.

Although I do not deny that the baby's mind-forming potentials and programmings belong to the growth potential in general and may as such in unknown ways exert pressure for manifestation, it seems that they get their dynamic motives, and their economic prerequisites for emergence and existence as mental phenomena, from such interactions with the environment as will bring them directly into the service of the discharge-demanding drive pressure. Thus, an economic and quantitative organismic necessity is needed to initiate the unfolding of the mind with its seemingly endless variation of qualities and secondary motives.

While all species-specific mental function-potentials seem to depend on an interaction with the environment for their activation and manifestation as mental phenomena, it seems that some of them are more fundamental (perception and memory) and require only a relatively simple activation which is almost certain to occur in the average environment of the human infant (the relief-bringing nursing activity of the mother). On the other hand, there are functional mental read-inesses which require much more complicated and vulnerable environ-mental interactions for their activation and emergence as mental func-tions, e.g., those requiring a model and becoming shaped through identifications. However, this state of affairs does not in itself make the former more "primarily autonomous" than the latter.

When the infant's mind-forming potentials have become mobilized, motivated, and cathected, the first percepts and their registrations as the first engrams represent the first contents of the mind and mark the emergence of its two fundamental functions, perception and memory, which henceforth will actively participate in all of its further struc-turalization. This is likely to proceed essentially as collecting un-differentiated experiential information about the sensory conditions of gratification, until the differentiation of the experiential world into self and object makes the structuralizing processes interactive even subjectively (Tähkä, 1987).

With the birth of the mind the mere physiological experience of organismic relief becomes a primitive mental experience of pleasure; thus, the prototype of an affect, just as the coincident undifferentiated sensory information experienced and registered, represents the pro-totypes of all later mental ideas. However, a further differentiation and development of affects and ideas cannot take place before the preconditions of *internalization* are filled in the child's experiential world.

The Concept of Internalization

Freud used the term internalization only in broad biological connec-tions (Compton, 1985). However, he was the first to describe certain specific processes of internalization, particularly in connection with mourning and depression (1917) as well as in the formation of the superego (1921, 1923, 1938). His is also the famous statement accord-ing to which "the character of the ego is a precipitate of abandoned object-cathexes" (1923, p. 29).

Hartmann and Loewenstein (1962) defined internalization as a transformation of external regulations into internal ones. Schafer (1968) expanded this to include the transformation of characteristics as well. Loewald (1962), who introduced the concept of degrees of internalization, defined internalization as a transformation of exter-nal relations into internal ones. Kernberg (1966) sees internalization essentially as a progressive collection and integration of "basic units" consisting of a self representation, an object representation, and an

affect disposition. Meissner (1981) refers to internalization as a movement of reality-derived structural elements in the direction of integration with the ego.

The basic question seems to be: What external aspects are transferred or transformed into what internal ones? It seems obvious that
the concept of internalization cannot be applied to the human world of
experience before there exists an experiential distinction between representations given the quality of interiority and those given the quality
of exteriority. Internalization can start as an experiential transaction
only when the primary crude differentiation between self and object
has taken place. The interaction and exchange between the experiencing self and the experienced object then leads to processes of internalization; i.e., what was formerly perceived as belonging to the object
will become something experienced inside the self or included in it.

Loewald (1962) proposed that since the infant's earliest undifferentiated registrations of his exchange with the outside world have not
experientially crossed the border between internal and external, those
processes should be called primary internalizations, as contrasted with
secondary internalizations that take place after the differentiation of
those basic dimensions of experience. This view, shared by Meissner
(1981), implied, in addition, that the experiential differentiation between internal and external would be *created* by hypothetical processes
of primary internalization and externalization.

However, the concepts of primary internalization and externalization can be used only in an "objective" sense, without any counterpart
in the infant's still undifferentiated subjective experience. If the psychoanalytic metapsychology should confine itself to concepts related to
mental experience, concepts implying experiential interiority and exteriority are logical misfits when undifferentiated levels of experience
are described. Interpersonal relations on that level are observed by us,
not yet experienced by the child.

Schafer (1972) argued that the term internalization should be
dropped as a pure spatial metaphor reflecting merely fantasies of
incorporation. He emphasized that because mental phenomena do not
occur in space, they do not have inside and outside and can move from
one place to another only in fantasy. By replacing "inner world"
(Hartmann, 1939) with "private world," Schafer wanted to avoid spatial terms and to stress the character of the latter as representing those
aspects of the mind that are not communicated or uncommunicable,
and therefore hidden or ignored, consciously or unconsciously. "Inside the self" is rejected by Schafer because the self for him is a purely

descriptive concept without systemic properties, which he, instead, ascribes to the ego.

My point of departure is different. Although the inner or internal (Freud, 1938) world is not an adequate term to describe the earliest modes of mental experience, after the differentiation of the representational world it is not only useful but indispensable as the experiential antithesis of the experienced outside world. In my conceptualization all mental processes occur in the world of experience and can be approached only as such.

Concepts such as the "inner world" and "internalization" correspond to the subjective experience of the human being after the differentiation of his experiential world into inside and outside, self and object. Interiority and exteriority are subjective experiences and discriminations taking place in the individual's mental world of experience. Internalization means transitions from experienced exteriority to experiencing and experienced interiority. Naturally, terms such as the inner world and internalization do not refer to any physical or spatial locality, but to an *experiential* locality that is not less real than the former. They represent the very *empiria* of the mind that we study as psychoanalysts and that cannot be escaped or transcended. While Schafer (1972) thinks that the mind is an abstraction similar to beauty or freedom, in my conceptualization it means the totality of subjective mental experience which certainly also includes those abstractions.

"Private" can hardly be substituted for "inner" in the way Schafer suggests. When a person communicates his thoughts and feelings, this does not in itself make them experientially less internal; he still feels that he speaks of and reveals his "inner world." What was communicated may no longer be private but still retains its subjective index of interiority. "Intrapsychic," especially in the more advanced phases of the development of the mind, refers to a much more organized and stable subjective experience than Schafer's "private world" in the sense of merely hiding and keeping silent.

Having defined internalization as an experiential transition or transformation of the aspects of the object world into the realm of the self, I must before proceeding discuss briefly the concepts of self and object.

SELF AND OBJECT

The self has been subject to increasing psychoanalytic interest since Hartmann (1950) introduced the concept of self representation as an antithesis to object representations. Hartmann defined self as a substructure of the ego, a view thenceforth shared by the majority of psychoanalytic authors (e.g., Sandler and Rosenblatt, 1962; Jacobson, 1964; Kernberg, 1966, 1982; Schafer, 1968). Kohut (1971, 1977) in his self psychology is not explicit in his treatment of the reciprocal relationship of these two concepts.

The self becomes mentally represented at the experiential division of the so far undifferentiated representational world. The level of organization of this primordial self experience is extremely low and will only gradually grow into the representational versatility required for the emergence of more detailed and lasting self images. These more advanced self images which normally develop into an experience of identity or self constancy are usually referred to when self representations have been defined as an idea that the subject has about his own person (Schafer, 1968, p. 28). However, a subject capable of experiencing itself as a subject—no matter how crude and primitive—is by definition a differentiated self with a representational existence in the individual's mental world of experience.

This brings us back to the relationship between the concepts of the ego and the self. If all constituents of the mind are seen as representational on some level of mental experience, statements such as "The construction of the representational world is a product of ego functions" or "the representational world . . . is a set of indications which guides the ego to appropriate adaptive or defensive activity" (Sandler and Rosenblatt, 1962, pp. 134, 136), clearly are not compatible with such a view. In these definitions an ego and its functions are postulated as nonrepresentational abstractions separate from the self which, instead, is given representational and therefore experiential properties. If my standpoint is accepted, it seems more appropriate to conclude that the self constitutes the experiential and functional manifestation of the mind after it has become capable of experiencing itself as separate from the outside world.

In part I of this study I suggested that the self has its origin when its first function, the hunger cry, becomes mentally represented through its ability to bring forth gratification (Tähkä, 1987). As emphasized above, mental functions and mental structure exist only when they are represented on some level of mental experience. Functional and structural cannot be kept separate from experiential and representational in the mental world of experience; on the contrary, they seem to be existentially interdependent.

Therefore, rather than regarding the self as a tool utilized by a hypothetical and nonempirical ego, I prefer to equate the self with the actively experiencing and functioning organization of the mind through which the individual is enabled to experience himself as existing and alive, as well as to observe an experientially separate outside world and to interact with it. The self then means the ever expanding and differentiating experiential subject with images of himself and objects of varying accuracy and duration, as well as with self-indexed functions which either antedate the birth of the self or are acquired through the processes of internalization.

The self is thus the structural organization into which the mind grows, thereby acquiring the sense of being a person in the world. Maintaining this sense of being alive, i.e., a subjective self experience, will henceforth be the individual's essential aim and the central motive for all further structuralization of his mind. All developments of the mind that follow occur through the self and are identical with those of the latter.

With the emergence of self experience the individual becomes capable of experiencing an outside world, observing it actively and interacting with it. *Object world* refers to the phenomena experienced as "not-me," separated from the self. The *external* ("real") *objects* are experienced as existing outside the self, whereas the so-called *object representations* are experientially located inside it.[1]

The experienced interaction of the self with the external objects will constantly test, influence, and modify the inner images of the objects, which are experienced as both gratifying and threatening, and with the proceeding structuralization increasingly as informative of so-called "reality." A total or selective cessation of this testing and modifying influence of the "real" object experience on the further development of the inner world of self and object images is responsible for the monotonously repetitive ways of experiencing, which in a more or less extensive and distorting form characterizes various levels of psychopathology, and which Strachey (1934) has called "closed representational worlds" to be reopened by the analytic work.

My use of the concept of self and object images thus has reference to inner ideas of self and objects, which are optimally subjected to continuous processes of differentiation and integration in a lifelong experiential interaction between the individual's self and object world. These processes are essentially processes of internalization.

---

1. Since all mental experiencing here means that phenomena are or become mentally represented, *object image* might be a better term than the accustomed object representation which does not satisfactorily distinguish between the experiences of "inner" and "outer" objects.

MOTIVATIONS OF INTERNALIZATION

The emergence of the human mind seems to be motivated by the necessity of coping with the energic pressures of the organism, and it leads to striving for mentally experienced pleasure and gratification. Provided that the seeking of gratification constitutes the primary motive for mental activity, preserving and improving the mental devices that have proved effective must become the most important secondary motives of the incipient mind. The development of the mind into an instrument increasingly effective in seeking and attaining gratification and pleasure both gives central importance to the preservation of the already established mental structure and leads to an ever expanding and ramifying network of derivative motives.

The first major structural achievement in the early formation of the mind is the emergence of the experiential differentiation between the self and the object world. I assume that the preservation of self experience will henceforth be the basic motive in all further developments of the mind, including processes of internalization.

As self and objects become differentiated from the so far undifferentiated mnemic registrations of gratificatory experiences, they will emerge as pure pleasure formations and can in the beginning exist only in that form in the infant's experiential world. There is no motivation for the states of frustration and organismic distress to become mentally represented before this differentiation, and they therefore are likely to remain in the realm of physiological experiencing (Tähkä, 1984b, 1987).

Before the experiential world develops further to include aggressively tinged images of "all-bad" objects, the inevitable frustration-aggression is bound to destroy repeatedly the newly won differentiation, which still rests solely on the experience of a self fully possessing and omnipotently controlling an object with an unlimited gratificatory capacity. It is probable that internalization starts in order to protect and preserve this ideal state of the self.

Even if internalization can be seen as a series of ways to deal with and compensate for the ongoing object loss with a concomitant emphasis on the "immortality" of the object (Schafer, 1968), there is hardly any doubt that the maintenance of a self experience is the primary concern of the primitive mind. Object, although spatially separate from the self, cannot in the beginning be experienced as anything but a means of gratification, self-evidently belonging to the self (although not included *in* the self). However, since the mental existence of a self is thus in the beginning dependent on complete experiential mastery over the gratifying object, the primordial self is obviously in need either of an illusion of a continuous presence of such an object or of taking over some of its gratificatory functions. These needs seem to constitute the immediate motives for internalization to get started.

Even if the experiential contents of these needs undergo changes during the maturation and development of the mind, strivings to establish an expanding inner world of objects as well as to improve the equipment of the self in ensuring gratification of its ramifying derivative wishes remain the central motives for all subsequent acts of internalization.

INTERNALIZATION AND STRUCTURALIZATION

I consider structuralization as synonymous with the building up of the mind in general and have proposed that everything that becomes mentally represented with some temporal duration belongs to the structure of the mind (Tähkä, 1987). This use of the concept of structure differs from its previous psychoanalytic definitions (e.g., Hartmann, 1939, 1950; Hartmann et al., 1946; Rapaport, 1951, 1957; Gill, 1963; Kernberg, 1976; Schafer, 1976; Schwartz, 1981) and needs to be better specified at this point.

While the earliest undifferentiated representations are considered to constitute the first structure of the mind, after the differentiation, i.e., when the subject has acquired a self experience, the existing and developing mental structure becomes and remains experientially self-indexed. Even if rudimentary in the beginning, the self experience brings with it a me-feeling that will thenceforth be attached to an ever increasing variety of functions, affective experiences, and images of both self and objects. These are experienced as included *in* the self or belonging *to* the self. Introjects, images, fantasies, and memories of the objects as well as all stored information of the object world in general constitute the latter category which, although referring to an outside world, remains self-indexed and experientially located in an inner world.

The subjective inner world is contrasted with an object world experienced spatially as outside the self. Since gratification is experientially connected with the differentiated object, the primary self will become increasingly motivated to mental operations that aim at transforming aspects of the experienced object world into experiences either included in or belonging to the self. These mental operations are the processes of internalization which constantly change the individual's subjective inner world both with respect to the self experience and the object world.

This lifelong development constitutes the very structuralization of the mind in a continual interaction with an experiential object world. After the primary differentiation, it becomes the development of a subject increasingly aware of himself as a subject and increasingly well informed about the experienced world of objects. As stated before, after the differentiation all further development of the mind is synonymous with that of the self, which has become the bearer of the individual's subjective world of mental experience. The experienced outside objects may *change,* but they do not *develop* as such—only our images of them and our ways of experiencing them do.

Internalization thus appears to be the very mechanism of structuralization after the differentiation of self and object, and consists in building up the individual's self-indexed mental equipment and inner world of representations. The various forms of manifestation during the different developmental stages will be scrutinized in the rest of this paper.

THE PROTECTIVE DICHOTOMIES

The subjective sense of being alive emerges with and is dependent on the dichotomy of the experiential world into self and object. I have suggested that this dichotomic experience, vitally important for the newly won self experience, is based solely on representations of pleasure and gratification and therefore becomes threatened by the frustration-aggression that inevitably emerges after the differentiation of self and object (Tähkä, 1987).

This basic dichotomic experience, indispensable for a personal existence, will from the beginning become protected by a series of other experiential dichotomies. The first of these is likely to consist of attempts to utilize the physiological level of experiencing to deal with tensions that would otherwise become mentally represented as representations of frustration and aggression. Individuals who during the first half year of their life have been forced to an exaggerated use of somatic channelization of accumulating drive energy are probably especially prone to continue to deal with painful tensions as "organismic distress" rather than moving toward their becoming mentally represented as affects and images.

Such a postponement of the "mentalization" of pain and frustration may leave behind a lasting paucity of representations of frustration with a concomitant tendency to react somatically in situations where so-called normal people would feel some variants of mentally experienced pain or anger. This state of affairs would at least partly explain the relative representational insufficiency or so-called "alexithymia" (Sifneos, 1973; Nemiah, 1975) of certain psychosomatic patients and their helpless resorting to psychologically empty physiological reactions in dealing with painful tensions in the organism.

While a prolonged utilization of the dichotomy between physiological and mental experiencing for the protection of the experiential differentiation of self and object tends to retard mental structuralization and leave it defective, the emergence of a new experiential dichotomy between "all-good" and "all-bad" object images (Klein, 1946) not only represents a specifically mental protection for the mentally experienced differentiation, but also provides an indispensable basis for all further structuralization of the mind.

The development of this first primitive experiential dichotomy between "good" and "bad" is motivated by the archaic annihilation ("de-differentiation") anxiety of a self still dependent for its existence on a fully gratified ideal state. Attempts to avoid the devastating emergence of frustration-aggression by re-creating the good object as a mentally felt presence are not sufficient for maintaining the experience of that ideal state as long as frustration and aggression themselves lack ideational mental representations. Once they have been created, the first "all-good" and "all-bad" object images leave the child's self experience considerably less at the mercy of the object's actual behavior.

As will be seen in the next section, new forms of protective dichotomies result from the utilization and vicissitudes of these new constituents of the primitive mind. But even in the later development of the mind it is not difficult to see how the basic existential necessity of an experiential differentiation between self and object world provides the basis for the general human preference of dichotomic approaches, valuations, and solutions.

INTROJECTION, PROJECTION, AND DENIAL

An introject is customarily defined as an experience of an object's presence inside the self representation (Schafer, 1968). It is the first image of the object that is experienced independent of the object's actual presence and thus constitutes the first product of internalization proper. *Introjection* refers to that mental process which brings about the experience of introjects and thus represents the first primitive way of thinking of the object.

Since according to my conceptualization the object can initially be

experienced only as an unlimited source of gratification, fully possessed and controlled by the primary self, the first introjects are likely
to represent attempts at the perpetuation of such experiencing (Tähkä, 1987). While hallucinations were the first attempts of the emerging
mind to control frustration and ensure gratification by re-creating
experiences of the latter, introjects are developmentally more advanced mental formations serving the same purpose.

The crucial difference between hallucinations and the felt presences
of objects is that the former can only repeat undifferentiated mnemic
registrations of gratificatory experiences with a minimum of control,
while in the latter the source of gratification has been recognized to be
an object, re-created and magically controlled in its introjective experience. Hallucinations thus represent the first attempts of the undifferentiated mind to regulate drive tension (Tähkä, 1984b, 1987),
while introjects constitute the first devices of the self to control the
object which has become both the bearer of gratification and the prerequisite of continued self experience.

The first introjective experiences probably are motivated by the dedifferentiation anxiety (Tähkä, 1987) mobilized by experiential lack of
a good object in a state of need. The experienced presence of an object
corresponding with that of the original ideal state thus becomes the
first condition for a preserved experience of differentiation in the
object's absence.

Introjects are images of a "functional object" (Tähkä, 1984a), the
bearer of the not yet internalized aspects of the child's future personality, including its tension-regulating and self-soothing functions.
Therefore, they can be controlled only magically in a passive experience, where introjective object images are expected to prove the continuous existence of the omnipotent self with its full control over gratification. Only after the establishment of self and object constancies
(Hartmann, 1952; Mahler et al., 1975) will it be possible to manipulate
object images freely in fantasy.

Object representations (images) are products of internalization and
constitute the store of an object world perceived as external. However,
the first object images are essentially substitutive in character and become only gradually more informative, the more further processes of
internalization will make it possible to experience the object's independent and self-determined existence.

When need arises, the self tends to experience the gratifying object's
presence. However, in the beginning it cannot be maintained for long
if the real gratification is postponed. Frustration is so far represented
only by aggressive affect and impetus for action; consequently, any

attempt to "force" the object to provide gratification and thus to save its "all-good" image will necessarily remain short-lived and be quickly replaced by pure destructiveness, which dissolves both the "all-good" object image and the self experience, still solely dependent on and justified by the experiential existence of the former (Tähkä, 1987).

To prevent this and to preserve differentiated self experience, separate ideational representations for frustration and aggression become indispensable and will be created out of the perceptions of the frustrating object. However, in contrast to the image of the all-gratifying object, which becomes activated as a felt presence in the state of need, the image of an all-frustrating object is in that situation kept experientially absent as far as possible. Consequently, the mounting aggression of the self in such a situation is ascribed or *projected* to the newly won all-frustrating object image and an attempt is made to keep it experientially absent, ignored, and disavowed. The last-mentioned attempt seems to be the first way in which primitive *denial* makes its appearance.

By projection I mean the experience of those aspects of self image which are incompatible with it or intolerable for its existence, as belonging to object image. It should be noted that projection specifically involves experiential and cathectic transitions from self image to object representation. Corresponding transitions from one object image to another are not projection but *displacement*.

Novick and Kelly (1970) distinguish between externalization of a self representation and externalization of a drive which they call projection proper. According to my conceptualization, in which drive is given only quantitative properties (Tähkä, 1987), a "pure" drive projection is not possible without the simultaneous projection of a self representation. The experience projected always involves a representation of the one whose experience it originally was. Thus, by projection a representation of the hating self becomes experientially a representation of the hating object and adds to the latter qualitative and quantitative aspects, peculiar to the way of hating of the former.

Nor can I share Novick and Kelly's view that projection would presuppose a considerable amount of structuralization, with fantasied dangers. The first danger of the self necessitating the first projective maneuvers is not fantasied, for as long as reality can be experienced only as a pleasure formation, frustration and aggression represent a very real danger for the existence of a separate self experience. Therefore, projection in the beginning of life should be regarded not as a "defense" but as an adaptive activity vitally important for the psychological survival of the child and for the further structuralization of his mind.

Although the "all-bad" object becomes through projection the bearer of the child's aggressive self and its worthless nonomnipotent aspects, incapable of bringing forth gratification, that object image is not a mere *product* of projection but stems basically from registered perceptions of the frustrating object. Mothers *do* frustrate as well as gratify their babies and although grossly distorted, both "all-bad" and "all-good" object images represent reality-based and adaptive information of the outside world at the developmental level under scrutiny.

Because of the dyadic exclusiveness of the primary object world and because the mother images inevitably belong to the infant's experiential orbit, the "all-bad" object image cannot yet be displaced onto a third person, as is possible in projective maneuvers later in life. Therefore, projection alone does not suffice to bring about an experiential absence of the perilous bad object. Primitive denial now seems to emerge to support the illusion of the object's exclusive "goodness."

It could be argued that the first attempt of the self to avoid mentally experienced unpleasure would be its denial. It may so be, provided that the primary denial is simply equated with a hypothetical capacity of the primordial self to resist the first object-related frustrations becoming mentally represented. However, a mere lack of representations can hardly be regarded as a mental activity and nothing can be denied before there is something to deny. If denial is considered to be directed against phenomena that are already represented mentally, experientially it amounts to an unawareness of the existence or meaning of those phenomena. It seems that such a decathexis of awareness of certain perceptions and representations becomes motivated only when an established "all-bad" object has to be kept from interfering with the original ideal way of experiencing self and object.

When fully established, introjection, projection, and denial have the common function of maintaining and protecting experience of this original ideal state. It then continues to exist as a relationship between the omnipotent self and the introjective presence of the all-gratifying mother's image, while the images of frustrated self and all-frustrating object are kept away by projection and denial. When successful, this constellation may represent the developmental core experience of the omnipotent elation regressively revived in *manic psychoses* later in life.

Since every frustration adds new experiential material, both "real" and projected, to the image of the "all-bad" object, it will grow the stronger, the more there is frustration in the interaction between the infant and his mother, while the "all-good" image will correspondingly weaken and its felt presence become threatened. However, in a situation where denial can no longer prevent the breaking through of the image of the "all-bad" object as a felt presence, its very existence seems now, paradoxically, to offer a new way of saving the experiential differentiation between self and object world.

The establishment of two opposite object images was originally motivated by a necessity to preserve differentiation as a purely pleasurable experience. However, when frustration has become represented, an object image has been created which in itself is not threatened by aggression; on the contrary, the greater the amount of aggression that is projected into the all-bad object, the stronger and the more persecutory it grows. Provided that the self can retain its experiential omnipotency as the possessor and controller of gratification, differentiated experience may be saved as existing between the self and the "all-bad" object.

This seems to become possible through a re-fusion of the self with the remaining image of the "all-good" object. This provides the self image with an unlimited capacity for gratification; everything that is pleasurable and gratifying will be experienced as magically produced by the self. Denial will be specifically directed against awareness that anything good would come from the object. In this partial loss of differentiation the image of the "all-good" object is lost and the object experience will thereafter completely rest on the retained image of the "all-bad" object. The experience of its persecutory presence will replace the "all-good" introject in its function of maintaining experiential differentiation between self and object.

Preserving a self experience is under these circumstances completely dependent on the retained omnipotence of the self image. This requires that all threatening representations of the self as frustrated and devalued are projectively ascribed to the image of the "all-bad" object. This constellation, in which the differentiated experience rests on a differentiation between the images of "all-good" self and "all-bad" object, cannot tolerate any flaws in the omnipotence of the self or in the object's exclusive malignancy.

This state of affairs where all good is kept inside and all bad outside bears a resemblance to Freud's (1915) postulation of a "purified pleasure ego" as a developmental stage where all that is pleasurable is incorporated in the self and all that is unpleasurable is ascribed to the external world. It also shows similarities to the "paranoid position" described by Melanie Klein (1946) from a different point of departure. Although representing a developmental cul-de-sac in itself, this experiential constellation provides an important emergency solution for the maintenance of experiential differentiation between self and object. As such it is passingly and fleetingly used by children before reaching self and object constancy, as well as by borderline patients with their incomplete and distorted structures. More long-lasting or chronic regression to this way of experiencing is seen in adult patients with *paranoid psychoses*.

Although the "paranoid"[2] solution thus appears to be an attempt to stay psychologically alive in situations involving excessive frustrations, it cannot be maintained if the gratifying object is lost even objectively. While the subjective experience of a good object is lost through a partial re-fusion, continuing experiences of gratification are necessary in order to maintain the omnipotence of the self as its felt provider. Even if the "paranoid" self dislocates the source of gratification, it cannot survive its actual cessation.

As contrasted with the "paranoid" solution, the experiential constellation that becomes regressively remobilized in *depressive psychoses* later in life seems specifically to represent an attempt of the self to survive psychologically a *loss* of the external object and thus also of the gratification customarily obtained from it. When the external object and the actual gratification provided by it are lost, the maintenance of the self experience is completely left to the inner world of representations, which does not yet provide many alternatives at the early stages of development.

When a prolonged absence of the customary gratification leads to the fading of the "all-good" introject with a corresponding strengthening in the image of the "all-bad" object, the self faces an acute emergency. Since the gratification from the external object is missing, the omnipotence of the self cannot be saved and maintained by an identification or re-fusion with the progressively weakening image of the "all-good" object. While the extensive loss of real gratification thus makes a "paranoid" solution impossible, the only way for the self to preserve differentiation in an experiential world, saturated by frustration and aggression, seems to be to identify with that part of the object representation which is not threatened but strengthened by the mounting aggression. After a global identification of the self with the image of the frustrating object, the experiential differentiation is maintained between a self turned bad and an endangered image of the good object. However, the longer in duration and the more total the loss of the gratifying external object, the less will there be left of the introject

2. I am aware that normal or more or less ubiquitous developmental phenomena should not be named after the pathological manifestations in which they may later in life become revived through regression. Therefore, expressions such as "paranoid" and "depressive" solutions are used here only hesitantly and in the absence of established alternatives.

of the good object and the more hateful and worthless will the self image grow. As identified with the frustrating object, the self absorbs all aggression and when the image of the good object can no longer be retained, concrete self destruction becomes a real danger.

Since the actual object losses of small children are, of necessity, usually compensated by new objects, their experiences of total loss of a gratifying external object tend to remain limited in time and scope. Although extreme forms of depression with suicidal behavior are therefore seldom seen in children, traumatic object losses in early childhood are likely to constitute the main mental predisposition to psychotic depressions of adult patients.

The depressive attempt to stay alive psychologically seems to presuppose some pre-established tolerance for frustrated and nonomnipotent self presentations. As will later be seen, this requires that the process of functionally selective identifications is well under way. A more stable establishment of the basic representational differentiation and a more enduring early structuralization seem to make the depressive patient more resistant to a regression to undifferentiated levels of experience than is the case with schizophrenic patients. The depressive patient's self can no longer resort to a "psychological suicide" but tends, instead, to destroy itself concretely when its experiential maintenance becomes impossible.

To sum up: in the "paranoid" solution the experience of the "all-good" object is lost through a partial re-fusion, both as internal and external, whereas the experience of the "all-bad" object remains preserved in both respects. The experience of gratification is not lost, although its experiential source has been transferred from the object to the self.

In the "depressive" solution the experience of the gratifying external object is lost for reasons independent of the child. In an attempt to save the inner image of a good object the bad object is experientially lost through identification, both externally and internally. What is left to preserve the differentiated experience is an inner relationship between the image of a self growing increasingly bad and the progressively fading image of the good object.

Unlike schizophrenia in which the experience of differentiation is regressively lost, the other major psychoses appear to show a regressive revival of the earliest attempts to preserve self experience by manipulating the representational world with primitive mental operations of introjection, projection, and denial. However, a further elaboration of the origins and dynamics of those states is beyond the scope of this presentation. Nor can the earlier psychoanalytic views, including the classical psychoanalytic studies of depression (Freud, 1917; Bibring, 1953; Joffe and Sandler, 1965; Jacobson, 1971) be reviewed at this point.

However, a few words should be said about the concept of *incorporation*. Without going into the history and various uses of this controversial concept (see Freud, 1905, 1915, 1917; Abraham, 1924; Lewin, 1950; Fenichel, 1953; Hartmann and Loewenstein, 1962; Jacobson, 1964; Schafer, 1968, 1972; Meissner, 1981), I want to state briefly my stand regarding its usefulness and eventual place in the phenomenology of internalization.

In his thorough and scholarly monograph on internalization Meissner (1981) presented incorporation as the primary and most primitive form of internalization, motivated by primitive wishes for union and leading to a dedifferentiation of self and object representations. According to Meissner, incorporation thus plays a role in severely regressed states.

According to my conceptualization, a prerequisite for the use of internalization as a term describing a subjective mental experience is that an experiential division between inside and outside exists in the subject's world of experience. Internalization is an experience of a differentiated self that results from something experienced as external becoming experienced as internal. The loss of differentiation destroys the possibilities for such an experience and can therefore be neither a form nor a result of internalization.

Secondly, I consider the primary motivation for all internalization to be the maintenance and protection of the established self experience. As I have tried to show in part I of this presentation, the so-called "symbiotic longings" cannot refer to experiences actually had and longed for by a differentiated self, but rather to the once experienced omnipotent harmony of the first differentiation, still uncontaminated by frustration and aggression (Tähkä, 1987). It is the last-mentioned experience that the early internalization strives to preserve, instead of seeking to replace it by undifferentiation. The dedifferentiation actually seems to take place only when it becomes economically impossible to maintain a self experience with the help of secondary structures achieved through internalization.

Incorporation in Meissner's sense thus appears to be a mere synonym for a regressive return to a subjectively prepsychological level of experience by a mind that has lost the prerequisites of experiencing itself as a person in a world and thus also the basic preconditions for internalization. It seems to me that the concept of incorporation, if at all useful, could be used attributively to refer to ideational contents of certain introjective experiences.

FUNCTIONAL RELATEDNESS

It seems likely that the early self experiences the gratifying object as its self-evident possession. The object and its services are felt to exist only for the child's sake and even if the gratifying, soothing, and mirroring functions of the former tend to be overestimated by the child as omnipotent,[3] these functions cannot yet be experienced as belonging to a self-determined somebody beyond the immediate control and possession of the self. It is not until the object can be experienced as having an inner world of its own as a result of the establishment of self and object constancy, that the object world ceases to belong experientially exclusively to the self.

The nature of the mother's functional services, experienced as self-evident, determines at any given moment the nature and affective color of the child's early object awareness. Depending on whether the mother's respective function is gratifying or frustrating, she is experienced by the child as "all-good" or "all-bad" with a corresponding and/or compensatory mobilization of the inner images about her. In the child's experiential world this early object is not yet somebody *with* functions but a much less differentiated somebody who *is* the function she is performing at a given moment (Tähkä, 1981, 1984a).

Since the child's early object experience is entirely dependent on the state of need, his experience of the mother is bound to oscillate between "all-good" and "all-bad." However, attention should be called to the risks inherent in the established use of the adultomorphic terms of "good" and "bad" at this early stage of development and object relatedness. Even if the gratifying nature of the mother's functional services may make the child experience them as omnipotent and primitively idealized, the nature of these services as self-evidently belonging to (although not included in) the self does not yet allow any experienced "goodness" of the object. As will be discussed in detail below, it seems that an interest in and a longing for the object as a person, i.e., a capacity for object love and hate with the corollary feelings of guilt and gratitude, become possible only with the establishment of self and

---

3. See Kohut's (1966) "idealized parent image" and Kernberg's (1976) "primitive idealization."

object constancy, and only then will "goodness" and "badness" become justified as terms describing the child's object experience.

In an attempt to discriminate between the levels of object relatedness before and after the establishment of self and object constancy, various terms and concepts have been suggested to illustrate the differences observed. Sandler and Rosenblatt (1962) refer to these differences in their proposed discrimination between changeable and temporary early images of self and object as contrasted with their more stable and permanent representations after achieved self and object constancy. Dorpat (1976) describes an earlier level of object relatedness, characterized by introjective experience and object relation conflicts as contrasted with a more advanced one with predominantly structural conflicts.

The nature of the early object as a self-evident possession of the self and its role as a substitute for the lacking structures of the child's future self (ego) has given rise to attempts to name that object experience according to these characteristics. A particularly infelicitous newcomer in this respect seems to be the widely used concept of "narcissistic object," inspired especially by Kohut's work. No matter whether narcissism is defined as a libidinal cathexis of the self (Hartmann, 1953), as a cathected state of the idealized self representations (Tähkä, 1981), or as a self-maintaining function of a mental activity (Stolorow and Lachmann, 1980), the attribute narcissistic pertains specifically to the self and to the interest invested in it. By definition, the cathexis of the object, cathected object representations, or mental activities aimed at maintaining object representations cannot be called narcissistic, regardless of how primitive the object awareness and how much the object still is experienced as belonging to the self's possession.

Kohut's concept (1971) of selfobject is defined as an object cathected with narcissistic libido and acceptable as such only if qualitatively different forms of libido are postulated. However, the concept could still be useful if it were redefined to mean specifically that level of object experience at which the object still performs such services for the child as the latter will later be able to take care of by himself, and at which the object can still be experienced only as a self-evident possession of the self. Without making it explicit, some recent authors seem to use the concept in accordance with this redefinition (e.g., Dorpat, 1976).

It seems to me that the most important characteristic of this early stage of object relatedness is its functional nature described above. Experientially the object is not yet an individual person but a group of functions, and this makes its affective color entirely dependent on the gratifying or frustrating nature of the object's respective function.

These functions of the object will normally, through identifications, to a great extent become functions of the self during the period of separation-individuation. During that period of structuralization the not yet internalized functions of the object continue to represent the dynamic core of the object relation, until the processes of functionally selective identification are sufficiently completed to allow experiences of object and self constancy to emerge as a new level of experiential differentiation and integration.

However, before this new level is achieved, the most pertinent attribute to describe the prevailing object relatedness appears to be *functional* (Tähkä, 1984a). I use the terms "functional object" and "functional object relatedness" to refer to the particular kind of object relationship predominant between differentiation and object constancy as well as to its persisting manifestations in "normal" and pathological object relations.

Patients with a borderline pathology have not reached self and object constancy. Unlike the neurotic patient's transference, which predominantly repeats repressed oedipal relations between an individual self and an individual object, the phase-specific repetition of the borderline patient activates essentially functional levels of relatedness. As a functional object the analyst comes to represent noninternalized parts of the patient's defective self that cannot be relinquished through mourning or comparable processes of working through. Representing still indispensable outside services, a lost functional object can only be substituted for by a new one or be replaced bit by bit by functionally selective identifications (Tähkä, 1979, 1984a, 1984b). No matter whether a preoedipal child or a borderline patient is concerned, it is this process of identification that seems to be indispensable to the development from a functional and introjective relatedness with objects to an individual's relationship with other individuals.

FUNCTIONALLY SELECTIVE IDENTIFICATIONS

The most specifically human readinesses seem to need human models and identifications in order to become mentally represented as functions and characteristics experienced as one's own. Therefore, identification is by far the most important process in the structuralization of personality.

Identification is here defined as a process of internalization through which functions and characteristics experienced as belonging to the object become functions and characteristics of the self. That this molding and building up of the self by using the object as a model are essential in identification corresponds with the use of the concept by most psychoanalytic authors (Freud, 1921; Moore and Fine, 1968; Laplanche and Pontalis, 1973).

Although the idea that the early identifications differ from those occurring in the oedipal period was already indicated by Freud (1917) in his discrimination between narcissistic and hysterical identifications, his main interest was in the identifications related to the oedipal situation and superego formation (Freud, 1923, 1933).

Most authors after Freud shared his interest in oedipal and superego identifications, which were generally regarded as the prototypes of identification. Thus, the described motives for and results of Jacobson's (1964) "selective ego identifications" mostly correspond with those of typical oedipal identifications; Schafer (1968) gave the latter the major structuralizing importance as compared with the earlier identifications. Hendrick's (1951) pioneering thoughts of the early ego identifications that lead to the establishment of central executive functions of the ego have only recently begun to attract the attention they deserve. The same holds true for Loewald's (1962) discrimination between preoedipal and oedipal identifications, the former being essentially structural elements of the ego, the latter those of the superego.

I assume that the structuralization of the mind which changes the essentially introjective-projective and functional experience into that of self and object constancy takes place through a multitude of identifications with the introjects and with the external object's observed functions. Thus, it is essentially the process of ongoing identification that is considered to make possible the developmental journey Mahler (1968) has called separation-individuation.

I have called the identifications preceding and leading to experiences of individual identity and individual objects *functionally selective* as contrasted with the *judgmentally selective* oedipal identifications (Tähkä, 1984b). The former essentially bring new *functions* into the self using the functional object or its introjective experience as a model, while the latter seem mainly to add *characteristics* to the self with the individual oedipal objects as conscious paragons.

MOTIVES AND PREREQUISITES FOR FUNCTIONALLY SELECTIVE IDENTIFICATIONS

The primary motive for the processes of functionally selective identification seems still to be the need to restore the ideal state of the self as the owner and controller of gratification. However, as contrasted to the passively experienced and magically controlled introjective presences, functionally selective identifications furnish the self with means of active control in its striving for gratification as well as in dealing with frustration. Separation/annihilation anxiety still predominates over the stage of functional relatedness and is in normal development dealt with through a gradual assimilation of the object's functions into the self in a process of bit by bit identifications with them. Other negative affects, envy and shame, have their advent and contribute as important motives to the ongoing processes of functionally selective identification during the period of separation-individuation.

Thus, the primary aim of identification is not considered to be restoration of symbiosis (Jacobson, 1964) but, on the contrary, its avoidance. According to my conceptualization, all internalization is secondary to the primary differentiation of self and object and leads normally to an ever increasing differentiation between these two. Although internalizations can be lost through regression, either partially as circumscribed re-externalizations, or extensively as in the loss of differentiation, the results of these regressive movements do not represent more basic forms of internalization, but rather demonstrate the insufficiency of the mind in retaining internalizations once acquired.

For the initiation and continuation of the functionally selective identifications four basic prerequisites seem to be necessary (Tähkä, 1979, 1984a, 1984b):

1. The general climate of the mother-child relation must be safe enough to enable the child to abandon the function of the mother that is to be identified with. Taking over the object's function in the form of identification implies that a partial loss of the functional object and a corresponding frustrated self representation have to be tolerated to some extent before the lost function can be replaced by a new function of the self.

The introjective presences that emerge to protect the child's self experience are representatives of the mother's various functional services. The more adequately synchronized the mother's share in the interaction with her child, the more varied will be the latter's stock of soothing and security-inducing introjects, provided, of course, that the mother also adequately takes care of the necessary direct gratification of the child's needs. In such circumstances there are several alternative experiences of tranquilizing inner presences available in the case of the mother's absence or frustrating behavior. The child is not desperately dependent on only a few good introjects and thus not constantly threatened by a loss of differentiation.

Adequate gratification and sufficient anxiety-ameliorating introjective alternatives thus appear to provide the safe enough general climate in which the child's self can afford to give up the object's functional services one at a time and make them functions of his own.

2. The object must provide primitively idealized functional models for the identifications, useful enough in tension regulation and in dealing with the external world.

It seems probable that omnipotence is initially concentrated in the archaic self feeling, whereas the functional object's importance in its maintenance is hardly recognized. While the first object primarily tends to be a mere means of direct gratification, its introjective experiencing does not provide such a gratification. Instead, while promising gratification in the future, the functional introjects become drive-controlling structures which help the self to wait and postpone gratification. As the felt importance of the soothing and anxiety-controlling introject grows, there probably will be a shift of emphasis toward these representations in the experienced omnipotence. In contrast to what is often maintained, this cannot yet mean an experiential sharing in the object's omnipotence; rather it implies an *omnipotence of ownership:* "I am omnipotent because I possess an omnipotent object." This shift of emphasis in the omnipotence toward the representations of the functional object seems to be necessary to provide these representations with the primitive idealization needed for the functionally selective identifications to become started.

While introjects seem to provide models for the tension-regulating and self-soothing inner functions, the emergence and practice of the executive functions and motor skills directly related to the world experienced as external seem mostly to become established with the external object as a functional model.

The child's growing awareness of the big size, strength, and powerful nature of the object's various functional manifestations makes the child idealize primitively these functions, but it also exposes him increasingly to experiences of primitive envy and shame as new variations of the affective experience of the self.

In functionally selective identifications with the external object, an important intermediate stage appears to be *imitation,* the significance of which as a forerunner of identification has been stressed by several previous authors (e.g., de Saussure, 1939; Jacobson, 1959, 1964; Schafer, 1968; Gaddini, 1969).

3. The frustrations that initiate the identification with a particular function of the object should be in tolerable limits instead of leading to overwhelming dedifferentiation anxiety or devastating experiences of shame.

4. There should be an adequately approving mirroring from the

object to encourage the final identification and to furnish the new function with a lasting value.

It would be tempting to postulate that the "pleasure of enjoying one's abilities" (Fenichel, 1945) or "pleasure in mastery" (Hendrick, 1951) would directly reflect the elated feeling of a self, now possessing the functional object's function, originally experienced as omnipotent. However, observational data, especially those from clinical work with borderline patients, do not support this overly simple model. Although it is true that the new functions of the self, acquired through identification, to various extents become heirs to the object's omnipotence, the idealization does not follow with the function without an additional identification with the mother's approving and admiring attitude regarding the practice and use of that particular function.

This approving and admiring function of the mother is one facet of the phenomenon of mirroring, which has been discussed and its developmental importance stressed by several authors (e.g., Loewald, 1960; Winnicott, 1967, 1971; Modell, 1968; Kohut, 1971; Spruiell, 1974; Mahler and McDewitt, 1982; Volkan, 1982). Mirroring is here defined as the totality of the ways in which the mother communicates to her child how she regards the child's respective functioning. It seems that this mirroring function of the mother becomes the model for a second identification, the nature of which largely determines how much of the original idealization of the functional object will be reflected back to the newly acquired function of the child's self.

A functionally selective identification thus appears to be a biphasic process that includes an initial identification with the object's function *and* a subsequent identification with the object's way of mirroring the child as the owner and exerciser of that function.

An established presence of basic safety, appropriate models, tolerable frustrations, and adequate mirroring appears to be equally necessary in the treatment of patients with a borderline pathology before belated processes of functionally selective identifications, essential in their treatment, will become possible (Tähkä, 1974, 1979, 1984b).

NARCISSISM RECONSIDERED

The question that inevitably arises at this point is: how do the vicissitudes of the early idealization fit in with the concept of *narcissism* and its primary and secondary forms as discussed by Freud (1914)?

It is not possible here to review the various ways in which the concept of narcissism has been defined and used. It should be stated, however, that if the dualistic drive theory is dropped (e.g., Tähkä, 1987),

Hartmann's (1953) classical definition of narcissism as a libidinal cathexis of the self is no longer useful. "Libidinal" cannot then be ascribed to any particular *quality* of the drive but can refer only to a "self-loving" *function* of the self. However, since love proper is not possible before the establishment of self and object constancy, positive affective attitudes during functional relatedness can obviously only be some variations of infantile omnipotence and primitive idealization.

If the term narcissism is seen as synonymous with the valuation by the self of itself and its functions and characteristics, Freud's original term *primary narcissism* could be understood as referring to the self-evident and limitless omnipotence of the newly differentiated primary self. This primary omnipotence equals the initial, experientially self-evident ability of the self to provide pleasure and gratification. However, accumulating experience connects this gratification increasingly to the functional object, both as such and as introject. This shift of emphasis makes the self increasingly dependent on the experiential omnipotence of the object's functions and on their full control and possession.

Functionally selective identifications with these primitively idealized functions of the object create in the self functions according to the models provided by the former. However, since no "idealizing libido" is postulated here to follow automatically with these functions that so far *have never been valuated as functions of the self*, this valuation has to be acquired through an additional identification with the valuating function of the object regarding the function internalized. The nature of the mother's mirroring function and the child's identification with it thus seem to determine the degree and quality of the future valuation by the child's self of the function in question. This estimation by the self of itself and its functions acquired through identifications with the mother's mirroring function can then be regarded as the first manifestation of the child's *secondary narcissism*.

Primary narcissism would thus represent the original omnipotence of the self, while secondary narcissism would refer to the nature and degree of the self-valuating and self-estimating functions. Primary narcissism would then refer to the self-esteem that emerges with and largely equals the primary self-experience, while secondary narcissism would refer to all self-estimation acquired through internalization.

CONSEQUENCES OF FUNCTIONALLY SELECTIVE IDENTIFICATIONS

The first sign indicating that functionally selective identifications have become initiated is a gradual increase in the changing of passivity into activity (Freud, 1920); i.e., the child starts to take care by himself of what the mother has so far done to him and for him. As a function-specific frustration gives rise to a function-specific (functionally selective) identification, the result will be the emergence of a corresponding functional capacity in the self with corresponding changes in the representations of self and object. After an established identification, failures of the mother in that particular function no longer lead to frustrations, since the arousal of the original need will now activate the child's own, newly acquired function. Aggressive manifestations formerly mobilized by those frustrations have disappeared, and the energy used for and discharged in those reactions can now be used for other purposes, for instance, to energize the use of the new function gained through identification. This change probably covers most of what is usually called the *neutralization of aggression* (Hartmann, 1950, 1955). However, no changes in the energy itself are postulated here, while that which is energized has undergone a structural alteration (Tähkä, 1984a, 1984b).

The most dramatic consequences of functionally selective identifications for the child's mental world of experience are undoubtedly those changes in his ways of experiencing the objects and himself which lead to the transformation of the functional object into an individual one, as well as to the replacement of a self feeling depending on the state of need, by an experience of individual identity.

A functionally selective identification makes the child self-sustaining in regard to the function that has become a part of his self. At this point he has become independent of the mother, who in regard to this function has ceased to represent a missing part of his future self. Since the function now is included in the self, its gratifying or frustrating performance no longer results in an oscillation of the object experience between "all-good" and "all-bad." In this particular respect the object has ceased to be functional and has become postambivalent in Abraham's (1924) sense. Functionally selective identifications thus eliminate, bit by bit, the functional representation of the object with its black-and-white ambivalence. Rather than through a fusion of opposite representations (Kernberg, 1966, 1976), the experiences of "splitting" and primitive ambivalence would thus recede through changes in the representational world caused by processes of internalization.[4]

It seems that the role of identification as a bond to the object is

4. Kohut's (1966, 1971) "transmuting internalization," elaborated further by Tolpin (1971), shows some important similarities with the process of functionally selective identifications presented here. However, because of equally important differences in understanding the process and its results, as well as in the theoretical premises, the two views cannot be compared in this connection.

disproportionately stressed in the literature as compared with its differentiating effects on the individual's way of experiencing himself and his object world. Unlike an introject, identification does not preserve a mentally experienced relationship with the object (Schafer, 1968) but transforms aspects of it into structures of the self that have historical but no longer experiential connections with the object. The structure created by functionally selective identifications represents the memory of the functional object as a depersonified precipitate, its establishment being one of the explanations of *preoedipal amnesia*.

A functionally selective identification thus means a loss of the functional object in a particular aspect. As the child becomes self-sustaining in regard to one of the object's functions, the introjective and projective representations of the latter are no longer needed. When the object is no longer factually the sole bearer and controller of the function in question, the corresponding object representation loses its character as an introjective presence which can be controlled only magically. What is left is an *informative representation* of the object performing this function in a variety of ways. In contrast to introjective and projective representations, an informative object representation is actively controlled by the self and exists experientially on conditions of the latter. Instead of a passively experienced presence of the functional object, there is now an informative representation of an aspect of the object that can be recalled and dismissed from the mind at the subject's will. Experiences of the object as the performer of this particular function will henceforth be registered in and added to this informative representation. Correspondingly, the magical control of the introject becomes replaced by an informative representation of the self as the master of the function in question.

A functionally selective identification thus breaks down the functional representation of the object into a new functional capacity of the self on the one hand, and an informative object representation, manipulable in fantasy, on the other. However, before the absent object, as a whole, can be kept in mind on the subject's conditions, a multitude of informative representations have to become gathered through functionally selective identifications and integrated to form the representation of an individual, self-determined object, perceived and fantasied as one having an individual identity. It seems that in the same way as a sufficient mass of mnemic material stemming from early experiences of gratification is needed before the first crude configurations of self and object can become differentiated, the experiential emergence of identity and individual objects likewise seems to require a sufficient collection of informative representations acquired through functionally selective identifications.

Functionally selective identifications thus change the object representations from introjective into informative. While thinking of the functional object is possible only as a passive experience of its magically controlled presence, the informative object representations will after their integration allow self-controlled active thinking and fantasying of the absent object. Informative representations are prerequisites for conceptual thinking and thus for the secondary process level of psychic functioning, which becomes dependably possible and predominant after the established self and object constancies.

IDENTITY AND INDIVIDUAL OBJECT (SELF AND OBJECT CONSTANCY)

The emergence of a self experience with individual identity, as well as an awareness of objects with identities of their own, marks the second major reintegration of the experiential world in the early formation of the mind. While a person was born into a world through the primary differentiation of the experiential world in the second half of the first year, the *individual* will be born (Mahler et al., 1975) into a world of other individuals as a result of a multitude of functionally selective identifications at the approximate age of 3 years.

An individual *knows* who he is and that his world is shared by other individuals. This knowledge presupposes that he is able to *think* of himself and of others instead of merely experiencing them or their felt presence. This, in turn, becomes dependably possible only when integrated overall configurations of informative self and object world have been synthesized out of the countless informative part representations created by functionally selective identifications.

Identity has been discussed by several psychoanalytic authors (e.g., Erikson, 1950, 1956; Eissler in Panel, 1958; Mahler, 1968; Greenacre, 1958; Lichtenstein, 1961, 1977; Jacobson, 1964; Kernberg, 1966, 1976). It has been defined in different ways and its emergence has correspondingly been differently located in the chronology of human development. In contrast to Kernberg's (1966) definition of identity as a process of internalization, I regard it as a result of such processes. Both identity and self constancy are here seen to refer to the way in which the self experiences itself after the integration of informative representations. A coherent and relatively stable informative self representation allows the self experience to retain a feeling of relative sameness, continuity, and predictability, regardless of the varying states of need. There is now an experiential "I," feeling sometimes good, sometimes bad, instead of a self experience equaling the ambivalently oscillating feeling states. A "reflective self representation" (Schafer, 1968) and *introspection* become possible only after the established self constancy.

The emergence of a permanent self with registered experiences which an experientially identical self can recall also marks the beginning of a dependable *sense of time* and *organized memory* (Hartocollis, 1983). While established experiences of identity and self constancy thus imply a discovery of oneself as a particular individual, with a private inner world, it is paralleled by a simultaneous discovery of objects as individuals, with their own inner worlds. A possessed world becomes a world shared with others.

The representation of an individual object emerges as an integration of its informative part representations created by processes of functionally selective identifications. The informative representation of the object is known to belong to the self as a mentally manipulable fantasy or memory of the external object that now can be thought of as absent and self-determined. Loss of experienced magical control over the external object, inherent in its change from functional to individual, has thus become compensated for by an active control of its inner representation.

Even if both mother and father may have participated in their child's care, all relationships during the stage of functional relatedness can be experienced by the child only as dyadic (Blos, 1985). However, with the emergence of object constancy, the object's new independent and self-determined existence in the child's world of experience will transform the object from a mere means to the very source of gratification, which has to be longed and actively sought for, as well as to be rivalled in a triadic relationship.

Loving another human being becomes possible only when she or he is experienced as an individual with an own inner world and motivations, and thus as being beyond one's immediate possession and control. Only this state of affairs enables and motivates conscious needing and longing for the object, as well as an intensive interest in and curiosity about the object's newly found inner world with a concomitantly developing capacity for empathic understanding. The child's discovery that the object's love is not self-evident but conditioned by his way of treating her will change the emphasis of his anxiety from the loss of object (and self) to that of the object's love. Attempts to please the object actively, increasing consideration of her feelings, normal guilt (Kernberg, 1976), and a need for reparation and reconciliation will now normally develop. The insight into the object's self-determined choices in loving initiates feelings of *gratitude,* just as the object constancy now enables *normal* idealization (Kernberg, 1980) of an individual object.

The birth of himself as an individual with subjective freedom of thought means a revolutionary change in the child's world of experience. Only some of the most obvious consequences of that change were listed above. They and other implications of this crucial developmental step will be discussed in part III of this study.

Summary

This is the second of three papers, in which the structuralization of the mind is investigated. I attempt to present a personal and coherent view of the building up of the mind during infancy and childhood.

While part I dealt with the developmental stages preceding the differentiation of self and objects, this part concentrates on phenomena and processes leading to the experiential emergence of identity and individual object.

BIBLIOGRAPHY

ABRAHAM, K. (1924). A short study of the development of the libido, viewed in the light of mental disorders. In *Selected Papers of Karl Abraham.* London: Hogarth Press, 1949, pp. 418–501.

BIBRING, E. (1953). The mechanism of depression. In *Affective Disorders,* ed. P. Greenacre. New York: Int. Univ. Press, pp. 13–48.

BLOS, P. (1985). *Son and Father.* New York: Free Press.

COMPTON, A. (1985). The concept of identification in the work of Freud, Ferenczi and Abraham. *Psychoanal. Q.,* 54:200–233.

DE SAUSSURE, R. (1939). Identification and substitution. *Int. J. Psychoanal.,* 20:465–470.

DORPAT, T. L. (1976). Structural conflict and object relations conflict. *J. Amer. Psychoanal. Assn.,* 24:855–874.

ERIKSON, E. H. (1950). *Childhood and Society.* New York: Norton.

———— (1956). The problem of ego identity. *J. Amer. Psychoanal. Assn.,* 4:56–121.

FENICHEL, O. (1945). *The Psychoanalytic Theory of Neurosis.* New York: Norton.

———— (1953). *The Collected Papers of Otto Fenichel,* First Series. New York: Norton.

FREUD, S. (1905). Three essays on the theory of sexuality. *S.E.,* 7:125–243.

———— (1914). On narcissism. *S.E.,* 14:67–102.

———— (1915). Instincts and their vicissitudes. *S.E.,* 14:117–140.

_____ (1917). Mourning and melancholia. *S.E.*, 14:237–260.

_____ (1920). Beyond the pleasure principle. *S.E.*, 18:3–64.

_____ (1921). Group psychology and the analysis of the ego. *S.E.*, 18:65–143.

_____ (1923). The ego and the id. *S.E.*, 19:3–66.

_____ (1933). New introductory lectures on psycho-analysis. *S.E.*, 22:1–182.

_____ (1938). An outline of psycho-analysis. *S.E.*, 23:139–207.

GADDINI, E. (1969). On imitation. *Int. J. Psychoanal.*, 50:475–484.

GILL, M. M. (1963). *Topography and Systems in Psychoanalytic Theory.* Psychol. Issues, monogr. 10. New York: Int. Univ. Press.

GREENACRE, P. (1958). Early physical determinants in the development of the sense of identity. *J. Amer. Psychoanal. Assn.*, 6:612–627.

HARTMANN, H. (1939). *Ego Psychology and the Problem of Adaptation.* New York: Int. Univ. Press, 1958.

_____ (1950). Comment on the psychoanalytic theory of the ego. *Psychoanal. Study Child*, 5:74–96.

_____ (1952). The mutual influences in the development of ego and id. *Psychoanal. Study Child*, 7:9–30.

_____ (1953). Contributions to the metapsychology of schizophrenia. *Psychoanal. Study Child*, 8:177–198.

_____ (1955). Notes on the theory of sublimation. *Psychoanal. Study Child*, 10:9–29.

_____ KRIS, E., & LOEWENSTEIN, R. M. (1946). Comments on the formation of psychic structure. *Psychoanal. Study Child*, 2:11–38.

_____ & LOEWENSTEIN, R. M. (1962). Notes on the superego. *Psychoanal. Study Child*, 17:42–81.

HARTOCOLLIS, P. (1983). *Time and Timelessness.* New York: Int. Univ. Press.

HENDRICK, I. (1951). Early development of the ego. *Psychoanal. Q.*, 20:44–61.

JACOBSON, E. (1954). The self and the object world. *Psychoanal. Study Child*, 9:75–127.

_____ (1964). *The Self and the Object World.* New York: Int. Univ. Press.

_____ (1971). *Depression.* New York: Int. Univ. Press.

JOFFE, W. G. & SANDLER, J. (1965). Notes on pain, depression and individuation. *Psychoanal. Study Child*, 20:394–424.

KERNBERG, O. F. (1966). Structural derivatives of object relationships. *Int. J. Psychoanal.*, 47:236–253.

_____ (1976). *Object Relations Theory and Clinical Psychoanalysis.* New York: Aronson.

_____ (1980). *Internal World and External Reality.* New York: Aronson.

_____ (1982). Self, ego, affects and drives. *J. Amer. Psychoanal. Assn.*, 30:893–917.

KLEIN, M. (1946). Notes on some schizoid mechanisms. *Int. J. Psychoanal.*, 27:99–110.

KOHUT, H. (1966). Forms and transformations of narcissism. *J. Amer. Psychoanal. Assn.*, 14:243–272.

_____ (1971). *The Analysis of the Self.* New York: Int. Univ. Press.

_____ (1977). *The Restoration of the Self.* New York: Int. Univ. Press.

LAPLANCHE, J. & PONTALIS, J-B. (1967). *The Language of Psycho-Analysis.* London: Hogarth Press, 1973.

LEWIN, B. D. (1950). *The Psychoanalysis of Elation.* New York: Norton.

LICHTENSTEIN, H. (1961). Identity and sexuality. *J. Amer. Psychoanal. Assn.,* 9:179–260.

_____ (1977). *The Dilemma of Human Identity.* New York: Aronson.

LOEWALD, H. W. (1960). On the therapeutic action of psychoanalysis. *Int. J. Psychoanal.,* 41:16–33.

_____ (1962). Internalization, separation, mourning and superego. *Psychoanal. Q.,* 31:483–504.

MAHLER, M. S. (1968). *On Human Symbiosis and the Vicissitudes of Individuation.* New York: Int. Univ. Press.

_____ & McDEWITT, J. B. (1982). Thoughts on the emergence of the sense of self with particular emphasis on the body self. *J. Amer. Psychoanal. Assn.,* 30:827–848.

_____ PINE, F., & BERGMAN, A. (1975). *The Psychological Birth of the Human Infant.* New York: Basic Books.

MEISSNER, W. W. (1981). *Internalization in Psychoanalysis.* Psychol. Issues, monogr. 50. New York: Int. Univ. Press.

MODELL, A. H. (1968). *Object Love and Reality.* New York: Int. Univ. Press.

MOORE, B. E. & FINE, B. D. (1968). *A Glossary of Psychoanalytic Terms and Concepts.* New York: Amer. Psychoanal. Assn.

NEMIAH, J. C. (1975). Denial revisited. *Psychother. & Psychosom.,* 26:140–147.

NOVICK, J. & KELLY, K. (1970). Projection and externalization. *Psychoanal. Study Child,* 25:69–95.

PANEL (1958). Problems of identity. D. L. Rubinfine, reporter. *J. Amer. Psychoanal. Assn.,* 6:131–142.

RAPAPORT, D. (1951). The conceptual model of psychoanalysis. In *The Collected Papers of David Rapaport,* ed. M. M. Gill. New York: Basic Books, 1967, pp. 405–431.

_____ (1957). Cognitive structures. *Ibid.,* pp. 631–664.

_____ (1960). *The Structure of Psychoanalytic Theory.* Psychol. Issues, monogr. 6. New York: Int. Univ. Press.

SANDLER, J. & ROSENBLATT, B. (1962). The concept of the representational world. *Psychoanal. Study Child,* 17:128–145.

SCHAFER, R. (1968). *Aspects of Internalization.* New York: Int. Univ. Press.

_____ (1972). Internalization. *Psychoanal. Study Child,* 27:411–436.

_____ (1976). *A New Language for Psychoanalysis.* New Haven: Yale Univ. Press.

SCHWARTZ, F. (1981). Psychic structure. *Int. J. Psychoanal.,* 62:61–72.

SIFNEOS, P. (1973). The prevalence of "alexithymic" characteristics in psychosomatic patients. *Psychother. & Psychosom.,* 22:255–262.

SPRUIELL, V. (1974). Theories of the treatment of narcissistic personalities. *J. Amer. Psychoanal. Assn.,* 22:268–278.

STOLOROW, R. D. & LACHMANN, F. M. (1980). *Psychoanalysis of Developmental Arrests.* New York: Int. Univ. Press.

STRACHEY, J. (1934). The nature of the therapeutic action of psycho-analysis. *Int. J. Psychoanal.,* 15:127–159.

TOLPIN, M. (1971). On the beginnings of a cohesive self. *Psychoanal. Study Child,* 26:316–354.

TÄHKÄ, V. (1974). What is psychotherapy? *Psychiatria Fennica,* 5:163–170.

—— (1979). Psychotherapy as a phase-specific interaction. *Scand. Psychoanal. Rev.,* 2:113–132.

—— (1981). On internalization. Presented to Finnish Psychoanalytical Society.

—— (1984a). Dealing with object loss. *Scand. Psychoanal. Rev.,* 7:13–33.

—— (1984b). Psychoanalytic treatment as a developmental continuum. *Scand. Psychoanal. Rev.,* 7:133–159.

—— (1987). On the early formation of the mind: I. *Int. J. Psychoanal.,* 68:229–250.

VOLKAN, V. D. (1982). Identification and related psychic events. In *Curative Factors in Dynamic Psychotherapy,* ed. S. Slipp. New York: McGraw-Hill, pp. 153–170.

WINNICOTT, D. W. (1967). Mirror-role of mother and family in child development. In *The Predicament of the Family,* ed. P. Lomas. London: Hogarth Press, pp. 26–33.

—— (1971). *Playing and Reality.* London: Tavistock.

CLINICAL PERSPECTIVES ON TERMINATION

On the Fate of the Intrapsychic Image of the Psychoanalyst after Termination of the Analysis

MARTIN S. BERGMANN

SCATTERED IN THE LITERATURE ON TERMINATION ARE A NUMBER OF REF-
erences to the troubling problem that termination does not always lead
to resolution of the transference neurosis. This literature, however,
does not deal specifically with the fate of transference love after termination. I came upon it because over a number of years I have been
exploring the nature of love from a psychoanalytic point of view
(Bergmann, 1971, 1980, 1982, 1985–86, 1987).

Regardless of how prolonged the termination phase may be, on a
certain date every analysis comes to an abrupt ending. A relationship
that was rich in interpersonal transactions has to become an intrapsychic one. Try as we may to find the optimal moment for termination,
there is always something arbitrary in every ending. There is no analogue in real life to the experience of termination. No wonder that
analysands so often associate termination with death. Experience
shows that some analysands continue after the analysis to feel love for
their former analysts even if the analysis was a disappointing experience. Others acknowledge the good results, but nevertheless experience considerable hostility toward their former analyst which they cannot overcome. Considerations such as these as well as the fact that we
are often dealing with the second or even third analysis have led me to
the conclusion that we have to reexamine the nature of transference
love and the problem of the resolution of the transference.

Clinical professor of psychology, New York University postdoctoral program.

Read at a symposium on "Clinical Perspectives on Termination," Western New En-
gland Psychoanalytic Society, October 25, 1986; Division for Psychoanalysis (39) of the
American Psychological Association, April 2, 1987; and the International Congress of
Psychoanalysis, Montreal, July 30, 1987.

In a previous publication (1985–86), I dealt with the difference between transference love and love in real life. I suggested that Freud did discover a technique by which a special kind of love, called transference love, could be elicited. There I said (1985–86):

Let us stop to ponder the magnitude of Freud's discovery. For centuries men and women have searched for mandrake roots and other substances from which a love potion could be brewed. And then a Jewish Viennese physician uncovered love's secret. There is indeed a way in which one human being can make another fall in love and the prescription is astonishingly simple: (1) Keep the environment as constant as possible. Let the person whose love you wish to elicit speak freely about everything that comes to his or her mind. (2) Intrude as little as possible into the evolving feelings and memories and, above all, do not disturb the flow of childhood memories. (3) Be particularly attentive to the recall of forgotten or repressed past loves. Give the repressed love feelings a chance to be re-experienced. (4) Show the person whose love you wish to elicit that after every disappointment in love he or she developed defenses against future love. Illustrate how the fear of re-experiencing a new love has become transformed into defensive character traits and symptoms and how these are used to maintain a barrier of suspicion and mistrust. (5) If this method is followed over a period of time, the love evoked will turn toward the person who has liberated these love feelings from repression [p. 30].

In presenting the material this way, I may have inadvertently created the impression that Freud deliberately set out to elicit transference love, but this was not the case. We know that in 1895 Freud did not welcome transference but tried to remove it as a "false connection" which interfered with the recollection of the trauma that Freud at that time thought was responsible for the hysterical symptoms. Eventually Freud recognized the psychic power of transference love and pressed it into the service of treatment. This happened, as Freud put it, after "following a dim pre-sentiment, I decided to replace hypnosis by free association" (1914b, p. 19).

In the *Gradiva* (1907) Freud states that the psychoanalytic cure is a cure through love.

The process of cure is accomplished in a relapse into love, if we combine all the many components of the sexual instinct under the term 'love'; and such a relapse is indispensable, for the symptoms on account of which the treatment has been undertaken are nothing other than precipitates of earlier struggles connected with repression or the return of the repressed, and they can only be resolved and washed away by a fresh high tide of the same passion [p. 90].

To Freud's views on love I added that they were entirely directed to the past. Freud ignored the place of hope in analysis and the phenomenon of loving. In my opinion, hope is a crucial ingredient in every love. Hope consists in the unconscious, sometimes even conscious, belief that the lover will repair the damage that was done by the earlier love objects. Much of the bliss of love is the anticipation of this repair. Because the lover is unconsciously expected to be a healer, the healer in turn can be put in the place of the lover.

When Freud wrote his papers on love (1910, 1912a, 1918), he was still working with a topographic point of view. Seen topographically, transference love does not differ greatly from love in real life. At first sight the advantages seem to be entirely on the side of love in real life, since it permits sexual gratification and reciprocity. On the other side of the ledger, transference love evolves in a situation where the analysand need not deal significantly with a real object in the outer world; he and his life alone are all that matters. The realistic personality of the analyst enters far less into the evolution of transference love than a lover in real life. The role of fantasy in transference love is correspondingly greater. Methodically, the analyst works on establishing trust and does his utmost to maintain the trust that has been elicited. As a result, many people incapable of loving in real life become capable of developing transference love.

When all goes well and in the course of treatment growth is resumed, one hopes that a point will be reached when the analysand will spontaneously yearn to exchange the now obsolete transference love for love in real life. In practice, however, the transition from transference love to love in real life is often difficult and sometimes never takes place, leaving the analysand dependent on transference love as the only love the analysand has known. If this happens to someone who becomes a therapist, he will be inclined to put more trust in transference love than in love in real life and may then seek to transform a transference relationship into a real-life relationship.

In the course of an analysis, Freud (1910, 1912a) suggested, one uncovers the preconditions for loving that are unique to every person. Some of these preconditions in a neurosis can become very narrow. Freud cites the example of a man always falling in love with a woman who belongs to another man. When Freud wrote about difficulties in loving, for example, the difficulty many men and women have in combining the capacity to love with passionate and uninhibited sexuality, he had conflicts within the oedipus complex in mind as the most serious obstacle to full, consistent love.

I have learned to look upon love as an amalgam of preoedipal and oedipal strivings. In the transference, we obtain two distinct types of loving. Preoedipal love is dyadic, diffuse, pregenital in aim; oedipal love is triadic, contains the pain of jealousy, and is genital. Difficulties on the oedipal level appear in the inability to fuse love with sexual passion. Difficulties on the preoedipal level appear in the fear of being taken over by or merged with the love object. Such men and women have to curtail contact; they need space for themselves away from the loved one. A split between oedipal and preoedipal can express itself also in bisexuality.

To Freud's concept of preconditions for loving I added (1987) that the preconditions can also be flexible and be based on different infantile prototypes, with each new love representing the activation of a new infantile prototype. The psychoanalytic process itself, by uncovering such hitherto repressed prototypes, often makes new prototypes available so that the love one develops for a person, during or after treatment, is based on different conditions than those that governed objects chosen before treatment. Even in real life, a meaningful love relationship may bring about a change in the future preconditions for loving, unless a fixation has taken place where every new love is only a replica of the old and therefore follows the same predestined course dictated by the repetition compulsion.

I have previously (1980) suggested that the integrative functions of the ego have still another function to fulfill, that is, the object selected for love should represent most, and we hope all, the significant love objects of infancy. When this is not possible, more than one love object will be needed at the same time or in rapid succession. In the course of a psychoanalysis one may have the opportunity to observe a number of instances of falling in love, each based on one particular infantile prototype. If the representations of one infantile love object have not been involved in the object selection, they will seek another object. These observations also are relevant to the problem of transference love after the termination of analysis.

The implications for termination are that if the analyst stood for the uncovered, early, libidinal objects, the analysand may not be capable of finding a replacement for the analyst in the real world. Every early object was originally cathected with its unique mixture of love and hate. It is reasonable to assume that some of these transferred feelings will continue to cling to the analyst, forming a residue that cannot be eliminated. To be capable of transference love is not the same as being capable of love in real life.

TRANSFERENCE NEUROSIS AND THE RESOLUTION OF THE TRANSFERENCE

Freud (1914a) was optimistic in his belief that neurosis can be transformed into a transference neurosis.

> . . . we regularly succeed in giving all the symptoms of the illness a new transference meaning and in replacing his ordinary neurosis by a 'transference-neurosis' of which he can be cured by the therapeutic work. The transference thus creates an intermediate region between illness and real life through which the transition from the one to the other is made [p. 154].

In the 1950s, this point of view became the cornerstone of psychoanalytic technique. In his contribution to the symposium on "Variations in Classical Psycho-Analytic Technique," Greenson (1958) said, "What is unique about psycho-analysis is that we handle this situation in such a way as to facilitate the patient's development of a full-blown transference neurosis" (p. 200). In 1954, Gill stated, "Psychoanalysis is that technique which, employed by a neutral analyst, results in the development of a regressive transference neurosis and the ultimate resolution of this neurosis by techniques of interpretation alone" (p. 775). In the same spirit, Anna Freud (1959) affirmed that in a transference neurosis the original neurosis is given up and entirely replaced by the new neurotic formation in which the analyst has replaced the original objects in the patient's life. Thus Freud's insights of 1914 became an article of faith in the 1950s. In the 1970s, the enthusiasm about the fostering of the transference neurosis began to wane. Timidly at first, Greenacre, in 1959, said: "I have myself been a little questioning of the blanket term 'transference neurosis,' which can sometimes be misleading. I would prefer to speak of *active transference-neurotic manifestations*" (p. 485f.).

Greenacre wished to curb the power of the transference neurosis and preserve the observing ego, the site of the therapeutic alliance. She stressed the importance of maintaining the autonomy of the analysand (p. 487). Greenacre also found that incompletely analyzed transference attitudes produce excessive pressures on other life relationships, onto which they may be displaced postanalytically. Ominously she added that unanalyzed transference residuals seem to amalgamate rather than disperse neurotic attitudes (p. 485).

Thus was set in motion an important change in direction in psychoanalytic technique. In 1971, Blum stated,

> Transference neurosis has an oedipal core, but is not always oedipal in content. There is an intermingling of developmental phases without rigid stratification. Classical analysis requires sustained, intense transference ("a transference neurosis"), but also maintenance of the therapeutic alliance and attunement to reality [p. 50]

What began as a dissent by Greenacre in 1959 was by 1971 in the mainstream of American psychoanalysis. We should note that the case against transference neurosis moves on two levels. First, it is never as complete as Freud and the analysts who followed him enthusiastically thought; and second, it is not desirable because the transference neurosis endangers the observing capacities of the ego.

The transformation of the concept of transference neurosis can be followed in the writings of Loewald. In 1962, Loewald observed: "An analysis is itself a prime example of seeking a substitute for the lost love objects, and the analyst in the transference promotes such substitution. The goal, however, is to resolve the transference neurosis, a revival of the infantile neurosis" (p. 261f.). In 1971, Loewald described transference differently:

> We may regard [transference neurosis] as denoting the retransformation of a psychic illness which originated in pathogenic interactions with the important persons in the child's environment, into an interactional process with a new person, the analyst, in which the pathological infantile interactions and their intrapsychic consequences may become transparent and accessible to change by virtue of the analyst's objectivity and of the emergence of novel interactional possibilities [p. 309].

In the 1962 formulation, the emphasis is on the transference neurosis as a substitute for the lost love objects; the goal is the resolution of the transference neurosis. In the 1971 formulation, the emphasis is on an interactional process with a new person which in turn makes possible novel interactional possibilities. "Resolution of the transference" no longer appears. In his use of "new interactional possibilities" the impact of object relationship theory is discernible.

RESOLUTION OF THE TRANSFERENCE—THE CLASSICAL POSITION

By comparison with the literature on transference neurosis, much less has been said on the resolution of the transference. The term does not appear in the index to the *Standard Edition* of Freud's work. To my knowledge, Freud used it for the first time in 1912 when he counseled against sharing one's own private life with the analysand. "The resolution of the transference, too—one of the main tasks of treatment—is made more difficult by an intimate attitude on the doctor's part, so that any gain there made at the beginning is more than outweighed at the end" (1912b, p. 118).

The German word Freud actually used is *Lösung,* which implies solution, the way a riddle is solved. "Resolve" is a metaphor that suggests settling of conflicts. It is stronger than "solution." It has both a stronger and more utopian connotation. When we are dealing with these translations from the German, we become once more aware of the metaphorical nature of so many psychoanalytic concepts. Ultimately these concepts are rich in connotation but lack clear denotation. Freud's term solution has its own difficulties. It applies to a riddle, to a scientific puzzle, but not to a deep, ongoing human relationship.

"Resolution of the transference" was, in my opinion, modeled on the concept "Dissolution of the Oedipus Complex" (Freud, 1924). Since then it has become evident that the oedipus complex is rarely if ever dissolved. All we can hope for is that it no longer forms the nucleus of a neurosis. We are satisfied when the oedipus complex has been rechanneled, sublimated, and rendered productive. If we take into account the differences, the same holds true for the resolution of the transference.

Another term often used in this discussion is "transference residue." I believe it was first coined by Brunswick (1928), partially to mitigate the shock that the Wolf-Man temporarily developed a hypochondriacal psychosis when he was under her care. What happened to him could have both alerted and alarmed psychoanalysts at that time, for it demonstrated the immense power still latent in the transference many years after termination, but psychoanalysis was not at that time secure enough to ponder the implications of what happened to the Wolf-Man, who was analyzed by Freud himself.

We will have to await the opening of the Freud Archives to learn the extent to which Freud's analysands actually resolved the transference neurosis. I have had access to a correspondence between Freud and his former analysand, Kata Levy. The correspondence takes place in 1920 and is intimate.[1] Freud shared with her personal happenings in his life, including the mourning over the death of his daughter Sophie. Mrs. Levy in turn continues to consult him about various questions in her life. Freud is continuously encouraging, urging her to be both clever and courageous.

1. Freud to Kata Levy (August 18, 1929), Freud Collection, B9, Library of Congress. I wish to express my thanks to Peter Gay, who made it possible for me to read this correspondence.

On August 18, 1920, he wrote:

> I cannot tell you how it relieves me to be able to write to you in a simple,
> warm-hearted way without the educational rudeness that prevailed
> during the analysis, without having to hide my warm-hearted friend-
> ship for you, a friendship you should never have doubted [my tr.].

To judge from this one relationship as well as from what we know of
Freud's relationship to his former analysands who became professional
analysts, one would have to say that at least in the case of some patients
the analysis was transformed into an abiding friendship.

The standard books on technique, such as those by Glover (1955)
and Greenson (1967), have little to say about the resolution of the
transference neurosis. Menninger (1958), however, has offered a description of an ideal resolution of the transference in a classical analysis. This is what the hypothetical patient says:

> He has reacted to the analyst as if he were his mother, his father, his
> brother, his teacher, his sister, his wife. Gradually these illusions have
> tended to fade in intensity. The analyst becomes more and more just
> the analyst, "that doctor who has patiently listened to me." The patient
> begins to be a little bit more considerate of the analyst as a person for his
> (i.e., the analyst's) own sake. This objectivity toward the analyst in-
> creases and the magic omnipotence of the great man begins to dimin-
> ish. In fantasy this is sometimes conceived of as his death; in a more
> constructive formulation it represents replacement by a friend, a friend
> with his own infirmities, his own interests, his own problems, but with a
> record of consistent and faithful efforts to be helpful. In this way the
> termination of an analysis often carries with it the thought expressed by
> Tennyson: "I hope to see my Pilot face to face, when I have crossed the
> bar" [p. 172f.].

The reader will note the allusion to death and God as the pilot. The
quote hardly fits the optimistic view Menninger was consciously trying
to convey.

This type of termination has been reported in the literature. I found
a good example in a case history that was published by Berg in 1947. It
sounds a shade less ideal than the one described by Menninger, but it
fits the classical pattern. I quote from Berg's patient:

> It has been a hell of an experience. The hell has been my blind, stupid,
> and insistent attempt to make you take the place of the missing mother,
> as I previously tried to make you take the place of the missing father. I
> have nearly broken myself trying blindly and persistently to make you
> not only into that essential companion and guide, to tag myself onto you
> like a baby to its mother, but most ridiculously of all to coerce you into

stimulating and gratifying all my emotional and instinctual needs. Of course, I did not realize while I was doing it that this was my persistent endeavor, and that my sulks, pretended indifference, and other defenses, and particularly my hatred and temper were because you would not play. . . . The hell has been having to abandon these futile attempts . . . with my release from their blind compulsive force, instead of that persistent baby forever needing a daddy or a mummy to tag itself onto [p. 218f.].

The analysand is angry at his neurosis and contemptuous of what he has been. He gets little appreciation from his ego ideal for having undertaken the difficult psychoanalytic voyage. Under the rule of abstinence, he gets little comfort from the analyst at this stage.

To give a third example, Dewald (1972) states that nonpsychoanalytic therapies restrict their efforts to changing derivative psychic structures while psychoanalysis, because it eliminates the repression barrier and fosters the recall of the infantile neurosis, reorganizes core psychic structures. It is the working through of the transference neurosis that modifies the core structures. I cite a description of the termination moment given by Dewald.

A young married woman in the terminal phase of her analysis was working through her grief and mourning over termination and was increasingly confident of herself and her relationship to her husband and his love for her. "There's nothing here for me anymore. You're a doctor and you've treated a patient and I love you for it, but I'm in complete control of myself and I don't need you. All good things have to come to an end and they can't go on forever." She went on to describe her awareness that there had been no real love relationship between us, that the entire experience had occurred in her own mind, and that since she did not know me in reality, she was no longer able to convince herself that she loved me. And with a transient feeling of disloyalty to me, she indicated that she now felt her husband to be more virile, attractive, and sexually appealing than I [p. 322].

Such experiences were not unjustifiably described as a weaning experience—weaning away from neurotic expectations, an expulsion from a false Garden of Eden into the real world in which the patient is now equipped to find what he or she needs. Implicit in the classical theory of cure was the assumption that having realized the nature of the neurotic attachment to the parental figures, the new ego will be strong enough to resist the power exerted by those prototypes. What Menninger's, Berg's, and Dewald's patients are talking about is a new ego state—the ego state of insight. However, we cannot be sure whether in the course of life the new insight or the power of the old prototypes will from now on determine what the course of life will be. It was a psychoanalytic article of faith that insight will prevail. It was not a genuine clinical finding.

What about the fate of the internalized image of the analyst after termination? Neither Menninger, Berg, nor Dewald pursued the problem, but we can well imagine that the relationship to the analyst is bound to remain an ambivalent one, a mixture of gratitude for the guidance and a less positive feeling for the evident human imperfections revealed by the analyst as a real person.

The two concepts, transference neurosis and the resolution of the transference, remain complementary concepts. If psychoanalysts can foster a transference neurosis but are helpless at resolving the transference they themselves have created, they may well be in the position of the sorcerer's apprentice who can begin a process that he cannot bring to conclusion.

DISSENT FROM THE CLASSICAL POSITION

In 1950 Macalpine observed that the resolution of the transference has been regarded as proof that suggestion plays no part in psychoanalysis, "but its ultimate resolution or even its ultimate fate is not clearly understood. Whenever it is finally resolved, it is during an ill-defined period after termination of analysis. By this feature it escapes strict scientific observation" (p. 534).

To my knowledge, the first to recognize that the transference may not always be resolvable was Annie Reich (1958), who said, "Sometimes his [the patient's] relation to the analyst may become the first really reliable object relationship in the patient's life, a contingency which of course entails the danger that it may seriously interfere with the possibility of the transference ever being analysed" (p. 230). By "analysed" Reich surely meant analyzed to the point of transference resolution. She did not specify what this danger entails.

A pessimistic appraisal based on the inability to resolve the transference was stated by Kubie (1968). He pointed out that psychoanalysts have assumed that the transference neurosis is resolvable if, during the analysis, (1) the analyst assiduously analyzes the transference; (2) if he scrupulously remains incognito; (3) if he maintains a watchful eye on his countertransference. However, he doubted that even strict adherence to these principles will guarantee the eventual resolution of the transference. "I have been impressed by many observations of how transference processes, which had been essential for both exploratory and therapeutic progress of the analysis could toward the end seem to turn upon the analytic process and destroy it" (p. 331).

Credit for the breakthrough in the area under discussion goes to Pfeffer, who in a series of papers summarized in 1963 reported follow-up studies after the termination of treatment. These follow-up studies were conducted by an analyst other than the treating analyst. Some of the findings came as a surprise.

> . . . the patient appears to deal with the follow-up study as though it were analysis and deals with the follow-up analyst as though he were his treating analyst. Second, the patient manifests either an intensification of residual symptoms or a recurrence of the symptoms for which analysis was first sought. . . . After the analysis the patient retains an important and complicated intrapsychic representation of the analyst. This representation of the analyst is connected not only with the transference residue but also, in an important way, with the resolved portion of the transference neurosis [p. 230].
> . . . conflicts underlying symptoms are not actually shattered or obliterated by analysis but rather are only better mastered with new and more adequate solutions [p. 234].
> [The patient] relives the separation which could not be altogether analyzed since the patient was not in analysis to do so even though the meaning of termination may have been partially analyzed in anticipation [p. 239].

Pfeffer's study showed that at least for the population he was dealing with, resolution of the transference did not represent clinical reality. Another study by Haskell et al. (1976) confirmed the powerful readiness for transference relationship in follow-up studies.

Loewald (1978) suggests that every termination has parricidal implications. It therefore generates a great deal of aggression and guilt in the analysand. While these feelings can be made conscious and worked over in the analysis, Loewald does not believe that they lose their potency, which remains after termination.

THE IMPACT OF OBJECT RELATIONS THEORIES

There is still another line of thought relevant to this subject. We need to examine the data from the perspective of our growing understanding of the impact on the psychic structure of early interactions between the infant and those who care for him. Freud and the classical analysts who worked within the model he created centered their attention on the analysand's repressed fantasy system and particularly on the fantasies associated with the oedipus complex. Freud did not think that it was possible or particularly relevant to reconstruct the actual relationship between the analysand as an infant and his parents. He was interested in the parents only insofar as the parents influenced the nature and severity of the superego. Ferenczi's paper (1933) on the confusion of tongues between parent and child is a notable exception.

In the 1940s, object relations theorists like Fairbairn and Balint redirected psychoanalytic interest when they suggested that the libido is object-seeking rather than pleasure-seeking. With this reformulation the great difference between "within the pleasure principle" and "beyond the pleasure principle" lost some of its significance, or at least appeared in a new light. If good enough parental objects are available to the infant, he will cathect them with pleasure. If the objects are sadistic or neglectful, the infant will eventually adjust to them by a narcissistic or masochistic personality structure and, if need be, by schizoid or schizophrenic solutions. When the analysis exposes the character of such parents behind the pathological defense mechanisms the patient has built up, the analyst becomes "the first reliable object" and as such acquires a position of psychic importance equivalent to that of the original parents. When this happens—and it happens to some extent in every analysis—we can no longer speak of the resolution of the transference.

DISCUSSION

Those analysts who concentrate exclusively on the analysis of fantasy systems can at the end of the analysis obtain results such as those reported by Dewald's patient. But even in Dewald's patient I suggested that the ego state that brought about the capacity to transfer the libido back to the husband is only one among many. At times of marital stress, she might feel that her love for the analyst was much more real than she imagined at the moment of termination.

As long as psychoanalysis was confined to the analysis of fantasy systems and analyses were comparatively short, it was still possible to hope that the significance of the analyst would diminish markedly after the end of the analysis. However, we cannot be sure, for unfortunately we have only the example of the Wolf-Man, and in his case there was no sign of the resolution of the transference.

We have to differentiate between interpretations that pertain to the analysand only and those that change his attitude toward the significant infantile objects in his life. It is one thing to draw attention to the analysand's depression and quite another to make him realize that his mother was depressed or that she was unable to allow him to separate because she regarded him as a part of herself. The more we uncover gross failures in the original love object in an analysand's life, the more likely it is that the analyst will replace the original parental objects as the major infantile prototype.

My experience has taught me that it is usually not possible to predict in what direction the image of the analyst will evolve after termination. In one case, the previous analyst became a persecutory image and a second analysis had to be undertaken for the patient to get mastery over the internalized image of the first analyst. When that patient terminated his first analysis, he had no foreknowledge that his feelings toward his former analyst would undergo so radical a transformation. Much will depend on whether the object representation of the analyst after the analysis remained cathected predominantly with love or with disappointment, whether a fixation on the analyst remained, or whether the analysand acquired the capacity to transfer from the analyst to objects in real life.

I do not wish to minimize the significance of internalization of the analyst's basic attitude toward the analysand. However, as already stated, I do not believe that internalization can, for most people, carry the full load of the object relationship that evolved in the course of an analysis.

I would now like to suggest that we look at the problem from a different metapsychological perspective. Every analysand enters analysis with some combination of primary process fantasies of what the analysis will accomplish and realistic secondary process realizable hopes. As the transference deepens and the transference neurosis gains in strength, the primary processes become increasingly important. However, the decision to terminate, if it is not faulty or premature, is by its very nature a secondary process decision. Indeed, the patients of Menninger, Berg, and Dewald I have quoted speak the sober language of the secondary processes when they decide to terminate. It is, however, unlikely that the primary processes which were so powerful in the course of analysis and worked in the direction of continuation of analysis have become so weakened that they will not search for a substitute for the analyst. Much, therefore, depends on the type of displacement that will take place after the analysis. A simple displacement will not suffice, for it will lead to a repetition of the past. Only if the displacement is based on an intrapsychic reorganization which was achieved in analysis can we hope for a new type of postpsychoanalytic relationship. Such a reorganization must take place whether the analysand finds a new love object or reorganizes a previously existing relationship. Some analysands cope with the new object representation by finding a love object who needs them the way they needed the analyst, while others hope to find a partner who will understand them the way the analyst did and in addition will be sexually gratifying. They fall in love with someone who reminds them of themselves as they were before the analysis began, while they themselves take on the role of the therapist. Whether such a solution is stable will depend on the genuineness of the identification.

A number of possibilities present themselves: (1) The postanalytic relationship continues in a dormant state, ready to cathect any suitable substitute for the analyst. These were the results that Pfeffer reported. Under such conditions it is likely that the analysand will resume analysis with the previous analyst or, if disappointed, with a new analyst. (2) The loss of the analyst leaves the analysand bereft, incapable of replacing the analyst with a new love object, or finding a way of transforming transference love into love in real life. The idealization of the analyst continues after the analysis, a prolonged mourning turns into a depression, and the analyst is considered irreplaceable. (3) A new object is found, modeled on the analyst, in whom a replica of the transference relationship is sought, with various degrees of success in real life. (4) A new love object is found representing a compromise between the original pathology-producing object and some features of the analyst. I wish to stress that compromise formations are not the same as integration. (5) The analyst is internalized through identification as the analysand's ego ideal. The analysand strives to become as much as possible like the analyst. Such former analysands tend to change their occupations to conform to the new ego ideal. (6) The process of working through was successful in liberating new integrative capacities in the analysand that either make it possible to transform his existing relationships or find a new love object based on the positive features of the significant love objects of his childhood, among whom the analyst, although not an infantile object, is nevertheless included.

Analysands during the termination phase often bring up feelings of anxiety or depression as to what will happen to them after termination. The traditional way of handling such a situation is to ask for further free association. This is still the method of choice, but the analysand's associations can become more productive if the analyst accepts as psychologically valid the anxiety of the termination phase and tries empathically to anticipate what life will be like for the analysand after termination. All too often we have to agree with the analysands who feel that while psychoanalysis solved many neurotic problems, it also created new ones.

I wish to close with a general observation. When Freud (1912a) used the mirror metaphor, when he urged the analyst to remain opaque to his patients and give only what has been projected, he created a new type of human relationship, designed to be self-liquidating. The analysand reaches a stage when he no longer needs the analyst, but the internalized image is not erased. When psychoanalysis was on the defensive and "falling in love with the doctor" scandalized the pre-World War I bourgeoisie, the concept of the resolution of the transference was a necessary one. What we need to aim at is not to resolve the transference neurosis but to make sure that it forms a productive inner structure in the life of the former analysand.

SUMMARY

The paper examined the psychoanalytic theory of love, the psychoanalytic theory of transference neurosis, and the concept of resolution of the transference insofar as they are relevant to the process of termination. "Resolution of the transference" is defensive in nature and no longer corresponds to the current psychoanalytic object relations theory, nor has it been confirmed by clinical data. Current psychoanalytic techniques typically lead to the analyst becoming a significant reliable object of the analysand. This fact makes resolution of the transference questionable. Internalization and identification with the analyst, though important, cannot carry the full burden of termination. Because the analyst remains important even after the analysis, ways must be sought to facilitate transference from the analyst to objects in the real world. Some difficulties in achieving this goal have been discussed.

BIBLIOGRAPHY

BERG, C. H. (1947). *Deep Analysis* New York: Norton.

BERGMANN, M. S. (1971). Psychoanalytic observations on the capacity to love. In *Separation-Individuation*, ed. J. B. McDevitt & C. F. Settlage. New York: Int. Univ. Press, pp. 15–40.

———— (1980). On the intrapsychic function of falling in love. *Psychoanal. Q.*, 49:56–77.

———— (1982). Platonic love, transference love, and love in real life. *J. Amer. Psychoanal. Assn.*, 30:87–111.

———— (1985–86). Transference love and love in real life. *Int. J. Psychoanal. Psychother.*, 11:27–45.

———— (1987). *The Anatomy of Loving.* New York: Columbia Univ. Press.

BLUM, H. P. (1971). On the conception and development of the transference neurosis. *J. Amer. Psychoanal. Assn.,* 19:41–53.

BREUER, J. & FREUD, S. (1895). Studies on hysteria. *S.E.,* 2.

BRUNSWICK, R. M. (1928). A supplement to Freud's history of infantile neurosis. In *The Psychoanalytic Reader,* ed. R. Fliess. New York: Int. Univ. Press, 1948, pp. 86–126.

DEWALD, P. A. (1972). The clinical assessment of structural change. *J. Amer. Psychoanal. Assn.,* 20:302–324.

FERENCZI, S. (1933). Confusion of tongues between adults and the children. In *Final Contributions to the Problems and Methods of Psycho-Analysis.* London: Hogarth Press, 1955, pp. 156–167.

FREUD, A. (1959). *The Psychoanalytic Treatment of Children.* New York: Int. Univ. Press.

FREUD, S. (1907). Delusions and dreams in Jensen's *Gradiva. S.E.,* 9:3–95.

——— (1910). A special type of object choice made by men. *S.E.,* 11:163–175.

——— (1912a). The dynamics of transference. *S.E.,* 12:97–108.

——— (1912b). Recommendations to physicians practising psycho-analysis. *S.E.,* 12:109–120.

——— (1914a). Remembering, repeating and working through. *S.E.,* 12:145–156.

——— (1914b). On the history of the psycho-analytic movement. *S.E.,* 14:7–66.

——— (1918). From the history of an infantile neurosis. *S.E.,* 17:3–123.

——— (1924). The dissolution of the oedipus complex. *S.E.,* 19:173–179.

GILL, M. M. (1954). Psychoanalysis and exploratory psychotherapy. *J. Amer. Psychoanal. Assn.,* 2:771–797.

GLOVER, E. (1955). *Principles of Psychoanalysis.* New York: Int. Univ. Press.

GREENACRE, P. (1959). Certain technical problems in the transference relationship. *J. Amer. Psychoanal. Assn.,* 7:484–502.

GREENSON, R. R. (1958). Variations in classical psychoanalytic technique. *Int. J. Psychoanal.,* 39:200–201.

——— (1967). *The Technique and Practice of Psychoanalysis.* New York: Int. Univ. Press.

HASKELL, N. F., BLACKER, K. H., & OREMLAND, J. D. (1976). The fate of the transference neurosis after termination of a successful analysis. *J. Amer. Psychoanal. Assn.,* 24:471–498.

KUBIE, L. S. (1968). Unsolved problems in the resolution of the transference. *Psychoanal. Q.,* 37:331–352.

LOEWALD, H. W. (1962). Internalization, separation, mourning, and the superego. In *Papers on Psychoanalysis.* New Haven: Yale Univ. Press, 1980, pp. 257–276.

——— (1971). The transference neurosis. *Ibid.,* pp. 302–314.

——— (1978). The waning of the oedipus complex. *Ibid.,* pp. 384–404.

MACALPINE, I. (1950). The development of the transference. *Psychoanal. Q.,* 19:501–539.

MENNINGER, K. A. (1958). *Theory of Psychoanalytic Technique.* New York: Basic Books.

PFEFFER, A. Z. (1963). The meaning of the analyst after analysis. *J. Amer. Psychoanal. Assn.,* 11:229–244.

REICH, A. (1958). A special variation on technique. *Int. J. Psychoanal.,* 39:230–234.

Termination Analyzable and Unanalyzable

HANS W. LOEWALD, M.D.

TERMINATION, AS UNDERSTOOD HERE, IS AN ENDING OF TREATMENT THAT is not crucially determined by extraneous factors in the patient's or therapist's life but appears as a natural organic outcome of the treatment process itself; it is, in that sense, not an interruption of treatment. Nor is it a product of acting out if by acting out we mean actions that run counter to the therapeutic engagement and its intended course. Therapy terminates at some given point in time, but that point is preceded and prepared for by a longer or shorter time period during therapy which is called the termination phase. My attention will be mainly focused on this phase.

Let me weave in here some general remarks. Distinctions and statements about termination, as compared with the rough and tumble of clinical work, with the ambiguities and multiple, overlapping determinants of psychic life, always sound more univocal and exclusive than the real thing. By the same token, clinical illustrations are so rich in meanings and open to various interpretations—often equally valid—that even experience-close generalizations do not easily emerge from them.

For convenience, the termination phase may be divided into two stages. There is a stage during which the patient with our help arrives at a decision whether or not to terminate. That first stage is initiated by various indications that the patient unconsciously or consciously approaches the question of terminating treatment with more than casual glances. The therapeutic process as seen by patient and therapist, sometimes seen more clearly by one than by the other, may show signs

Supervising analyst, Western New England Institute for Psychoanalysis, and clinical professor emeritus, Yale University School of Medicine, New Haven.

Read at a symposium on "Clinical Perspectives on Termination," Western New England Psychoanalytic Society, October 25, 1986.

of nearing a measure of completion or of diminishing returns. A second stage is ushered in when patient and therapist eventually agree that the patient, if only in disguised form, has been seriously and rather consistently thinking about actually ending treatment, and that termination in a fairly near future makes sense and promises to be beneficial. Now the impending, actual, permanent separation, the factual ending of the therapeutic relationship, tends to become a dominant or recurrent theme of experience to be scrutinized—and this while the patient is still engaged in that very relationship. Often patients complain that the therapist *makes* this into a stage in treatment; they may want to have termination be an event pure and simple, the less said about it the better, and/or make it into a nonevent by recoiling from the idea of stopping. They may see this stage as the therapist's devilish device to prolong treatment, or alternatively as a device to insist on termination, even to rub salt into the wound.

During the termination phase we are not dealing only with separation experiences of the patient's past and their impact on current-life relationships, and not only with the here-and-now of their revivals and reverberations in the therapeutic transference situation, poignant and involving as these are. We are also dealing with the anticipated here-and-now in a new dimension: the actual separation of patient and therapist. By contrast to the reality of the transference, although deeply imbued with it, the two participants, especially during the second stage, plan to take themselves out of the transference situation into a factual parting of the ways. The termination is to be understood in its transference dimensions, in the context and under the influence of the patient's life history, but there remains the irreducible fact that precisely this form of experiencing and understanding itself is about to end, is itself about to become part of the historical past. Never mind that the therapeutic effect of treatment seems to depend so much on the treatment experience becoming part of the patient's living past. During therapy, we say, everything is grist for the mill; but what if the mill itself is to be dismantled? With the therapist's cooperation the patient is pulling the prerequisites for further common work out from under his own feet. To what extent is termination analyzable?

The most important aspect of the termination of a therapeutic relationship is the work of mourning. Mourning in its full sense involves the gradual relinquishment of a cherished relationship with another person, and its internalization. By internalization I do not simply mean remembering the person and the relationship in thoughts, images, and fantasies. I mean an increasing dissolution of the relationship as one with an external object—whether present or imagined—leading to an absorption into the very fabric of the subject. It has been described as a kind of identification, as contrasted with an object relationship. These internalizations often coexist with conscious recollections of what is lost. What is lost is being reconstituted in a movement of self-transformation. The development of the superego as an internal structure, during the dissolution of the oedipus complex, is a prominent example of that kind of transformation.

Facing the impending renunciation and loss creates a new distance between patient and therapist as well as a new closeness brought about by the pressure of termination. Maintaining and tolerating an optimal degree of closeness and distance in a meaningful relationship are inherent tasks from the very beginning of treatment. An important goal of psychoanalysis and psychoanalytic psychotherapy, greater inner freedom and further individuation, is pursued from the start. Termination in that sense is always in the offing. I emphasize this because I believe that termination of treatment has to be seen in this larger context of coming to terms with individuality and its freedom and limitations. Of course, there are patients who first need to learn something about closeness in a therapeutic relationship, about intimacy in which their autonomy is not totally endangered by fusion with or surrender to the therapist. There are others, or other sides of the same patients, who need first to learn that over time closeness is not destroyed by experiences or prospects of distance and of frustrations spelling for them total isolation or worse. There are patients who remain unable to learn or relearn something useful about this middleground of intimacy-in-distance; they are likely to stop or, if possible, to go on indefinitely. Many psychotic and certain borderline patients, while benefiting from treatment in various ways, stop at some point but do not go through a termination phase; not infrequently they require tangible evidence, from time to time, for instance, by means of long distance phone calls, that the therapist is still around.

I come back to termination as an exercise, if you will, in coming to terms with individuation, and to how this is at play from the beginning of treatment—with a vengeance, as you will see, in the following clinical example. A male patient, having started analysis with a male analyst just a few weeks before, dreamed that he stayed in an inn and was being pursued by robbers; an analyst, robust and aggressive (who was not the patient's analyst), offered help, but the dreamer told him that he could handle things very well by himself. Much could be said about this dream, including the patient's sexual-aggressive fear/wishes in regard to his analyst. Here I want to underline only the patient's protestations of self-sufficiency, indicating a propensity to stop the analysis. He did not speak and, I believe, did not consciously think of terminating or stopping the analysis; he enacted this in a dream. For good reasons he was proud of his relative emancipation as an individual and of his competence, but he was afraid of losing his balance by dependent closeness to his analyst. That he continued analysis may be taken as a sign that the threats were not overwhelming and that the reworking of old conflicts in the transference might be beneficial. Problems of mourning had been prominent in his life history.

This dream demonstrated very early resistance against analysis. I wish to comment here on resistance during the termination phase itself. We may distinguish between resistance against continuing the treatment and resistance against ending it. As to the former: continued or intensified emotional involvement with the therapist may be resisted, together with a growing aversion to continued efforts of turning inward and self-understanding. The idea of termination may become persistent when deeply unconscious problems are touched on by the patient that seem too troublesome and painful, conflicts often recognizable in the transference situation so that their coming to the surface threatens even deeper, more extended emotional involvement with the therapist. In terms of a patient's mental welfare, enacting independence by withdrawing from therapy and therapist may be premature, and a decision to take that course may be ill-advised. On the other hand, resistance to further treatment may be a sign of increased genuine independence, of healthy emancipation from the therapist as well as from the therapeutic process itself; regardless of involvement with the particular therapist, psychotherapy or analysis may no longer be needed, even though still appealing, hard to forego, and perhaps useful again at some future time.

Most often the motives for the patient's inclination to terminate are mixed, and frequently it is no easy task for the therapist to assess the balance of forces. I would include here also the therapist's realistic appraisal of the weight of external factors that may favor or seem to compel termination. Once termination is seriously considered, the therapist—I am speaking particularly now of psychoanalysis—in his own deliberations with one foot has to step out of the analytic process and take into account, in a different way than usual, the overall picture of the patient's life situation at the time. What we call external factors, for example, moving to another location, a new job, a new love relationship, marriage, changed financial commitments or obligations, may mainly be pretexts for avoiding further therapeutic work. But such changes may be mainly results of therapeutic work accomplished, signs of a significant measure of achieved autonomy. Even though analysis in a certain sense is interminable, life is finite, and analysis has to end at a given point, if it is to be a guide and a rehearsal for a better life and not an end in itself. (Concerning this last statement, we may wonder what it implies for the life of an analyst, one for whom analysis has more or less become an end in itself; but that is beyond the scope of the panel's topic as I understand it.) Reverberations of the therapeutic encounter and rehearsal continue after termination in one way or another, sometimes in the form of an internal dialogue similar to the patient-therapist dialogue but more or less depersonalized. If it becomes necessary at some future time, therapy may be resumed if circumstances permit.

The therapist takes the patient's contributions to an assessment into account; but I wish to emphasize that it is the therapist's responsibility, and an aspect of his competency, to make an objective assessment of the balance of motives mentioned earlier, so as to agree or disagree with the patient about termination. The final decision is the patient's. With hysterically inclined patients we need to be on guard against precipitous decisions; with patients of a more obsessional disposition we have to watch out for their indecisiveness and procrastinations. I believe that these dispositions play a role in both neurotic and more severe mental disturbances. The therapist's recommendations tend to be taken by the patient as commands, even by those patients we deem ready for beginning the final termination process. There is an element of submission to authority and of rebellion against authority, in whichever direction the therapist's consent or explicit recommendation goes. The patient, if well enough advanced, will himself be aware of these impulses and take them into account. The therapist certainly must give them their due without becoming immobilized by them. In other words, the therapist, when all is said and done, must take the risks involved in his consent or recommendation, as is true for all other interventions too.

Otto Rank, in his later years, in connection with his birth trauma theory, advocated setting a time limit at the beginning of treatment (he greatly influenced the orientation of the Pennsylvania school of social work in the 40s and 50s). Apparently he believed that the main task in therapy was the conscious experience and understanding of termination and separation itself, and that the acknowledged definite prospect of it provided the necessary pressure to make treatment terminable. It is hard to quarrel with the notion—the observation can be made many times—that impending termination often creates its own momentum, enhancing therapeutic work not only on termination but on many aspects of the patient's life and its history of separation issues. But I do not believe that in most cases the inward-looking, unhurried, and in that sense timeless work of analysis can be done well if the pressure of time is high from the start. Time pressure, as we know from impending separations before vacation and other interruptions, can temporarily promote as well as impede the therapeutic process. Especially in early treatment phases impending interruptions tend to be impediments: often patients become too depressed or angry or aloof, acting in disruptive ways; they may retaliate, for example, by starting their own vacations earlier than the therapist, returning later; there are stubborn silences, unremitting expressions of anger that do not allow for useful analytic work at the time. After interruptions, when treatment is resumed, such moves have a chance to be interpreted as enactments of powerful feelings.

I am turning to *resistance against termination*. I should like to emphasize that the term "resistance" in psychoanalytic parlance signifies an impulse or movement against the therapeutic process and/or the therapist, but that the motives for resistance are multiple and may include a patient's strivings for self-affirmation as positive and valuable ingredients. These may be dominant not only in his urge to terminate, but also in another way if he wishes to continue treatment. As he considers ending treatment, a patient may rightly decide that he needs more of it. He may feel, for instance, that he now has a far better understanding of the origins, ramifications, and expressions of his problems, but that he still is not sufficiently able to manage them or that important areas of his psychic life have remained in limbo. He hopes that continued treatment will help him here. He may be right that only in that transference medium of emotional experience in shared insight further progress is apt to take place. If the therapist feels that by and large he is not dealing with rationalizations for prolonging a dependent relationship for its own sake, termination is set aside for the time being (although, once seriously considered, it has a way of not altogether disappearing from sight). The wish for continuing a dependent, perhaps sadomasochistic, relationship with the therapist is well known; here I shall not further comment on it. Its weight in patients' urgings for continuing and in actual prolongations of treatment is beyond question.

Let me briefly consider the difficulty of transforming intellectual into emotional and effective insight, to the extent to which it is a problem of internalization and individuation. Gaining emotional insight—insight that changes the person, not just his ideas and thoughts—is a movement wherein what the patient has learned, as interesting and cherished information, is absorbed into his very existence, is internalized in the strong sense of that word. The acquired knowledge *about* himself changes from remembered and reproducible information to reorganization of the self. This change spells separateness not just from a particular person, but the separateness of being more of an individual. By contrast, intellectual insight resides on the surface, remains part of the interface joining patient and therapist. Being more individuated means experiencing the loneliness and vulnerability, and the richness and freedom of individual existence. I should add that intellectual insight has a positive potential; it often represents early steps on the path to more penetrating insight.

How do we decide which are the patient's dominant or decisive motives for or against termination? A quote from general Karl von Clausewitz's remarks on military genius comes to my mind: "War is the realm of uncertainty: three-quarters of the factors on which action in war is based are wrapped in a fog of greater or lesser uncertainty. A sensitive and discriminating judgment is called for, a skilled intelligence to scent out the truth . . . and the courage to follow this faint light wherever it may lead." Psychotherapy is not war, but we are similarly confronted with the uncertainties and complexities of multiple motivations, on which eventually we must base our actions and interventions, especially when it comes to termination of treatment. And geniuses are a rare breed indeed. Are there any guidelines to help us scent out the truth regarding the patient's motives for or against ending treatment? A patient may, consciously or unconsciously, broach the issue of termination with some consistency when convincing therapeutic work has been going on for some length of time, convincing, that is, to both partners. In that case it is more likely his healthy side that speaks here. We must also consider that he may try to silence that healthier voice by protesting the opposite, bringing termination up as something not at all on his mind or to be considered. The context in which the topic comes up gives us valuable clues. If he is in a hostile phase vis-à-vis the therapist, it is likely that we are dealing with angry withdrawal. As mentioned earlier, the hostility often is combined with or based on the fact of his approaching issues of his psychic life from which he recoils. Even if this does not lead to anger at the therapist, ending treatment becomes tempting, and the therapist will be on his guard against premature closure. The therapist also must try to assess the patient's capacity for facing those more disturbing conflicts without getting overpowered by them and becoming sicker. In some cases the possibility may be considered that only during or after such breakdown deeper psychotherapeutic work becomes feasible. Whether to take the risks inherent in following that course, the therapist ultimately must decide for himself. A patient's vacillations between terminating and not terminating often have aspects of testing the therapist's interest, love, commitment. If termination comes up after an interruption, the therapist should take into account his own inner distance during that time, and his own pace, perhaps remoteness, as treatment is resumed; these may cloud his judgment concerning termination. Patients after a vacation may desperately cling to the therapist and the sessions, even though termination had been discussed at length and convincingly before the vacation. We would take into consideration that this may be a patient's attempt at undoing, triggered by the interruption, that needs to be interpreted accordingly.

The patient's communications regarding termination often are, at least at first, not expressed as conscious thoughts and feelings. He does not speak of termination. For instance, he repeatedly dreams of departures, travels to far-away places; he finds himself in lonely regions, at funerals, or in a new or refurbished home. He may keep on dreaming of meeting the therapist outside the office, on social occasions; or he has more persistent fantasies of that nature. The verbal material may more frequently and intensely refer to current and past relationships involving changes in himself or experiences of separation and loss by death, but also happy reunions and encounters. Or the patient begins seriously to consider new jobs, moving to another city, and the like, which would prevent him from continuing treatment without mentioning that. All this is particularly pertinent to analysis where verbal interactions and discussions of practical issues between therapist and patient are less frequent and the spontaneous flow of associations and their unconscious focus are more easily observable. The analyst, if the overall context of the treatment process suggests it, hears allusions to or expressions of thoughts of nearing actual termination in the material. When he interprets it in those terms, patients often are taken aback and alarmed as they may be by interpretations of other unacknowledged motivations and connections, interpretations that bring repressed or vaguely felt, unformulated ideas and intentions to the surface.

It is not uncommon that under the realistic pressure of the termination phase oedipal and earlier separation-individuation problems become more vivid and in a new way available for interpretative work and for mastery of conflicts. I have gained the impression that what we call the transference neurosis often comes to full bloom just during that phase. On the basis of all the preceding work, with the actual ending of therapy in sight, what the patient has experienced in the past and learned about himself becomes more acutely alive and meaningful. This expresses itself in his vacillations about termination—a new edition of early dilemmas—and in his increased readiness to work on oedipal and preoedipal problems as issues of his now present past. It is as if in a "good enough" termination phase that mutual correspondence and interdependence of his past and present really begin to sink in, an integration that makes for change. I believe that in psychotherapy other than formal analysis something comparable can take place.

Let me switch back to resistance against mourning the actual separation from the therapist in the near future, and especially in the latter's live presence. Even though the loss of the therapist and the ending of treatment in the last stage of termination are anticipated certainties, they have not yet taken place. Mourning in advance, as in analogous life situations, seems to hasten the arrival of the loss of the therapist or prematurely make it a reality, as though mourning in some way gives it the stamp of truth, even of approval, of the therapist's death. Powerful feelings of guilt may arise, guilt of murdering the therapist by mourning before the fact, perhaps in that act destroying oneself too. Seen in that light, a sense of being abandoned by the therapist—despite convincing evidence that the patient wants to leave—is more tolerable: responsibility shifts from patient to therapist. But the reality of impending separation remains, and with it often the sense that conscious mourning, with the object of mourning present and listening, amounts to the enacted destruction of living persons, and is not a relinquishment of fantasy ties after the event, as Freud (1917) has discussed it in "Mourning and Melancholia." I have suggested how verbalized mourning of termination may be fraught with conflicts that one can touch on and name. Due to the meanings of the actual ending, however, deeper work on mastering the real event must be left to the now strengthened and revitalized own capacities of the patient.

As this leads back to internalization, I like to give an example of internalizing processes manifested on a sexual-instinctual level during termination. Many years ago I described a group of male analysands who were terminating analysis with male analysts (Loewald, 1980). While occasionally they had dealt with homosexual conflicts in the course of analysis, these had not significantly troubled them, nor did they seem to require specially focused analytic work; paranoid problems were minimal or absent. During the termination phase these patients became acutely aware of passive homosexual fantasies in relation to the analyst, such as anal intercourse with him, fellatio, and pregnancy fantasies, often together with or followed by somatic symptoms like intestinal or throat discomfort, abdominal bloating, nausea. In one way these experiences are an example showing the crystallization of aspects of the transference neurosis during termination. Here I want to comment on them as manifestations of internalizing aspects of mourning. Unconsciously the analyst's influence is taken as desired/rejected intrusion, loved and hated, and the analytic process, under the pressure of the termination experiences in particular, again becomes a libidinal-aggressive transaction. Transforming these transactions into intrapsychic ones that no longer have the nature of object relations but are becoming elements of the patient's character, of his self (if you prefer that designation), is what I call internalizing. During the termination phase this movement toward emancipation becomes predominant, together with and contradicted by urges not to give up the relationship with the therapist. The patient sees the therapist, and himself as well, as an enemy and as a promoter of emancipation. While the above-described fantasies signal and concretize internalization dilemmas, they also, as fantasies of object relations, indicate the patient's wish to hold on to the satisfactions of a libidinal object relation with the therapist and to avoid the loneliness when it is dissolved. That internalization does not preclude object relations, even though termination stops contact with the therapist as therapist, that indeed internalization rather expands object relations and raises them to new levels—of that patients often are not fully aware at the point of termination. Needless to say, women show the same or similar dynamics, and both genders with therapists of both genders, although in different permutations and with different accents and nuances that carry considerable weight.

A few comments on some practical matters. I have said that in the initial phase of termination an agreement between patient and therapist is eventually reached that ending of treatment in the near future is indicated. Actually this is not always what happens. The patient may insist that he needs further treatment, while the therapist is persuaded that all has been done that could be done, at least with this therapist. Or the patient has reasons, convincing to him, to bring treatment to an end while the therapist is reasonably convinced that continued treatment with himself would be beneficial and desirable. The final decision here is, of course, up to the patient. But what if the patient insists on continued treatment with his familiar therapist? Should the therapist consent, against his judgment to the contrary? There are times when a patient's perseverance might prevail, given the uncertainty of predictions, perhaps a therapist's own inclinations, if pressed, to give the endeavor another chance. But there are other times when such a course is not indicated, for example, when the therapist is firmly convinced that a patient, pressed by the prospect of actual separation, clings to the personal relationship with him under the guise of forlorn hopes for further therapeutic benefits. The patient being faced with ineluctable facts and living through the definitive termination stage, which shades into the period after ending treatment as a part of the termination process—these experiences may be necessary to clinch the case. With such patients the final decision, in my view, is up to the therapist, painful as it is likely to be for the patient, and the therapist too.

The agreement between patient and therapist to terminate may be explicitly tentative (including the date) for a while and later made final. Then again, in order to forestall endless procrastinations, it may be best to set a firm limit. If a death in the family occurs, one may have to postpone the actual ending. Some patients and therapists prefer to stop in conjunction with the onset of vacations. Others feel that termination and the date of stopping should not be influenced by these considerations, should instead be highlighted by avoiding that conjunction. I find it impossible to have hard and fast rules about this. It is difficult to disregard the practicalities of life when it comes to the practical matter of ending treatment. To have the start of a vacation, even the end of a work week, coincide with ending treatment presents itself as an acceptable natural solution. To be sure, this tends to play into a patient's fantasy that he is being forced out of therapy; or it may play into his fantasy that the end is merely an interruption. Undoubtedly, the therapist's own scheduling interests should not be a determining factor. But the natural accustomed rhythm of the whole treatment process often speaks in favor of ending when a long-held-to, though previously only temporary, stopping point is reached. This may also provide an added incentive for the patient to cut the tie, based on memories of prior experiences. A therapist may, on the other hand, suggest a few months of treatment after vacation—provided that ending itself is not put into question—if that promises that important further work on termination issues may be accomplished after the break.

Having talked a good deal about internalization as an element of mourning, I wish to point to another dimension of internalization. Internalization is not solely a matter of internally reconstituting a renounced object relationship (as in mourning and in superego formation); it has a component of another kind. As in early development in particular, there is an element of smooth transition and passage between partners, something seamless, without a sense of loss and grief. What is taken in is more of the nature of a gift, or is becoming a trait or an attitude and stance now held in common. Freud (1921) spoke of similar phenomena when he first outlined his thoughts on the ego

166 *Hans W. Loewald*

ideal. The internalization phase of mourning is leavened with such nonseparative elements. It is well to take this into account, especially during the termination phase. I shun the word "model" because it so much suggests something to reach for or emulate, whereas here something is being attained and shared. The therapist's presence and interpretative participation in the mourning process not only help to make mourning a conscious experience. As tangible manifestation of communality in mourning it tends to put in relief, once more toward the end, those nonmourning elements of internalization.

BIBLIOGRAPHY

FREUD, S. (1917). Mourning and melancholia. *S.E.*, 14:217–235.
——— (1921). Group psychology and the analysis of the ego. *S.E.*, 18:67–143.
——— (1937). Analysis terminable and interminable. *S.E.*, 23:209–253.
LOEWALD, H. W. (1980). Comments on some instinctual manifestations of superego formation. In *Papers on Psychoanalysis*. New Haven: Yale Univ. Press, pp. 326–341.

Sweating It Out

HANNA SEGAL, M.D.

I HAVE ENTITLED MY PAPER "SWEATING IT OUT" BECAUSE THIS PATIENT had had as one of his symptoms profuse and offensively smelling sweating—really smelling of fear—and the last few months of the analysis he again sweated a few times on the couch. And those last months one could say he was really "sweating it out." Freud once observed that at the end of the analysis patients sometimes revert temporarily to the early symptoms. This has not been frequently my experience. More often—and this was markedly the case with that patient—old themes are taken up. Anxieties are reawakened, defenses of the past remobilized in sessions, but not necessarily resulting in the reappearance of symptoms; as in this patient, termination was a time of working through, sweating it out, at times with a great deal of pain. What he had to work through was the final facing of separateness and separation with all the attendant anxieties and depression. The patient had always been exceedingly sensitive to separation. In the early years of his analysis he was regularly physically ill before or during holidays.

He was virtually symptom free over several years. When he started, his sexual life was in a mess. He was very perverse, mostly in fantasy, but also in acting out. He was, in turn, grandiose and feeling disintegrated by anxiety, occasionally transitorily hallucinating. In previously describing this patient, I emphasized his pathological and excessive use of projective identification and identified the moment when he came out of it, which was one of the turning points of his analysis. He is now very happily married with a family of two children, very successful in his profession, a very gifted and respected physicist.

He remained a fairly anxious person and is still inhibited in reading and writing, though in the last few years he started writing papers. (As a child he was so inhibited intellectually that he was discouraged from

Training and supervising analyst, British Psychoanalytical Institute, London.

Read at a symposium on "Clinical Perspectives on Termination," Western New England Psychoanalytic Society, October 25, 1986.

taking A levels—willing but not intelligent enough, was the school's verdict. In fact, he is very bright and once out of his difficulties, he achieved good academic status. But throughout his childhood and adolescence he was lost in a permanent daydream.

His reasons for staying in analysis were mainly his realization of remaining character weaknesses—for instance, a tendency to placation, and insufficient courage in standing up for his ideas and his fear of regressing, should he stop. He was very worried, for instance, about occasional recrudescences of nasty pornographic fantasies when thwarted or anxious. But underlying that was a fantasy that analysis was, or would end in, a marriage between us—a marriage in which he would fuse with me and eventually would become me. The only way of separating from me which would not expose him to jealousy or envy would be by becoming me. For instance, sometime before Easter (his analysis was to finish at the end of July) he had read Melanie Klein's *Narrative of a Child Analysis* (1961). He dreamed that he was writing Richard and felt embarrassed telling me the dream. Not being able to maintain that he was Mrs. Klein/me exposed him to recognizing violent feelings he found hard to bear. The day after the Richard dream he was worried because he bought boots with sheepskin linings. They were very expensive, and he felt guilty toward his family. But he also felt very guilty about the sheep—killing them to get into their skin. On the way to the session, mixed with thinking about the sheepskins, he realized he was also thinking about my funeral—how would it be? He thought he dreamed of metal coffins. He also noticed that passing a funeral, he again started to salivate as he always had in the past.

This cannibalistic fantasy (he had many others of that kind) was at the service of projective identification—biting his way into me to get into my skin. This was a defense against loss, but also, and predominantly, against envy. He recognized with a lot of pain that he just could not stand the thought of me being better known as an analyst than he was in his field and his own feeling that his papers were not up to mine, Klein's, or Freud's; he did not write Richard!

The patient had resorted again to projective identification so prominent at the beginning (becoming Mrs. Klein, getting into my skin). This led to the experience that the working through of his projective and cannibalistic wishes was felt by him as my expelling him from inside me. For several days he had been surly, feeling, as he told me, that all he wanted to do was to stay on the couch and to sulk. Then he brought the following dream:

He was late for a student who he felt was very rejecting of him. He was giving him a tutorial in a dreary basement. Then he drove out and it was, as he said, like a dream within a dream. He thought, "I know these crossroads. That's where I had a terrible fight with an obstetrician. I saw my head covered with blood. As I told you, it was like a dream within a dream." He associated to the student in the dream that he was also about to terminate his course. The student represented himself rejecting me, and his being late for the student represented his unwillingness to face that aspect of himself. Curiously, though at this stage he was very perceptive about his dreams, he had no associations to the crossroads with which he was familiar and his head being bloodied in his fight with the obstetrician. I suggested that the familiar crossroads were his fantasies of birth. He then realized that he was not sure if the blood was his own; in fact, his bloodied head reminded him of the childbirth of his first son—a forceps birth which was very traumatic. For a time brain damage was suspected. Following that he remembered another bit of the dream. The choice he had at the crossroads was one road leading to the downs full of rabbit holes. The other, probably the right one, led through a territory unknown to him. He associated to the end of the treatment and his choice of being born and facing the unknown future or trying to hide again inside the analysis like a womb or a rabbit hole—"To be or not to be." He often felt bitter about his cowardice, looking for holes to hide in.

For several days he struggled with this problem. He realized again something familiar from the past—that in my building he was all eyes, ears, nose, and had a fantasy that he knew everything that was going on in me and my house. He had a dream of being in bed with his mother, legitimately he said, as his father was out. There was some return of violent and cannibalistic fantasies. He once started the session by complaining of the district he lived in, which was a bit slummy, saying there was too much violence—"I can't afford to live there"—with a determination to move to Hampstead where I live. It was clear he felt he could not afford to separate off from me because of the violence which it stimulated in him. He talked to a friend who terminated analysis a year before and complained that R., her analyst, pushed her out, but kept her blue-eyed boys (two members of his professional team).

That night he dreamed that he was in analysis with R., but the session paradoxically lasted only 25 minutes. Then he was in a session with me. He was silent and I said, "It seems you don't want to be helped by me." He then experienced a wave of absolute fury and hatred and had a determination not to tell me anything. But then he did tell me in the dream whatever it was and the atmosphere in the session changed and he was full of affection. He obviously found it hard to give up his fantasy of his being my blue-eyed boy whom I would keep forever and, to begin with, was full of fury. He did not want to be helped because to be helped meant to be helped to finish his analysis and face both separation and his envy of being helped. In the dream, however, when he could get in touch with the feeling, he overcame the fury and love came back. The next night he dreamed that there was a house on the hill which looked very nice and of which he was very fond, but it was quite clear to him that the house wasn't his.

When he could face his separateness from me, the oedipal themes returned. For instance, just before Easter he dreamed of M. working in the British Museum Library and he hated him for working in *his* library. He has heard someone referring to M. and myself in the same breath. After Easter he had a dream of being a Polish insurgent that attacked violently someone whom he thought was a Polish oppressor on a railway track. He knew I was Polish. He associated the railway track with his return to analysis. But he also said that the Polish oppressor wasn't nearly as terrible as it was made out to be. The oppressive Polish Government did not compare, for instance, with Chile or South Africa. The oppressive, hated father he linked with his stepfather, whom he considered a tyrant. Soon thereafter, having been quite difficult, he became very affectionate and smiling. I had become his real father, but one felt to be easily homosexually seducible. His father had died when the boy was 12 and his mother remarried. He dreamed that when he was 16, his father returned. It turned out that his father hadn't died but merely left mother for another woman. He felt enormous love and relief. From various associations and his seductive smiles at me, it was clear that the other woman was himself. He was very upset at recognizing that at work he found himself again placating and seductive to dominant male figures. There had always been a difficulty with this patient to maintain a good father figure without homosexualizing it. There was a split between his stepfather and his father. He hated his stepfather who he felt was a tyrant. The father, on the other hand, was often felt (I think without very realistic grounds) as being open to homosexual seduction and alliance against women. This became crystal clear in those last months of treatment. He recognized that there was a great deal of strength, masculinity, and positive guidance that he received from his stepfather despite some of his rigidity and severity. On the other hand, his own father was less soft than in the patient's fantasy. The problem was of tolerating the jealousy or envy of a father who could be potent, good, and not homosexual.

He had a dream about a watch given to him by a very admired uncle. In the dream he had in the past paid an enormous repair bill to get it repaired. Now the bill was much smaller, but he realized that he was very reluctant to pay it. He boasted to somebody that he had a wonderful watch repairer, but that person told him, "Ah, but he's an alcoholic, he is no good." The analysis of the split between the father and the stepfather mobilized the envy of the potent analyst/father who could give him a watch (reality sense) and was a wonderful repairer. The watch and the repairer were both devalued. He was too mean to acknowledge the debt and repay it, though he acknowledged that the cost was not great. Meanness of a pathological nature was a marked feature of his character, which greatly altered in his analysis.

He recalled that there was another part of the dream, very vague, "having to do with loops on railway lines and going round the bend." He said he had messed up some appointments at work and didn't work very well. No wonder he thought he was going round the bend—became loopy—if he could not look after his analysis "watch."

In June I had to take a week off. Most primitive separation anxiety reappeared. He remembered dreams of two nights during the break. The first lot he thought was more positive, but the second one was a terrible nightmare. In the first dream he was in a desolate landscape in some exile. He was aware that his analyst had gone, but in the dream it meant that everything else was gone too, for instance, his place of work and his home. He felt desolate and anxious, but he also felt that somehow he could manage on what he had within himself. In the second dream that same night his little boy lost his milk tooth, but the new one was already there; so there was no gap, no pain. The little milk tooth was also like a drop of curdled milk. He thought those dreams meant that he could manage the weaning and the loss, even if it felt as if he had lost everything. I thought, however, that the end of the second dream contained a denial. There was no gap, no pain. But his dream later in the week, the patient said, was a terrible nightmare. In the first part he was conferring with a child oncologist, discussing a child who may have been mentally deficient or may have had a brain cancer. That reminded him of how he had always been convinced that he was mentally deficient and that his fear had left him in the last few years. But the second part of the dream was terrible. He was holding his baby son who was horribly mutilated. He was only a mouth. The patient could not feed him because he had no inside. He had no senses—no sight, no hearing, not even a sense of touch. The only way to save him and reunite him with himself was to give him to his mother. So it seemed that when I, the mother, went, all went with me, including most of himself. In this dream he came back to the most violent and primitive projective identification in which he put into me his sense organs, his insides, and left himself mentally deficient and unable to introject—he could not be fed. This dream recalled again severe mutilations to his mental apparatus which were prominent in the early years of his analysis and made him dread that he was mentally deficient or mad. The analysis of this was followed by a great deal of relief and improvement. In a later session he said that the paper which he thought he would never finish, to his surprise, was nearly done. He related a number of positive developments, including the fact that a mess he had made quarreling with the head of his department—one that made him anxious for several days and that he thought was irreparable—he quite easily cleared up as soon as he could admit his own mistake.

He had a dream, in which he was in a kind of mess, maybe a reference to the mess he made with the head. He went to the home of his friend, David. All the family was there. He was acutely aware that he was not a member of the family, but he was welcome. After a time he left David's home and felt very different—confident that he could clear up any difficulties. He associated that David was a very good leader and it was as though he himself, through staying in David's house, acquired this characteristic. He commented how different this dream was from many other dreams or fantasies in which he was invading David's house and ending by getting off, with him either excluding the wife or the wife excluding him. His dream was reminiscent of the one of the house on the hill which did not belong to him, but it included the whole family. It also emphasized that when he was not intrusive and possessive, then he felt welcome and free to choose what he wished to identify with. It signified a renewed withdrawal of intrusive projective identifications with sexual parents which underlay his perverse sexuality. But it also linked with his growing recognition that though I represented his parents, I was not even family. He was a visitor in my house. The analysis of that dream and associated thoughts eventually centered on a renewed mourning in relation to his father. Until he came to analysis he had not mourned his father at all after his death. He just became ill and even more withdrawn than he had been previously. In analysis he was able to mourn his father. But he told me now that he could never mourn his father completely so long as I was there because he had a father in me. It was only at the end of analysis that he could face that he really had no father.

In the last two weeks of analysis he was preoccupied with death. He always had a terror of death to the point of thinking that if there was death, then life was not worth living. Part of his avoidance of separateness was that separateness is the first intimation of death. He started a session saying, "I have two dreams about my death. In the first one

I learned that in 2017 the world will disappear. It wasn't through a catastrophe of nuclear explosions like in my previous dreams. It was just that the world will run out of fuel or life. The earth will get exhausted—or just entropy." He associated to the conversations with his father whom he often asked, "What will I be like in such and such a year?" And the father would tell him, "You will be grown up, or married, or old." But they never reached a point at which the father would say, "By then you will be dead." Neither had the courage to face it. His father died when he was 70. He himself will be 76 in 2017. Maybe, he said, he allowed himself the benefit of a new average life expectancy. But he seemed somewhat uneasy. In the second dream he was in bed and his wife with a child went up. He was left quite alone and resigned. He had let them go. There was an evolution in his thoughts about death. As he noted in his associations, he used to think of death as the result of destructiveness—atomic explosions. When we originally agreed on the date of termination, he had numerous dreams of war, atomic explosions, etc. In those dreams, death was a natural event; there was also an evolution as between the first and second dream. In the first dream he took the world with him. But in the second dream he was resigned to dying alone and allowing the others to live. The acceptance of the end of his analysis, birth, separateness, weaning, oedipal renunciation—all these were experiences allowing him to live as a separate individual, but they were also a preparation for death. I was to him also a representative of death. This was clear in the next session. He felt frightened of me and did not know why. Then it turned out that he was frightened because the date 2017 in the dream was a cheat and he knew it should have been 2010 and he did not tell me. (It had to do with a mistaken date in his driving license.) So he was still trying to cheat death, and cheating death and cheating me were the same thing.

What am I trying to say in this paper? Some may think that a patient who has such primitive fantasies and defenses and resists so much the ending is not ready to stop. That was what my patient often tried to make me think. I had few doubts that this decision was right. What are my criteria? Very broadly I could say that my criterion would be a sufficient move from the paranoid/schizoid position with predominance of splitting, projective identification, and fragmentation to the depressive position, with a better capacity to relate to internal and external objects. In the depressive position he has to face separateness, conflict, like in the dream of the session in which he hated me, and an integration of hatred. He has to bear loss and anxiety, like in the dream of the exile, and has to be able to internalize a good experience and learn from experience, like in his dream of the visit to David's house. Part of this working through is also an eventual acceptance of death— particularly at his age—just past mid-life.

The complete resolution of the depressive position is never achieved. It was the patient's fantasy that one day he would be free of fluctuations. In his mind that meant becoming like me—perfect. In fact, fluctuations remain throughout life. The assessment has to be about the severity and persistence of bad states of mind. In this patient the fact of ending reawakened the most primitive fantasies and defenses. But the situation was very different from that at the beginning of his analysis. The symptoms were minimal and the regressions were mostly contained in dreams, fantasies, and the sessions. He was not getting stuck at any point. He was very quick to perceive what was going on in him and could tolerate a lot of pain and anxiety. He would say, for instance, with great pain, "The moment your back is turned, I am up to my old tricks." Whereas in the past he had acted out in relationships and symptoms, he now could tolerate the knowledge of disturbing parts of himself. He had internalized sufficiently a good analytic experience to reestablish good internal objects and to internalize the psychoanalytic function of self-awareness. This is illustrated by one of his last dreams.

He dreamed of a gadget which had 5 U tubes. His association was to "you," meaning me—5 being 5 sessions. It also reminded him of a piece of equipment, a manometer that went wrong in Chernobyl. But it also reminded him of a gadget associated with his work as a very young man. A friend who was a hospital consultant was looking for ways to measure directly the blood pressure of vena cava in cases of suspected internal hemorrhage. He had an idea how it could be done and entrusted my patient with working out a suitable instrument, which he did very successfully; the very next day after the gadget was delivered by the workshop, it probably saved the life of a young man. Neither he nor the consultant ever published this result.

This last association was surprising. We were familiar with a pattern in which (before his analysis) he would become someone's blue-eyed boy and invariably failed to live up to his promise, abandoning or messing up any piece of research he was entrusted with. He never before had told me of this success. He had never made this result public to me or even to himself until now. I think that this U tube gadget is a manometer to warn him of possible disasters (Chernobyl) and is the analytic function he had internalized. And this is associated also with a rediscovery and reowning of constructive successful parts of himself.

He is the young man whose life has been saved—something he can now allow himself and me to know. It is published between us.

BIBLIOGRAPHY

KLEIN, M. (1961). *Narrative of a Child Analysis.* New York: Basic Books.
ROTHSTEIN, A., ed. (1985). *Models of the Mind.* New York: Int. Univ. Press.

DEVELOPMENT

The Development of Time Sense in Adolescence

CALVIN A. COLARUSSO, M.D.

THIS IS THE THIRD IN A SERIES OF PAPERS ABOUT TIME. IN IT I EXPLORE THE contributions of adolescence to a developmental line of time sense. As in the two preceding articles (Colarusso, 1979, 1987), my primary focus is the normal development of the subjective or intrapsychic sense of time, in contrast to objective or perceptual considerations. This developmental line is considered to be lifelong; the present focus on adolescence bridges the two earlier efforts about childhood and others yet to come on developmental aspects of time sense in adulthood. The data for my observations and hypotheses stem from analytic work with adolescents and young adults, and the discussion is divided into four sections: a brief recapitulation of time sense in childhood followed by similar considerations in early, middle, and late adolescence.

TIME SENSE IN CHILDHOOD

In my initial study of time sense from birth to object constancy (1979), I presented a developmental line of subjective time sense for the first three years of life. In earliest infancy, because of the undeveloped state of the ego, there is little organized time sense, little differentiation of past, present, and future or sense of duration. The existing precursors are homeostatic regulatory mechanisms and alternating sensations of frustration and gratification (Seaton, 1974) such as hunger and satiety as well as diurnal and physiological rhythms such as the heartbeat (Gifford, 1960) and breathing which convey kinesthetic sensations

Training and supervising analyst in child and adult psychoanalysis, and chairman of the Child Analytic Committee, San Diego Psychoanalytic Institute; clinical professor of psychiatry, University of California, San Diego; director, UCSD Child Psychiatry Fellowship Program.

basic to the differentiation of intervals (Fenichel, 1945). Almost immediately those innate factors become subsumed in the mother-child dialogue.

Through her power to control hunger and other painful sensations, the primary caretaker becomes *Mother Time,* the provider and manipulator of time. As the ego develops and activity supersedes passivity, the infant first imitates and later identifies with her, gradually internalizing the sense that time is in endless supply and can be controlled.

In the oral phase the rudiments of time sense are related to the mouth and stomach and the feeding relationship with mother; with the libidinal shift to the anal zone, the experience of time becomes centered in the lower end of the gastrointestinal tract, defecation, urination, and eventually toilet training. During the anal stage, time sense is related to anal libido and body products, the preoedipal mother and toilet training, the transitional object, the development of language, and the experience of object constancy. As his ego develops, the toddler gradually recognizes that he is dominated by mother (Brunswick, 1940) and through identification with her, he begins to experience a sense of control and domination over time which remains in the unconscious as a central component of time sense throughout life.

The transitional object (Winnicott, 1967) and mother during separation-individuation (Mahler, 1975) influence the evolving sense of time as the toddler interacts with them. Because the transitional object is controlled by the child through active mental and motoric action, he can manipulate the object itself and related fantasies, making them come and go and in the process manipulating past and present. The same temporal control is exercised over mother, particularly during the rapprochement phase, as the toddler repeatedly leaves her and returns.

Language development adds a conceptual dimension to time sense through the first use of terms like *soon, tomorrow, today, yesterday, now,* and *when.* Then the achievement of object constancy produces three important changes in the way in which the child experiences time: (1) time becomes more self-contained, internalized, and autonomous; (2) past, present, and future begin to have more continuity as psychic experience; and (3) the capacity for a sense of duration is established.

In "The Development of Time Sense: From Object Constancy to Adolescence" (1987), I traced the developmental line of subjective time sense through the oedipal phase and latency. I included Piaget's ideas on time in childhood: in the sensorimotor period (0 to 2 years) the child is restricted to mental responses that lead to direct interactions with the environment in the present; and during the period of concrete operations (2 to 11 years), which roughly encompasses the oedipal phase and latency, he is able to manipulate symbols that represent the environment and to involve them in complicated fantasies that include the past and the future as well as the present.

During the oedipal phase the oedipus complex and the infantile neurosis significantly alter the developing sense of time. External parental influence on time sense is primarily exerted through attitudes toward the child's impulses. This complements the internal constructions of *Father Time* and Mother Time. Meerloo (1948) conceived of Father Time as the oedipal castrator who controls time through his power over life and death. To this I added the notion of Father Time as the oedipal gratifier, the source of real and fantasized pleasure for his daughter in the midst of the positive oedipus complex, and for his son as the object of loving sexual feelings related to the negative oedipus complex. I suggested similar roles for Mother Time: influencing temporal attitudes as a gratifier or frustrator, as lover and competitor for her son or daughter. These internal constructions influence the affects associated with oedipal fantasies about past, present, and future and, particularly because of the phobic symptoms that are part of the infantile neurosis, feelings about day and night.

Latency is the first phase of development in which the child can actually tell time. Perhaps an even greater influence on subjective time sense during latency is the progressive internalization of moral demands and proscriptions in the superego. By refusing to allow oedipal fantasies into consciousness the superego renders the past vague, inaccessible, estranged, and increasingly unalterable. The future is now characterized by goals and expectations aspired to at the risk of feeling the superego's recriminations. Likewise the present is associated with an organized quality of deprivation and judgment. This attitude is experienced as coming from within in relation to such realistic demands as school performance and developing new skills and from without as exemplified by latency-age games which are replete with rules, penalties, and time restrictions.

TIME SENSE IN EARLY ADOLESCENCE

PUBERTY

Puberty may be defined as the wide-ranging physical, psychological, and social effects that surround the occurrence of the first menstrual period in the girl and the first ejaculation in the boy. Its effects on psychological development are well known, but its extremely powerful influence on the internal perception of time has not been previously described in detail. Puberty is actually a major demarcator of time sense, an indicator of significant psychobiological change which brings with it a sense of the passage of time, of movement from one developmental phase to another, and more specifically a sharp division of life into the physically/sexually immature past and the physically/sexually mature present.

Although young children continually redefine past and present as the result of conceptual and psychological development (for example, the internalization of moral demands in the superego and the ability to tell time, which occur during the oedipal phase and latency), earlier delineations pale in comparison to the forceful, inescapable effects of puberty. One 13-year-old, after announcing his first ejaculation, declared with considerable pride, "Today I am a man."

The connection between time and puberty is even more dramatic for girls because menstruation is described in temporal terms: the menstrual cycle, the monthly period, heavy days, light days, etc. Time becomes linked in these specifically adolescent ways with sexual functioning and procreation. Although it is not a central adolescent concern, he and she are now capable of replicating themselves, of achieving genetically a kind of immortality with which to conquer time and cheat death. Those issues will loom large indeed in the temporal perceptions of midlife.

During the oedipal phase the incest barrier was experienced by the child as created by time.

> Realizing that his or her body is an insurmountable handicap in his quest, the oedipal youngster longs for the time when he or she will be physically mature. If only the loved one would *wait* until that future time when the child has the adult sexual attributes and the strength to compete with and vanquish the oedipal competitor. According to Arlow (Panel, 1972), the incest barrier is an actual barrier imposed by time. The frustration is heightened by the simultaneous growing cognitive understanding of time. As these phase-specific cognitive and emotional factors become consciously and unconsciously elaborated and interrelated, time in the abstract is conceived of as a powerful frustrating force.
>
> In part, adolescent infatuation is a phase-specific attempt to win the oedipal love and master the narcissistic injury imposed by time. The new idealized love, a displaced personification of the oedipal object, will be possessed physically and emotionally, forever. At last physical immaturity and the barrier imposed by cruel time are conquered, hence the exhilaration and ecstasy of puppy love [Colarusso, 1987, p. 127].

So a major effect of puberty on subjective time sense is the destruction of a vital aspect of the incest barrier, namely, the child's youth and accompanying physical immaturity as compared to the adult's age and physical maturity. By removing the factor of physical immaturity from the equation, puberty gratifies long-standing oedipal wishes and makes the present exciting—and dangerous. Instead of being a powerful *frustrating* force, as it was during the oedipal phase, time now becomes the ultimate *gratifier*. The temporal pendulum has swung from one apex to the other. Equipped with a physically and sexually mature body, the teen-ager is now able to possess the oedipal object and vanquish the oedipal competitor.

Puberty is genetically programmed into the organism's biological clock. Both desired and dreaded, it can be anticipated, but its onset, progression, and effects cannot be controlled. This lack of control of the pace and speed of change is experienced narcissistically as highly injurious as well as exciting; the boy's mixed response to spontaneous erections and wet dreams and the girl's anxious response to the unpredictable onset and length of menstruation are examples. Further, puberty may occur "too early" or "too late." Roger, a 17-year-old junior in high school, had not yet experienced his adolescent growth spurt or first ejaculation. He felt inferior, a fish out of water, and was rejected by his peers. His life and our work centered around his temporal plea, "When am I going to grow up? When am I going to be ready to date girls?"

These attitudes stand in sharp contrast to those of a few years earlier during latency when physical and psychological growth were experienced as gradual and smooth, temporally and narcissistically gratifying. Nor do such biologically determined, time-sense-influencing experiences end with adolescence. After a brief respite in the 20s, the gradual onset of physical decline and retrogression, already in evidence in women in their 30s with regard to the running down of the biological clock for childbearing, becomes a dominant theme in midlife, a source of discomfort, disruption, and narcissistic injury, and again a central organizer of time sense.

TIME MODES IN EARLY ADOLESCENCE

Both Bonaparte and Erikson relate puberty to a unique adolescent experience, *time diffusion*. It occurs because "too many instincts are in ferment . . . powerful currents rise up from the organic depths of his being" (Bonaparte, 1940, p. 429) which keep the adolescent from experiencing an adult sense of time. In its milder forms, time diffusion "belongs to the psychopathology of everyday adolescence. It consists of a sense of great urgency and yet also of a loss of consideration for time as a dimension of living. The young person may feel simultaneously very young, and in fact baby-like, and old beyond rejuvenation" (Erikson, 1956, p. 82).

Puberty and time diffusion produce significant changes in the intrapsychic experience of the time modes of present, past, and future. These normative effects need to be differentiated clinically from the changes in temporal perception that are produced by trauma (Solnit, 1984; Terr, 1984).

The *present* is imbued with enormous sexual affect, with excitement, *urgency,* and anticipation. The experience of being flooded, overwhelmed, by sexual feeling at the moment of masturbatory climax diminishes the sense of duration—the connectedness of moment to moment—and contributes to the sense of time diffusion. The present is no longer predictable and measured, a vassal of the latency superego which counseled frustration and delay. It has become unpredictable, unreliable, corrupted, a sometimes willing captive of the insatiable id. A 14-year-old boy came to a late summer afternoon analytic session looking confused and exhausted. He had been alone most of the day "fighting with my penis, trying not to play with it. I lost . . . three times! Maybe I'll do better tomorrow; I've got no strength left today."

The early adolescent *future* is also transformed by puberty into a time of sexual *anticipation* and apprehension, self-definition and responsibility. Erikson (1956) noted that the adolescent experiences a decided disbelief in the possibility that the future may bring change and an equally powerful fear that it will. This ambivalence particularly influences the way in which future sense is experienced. Every adolescent "knows at least fleeting moments of being at odds with time itself. In its normal and transitory form, this new kind of mistrust quickly or gradually yields to outlooks permitting and demanding an intense investment in a future, or in a number of possible futures" (p. 97).

Increased knowledge and immersion in the peer group and physical maturity produce a strong sense of expectation that sexual involvement with another will occur soon. The anticipation is also coupled (partly defensively) with heightened frustration. Because of physical and psychological maturity, what is desired, longed for, is clearly recognized but still unattainable. As one 15-year-old put it, "I wish I was older. When I was a kid, I didn't know much about sex. I didn't know what I was missing, but now I do. On top of that I could *really* do it now. I'm ready, but I guess I'm still too young."

The presence of a physically mature body and the anticipation of adulthood also force the adolescent seriously to consider his place in the adult world in regard to career choice, leaving the family of origin, and finding new objects. This profound psychic reorganization is at the core of Loewald's (1962) concept of the "future ego" and Blos's (1962) ego ideal.

In early adolescence the *past* is disparaged as a time of physical and emotional immaturity which, because of the need to separate from the infantile objects—Blos's (1967) second individuation—begins to be experienced as distinct and remote. This initiates a process that reaches a peak in late adolescence (Seaton, 1974), resulting in all of childhood being defined as the past.

At the same time that the early childhood past is experienced consciously as fading, it is exerting a powerful unconscious influence on the adolescent process, particularly in regard to the reengagement of the preoedipal mother (Brunswick, 1940) and the return of the oedipus complex. The reworking of these basic developmental themes provides a potent link between past and present, rarely if ever experienced as intensively prior to this developmental stage.

To summarize, physical maturation creates a new, adult body with altered functions and appearance. This maturation process forces an intrapsychic reorganization of the way in which the three temporal modes are seen and experienced. Childhood's body and activity become synonymous with the past; the adolescent body, as it continues to mature and change, with the present; the emerging adult body, with the future. Clearly identified with the immature body, the past in particular is sharply distinguished from the present and the future.

MASTURBATION

This psychically organizing, psychobiological experience is related to time sense in adolescence as sucking and feeding were in infancy (Colarusso, 1979). Like hunger, the persistent periodic urge to masturbate has a significant effect on the way time is experienced. Rhythms and intervals become highly sexualized as the genital is stimulated slowly or rapidly in an attempt to control or heighten pleasure. Time itself is subjectively manipulated along with the genital in an attempt to speed up or delay the climax. Sexual differences are also conceptualized in temporal terms. The male is quickly aroused and rapidly spent after a climax; the female's response is more gradual in both regards. She experiences no interval of nonpleasure, no "refractory period" as he does, and is capable of serial climaxes. For both sexes the length of the climax has considerable significance. For the male a spatial aspect is involved as well, related to the quantity and projection of the ejaculate.

The three time modes are intimately involved in both aspects of masturbation: action and fantasy. During the act, sexual pleasure is experienced more intensely than ever before. The prospect of repeating the act in the near future is often contemplated during the present activity. Because of the weakening of the superego, long repressed wishes are thrust closer to consciousness. Thus the past, particularly the oedipal past, plays a more prominent role than was the case in latency. Past and the future are intimately combined in the present through the masturbatory fantasy which in the normal adolescent is an expression of (a) oedipal and preoedipal wishes; (b) fantasies and memories from the recent past about real and/or imagined sexual partners; and (c) plans for future experimentation and repetition.

MOTHER AND FATHER TIME

Through the oedipal phase of development, subjective time sense is closely related to interaction with the parents. With the introjection of the parents in the superego, Mother and Father Time become increasingly unconscious constructions (Colarusso, 1979, 1987). In adolescence, parents continue to have a powerful external influence on how their offspring use time. Battles over curfews and the "constructive" use of time are an integral part of the interaction because the adolescent often sees the parent as opposed to the use of time for instinctual gratification and independence.

While this real battle rages, significant change and conflict surround intrapsychic temporal representations. The upsurge of oedipal impulses resulting from puberty forces a deidealization and decathexis of parental introjects in both the ego and the superego, including the constructions Mother and Father Time. In part this explains the altercations over time between parent and adolescent and the weakening of the ego's ability to regulate the constructive, rational use of time. The process is part of the broader experience of unstable ego and superego functioning due to the decathexis of parental introjects. As this occurs, temporal regulation is increasingly transferred to the newly formed psychic structure, the ego ideal (Blos, 1962), and to the peer group.

The ego ideal becomes the repository of temporal attitudes of all kinds, but particularly those about the future. Time is increasingly related to preparations for adulthood, which for the most part involve delays in gratification: time for study and work and eventually for the responsible care of others. The sources for these attitudes are also the parents and other adults whose use of *most* of their time in the past and the present to work and care for others, particularly their children, adds a new dimension to parental influence on the continuous evolution of subjective time sense in the adolescent and young adult. The process of internalization of these parental attitudes is very similar to the interactions in infancy and childhood that led originally to the formation and elaboration of the constructs of Mother and Father Time.

The internal experience of frustration related to the emerging ego ideal sharply conflicts with wishes for immediate gratification resulting from the weakening of the superego and the transfer of time regulation to the peer group. Adolescent time is increasingly spent on "secret" activities with peers—on the telephone, at school, dances, parties, etc. For example, Jeff, a high school senior, spent an entire weekend at a friend's home (his parents were away) making out, drinking to the point of illness, and recuperating. Although only a few blocks from home, he managed with the help of his friends to keep his own parents in the dark. Jeff related the story with excitement and glee; for the moment the superego was overthrown, his parents deceived. He expressed his feelings in temporal terms. "It was the best time of my life. I've never had a better weekend. I can't wait to do it again. Well, maybe all of it but getting sick."

TIME SENSE IN MIDDLE ADOLESCENCE

INFATUATION AND LOVE

Adolescent infatuation alters both objective and subjective time sense. Interest in the objective world, in investing time and energy in obligations and responsibilities, is replaced by the desire to spend every possible moment with the beloved. This external shift mirrors an internal preoccupation which affects the way time is perceived and manipulated. Day and night are measured by the minutes or hours that must pass before the loved one is seen again. Powerful upsurges of feeling and fantasy temporarily diminish the capacity for duration—the ability to connect events in time—not unlike an electrical short circuit caused by a bolt of lightning. Time words become imbued with the affect of infatuation: "I can't wait to see you tonight," or "I'll always love you." The three temporal modes become vehicles for the expression of feelings about the all-consuming relationship. The present has meaning primarily in terms of whether the loved one is at hand or absent; the past is defined as the time of emptiness before he or she was discovered; the future, as a time of anticipated pleasure together.

Masturbation, with conscious fantasies about the love object, is consuming. Prior to and early in adolescence the fantasies were vague or absent because of their relationship to incestuous objects and the lack of intrapsychic separation; here in middle adolescence they are often elaborate. This new element adds specificity and intensity to the temporal aspects of masturbation described in the preceding section.

In addition to providing a framework in which to rework critical developmental issues from the past and present, adolescent infatuation also points the way to the future. "Does a loss of the sense of time, a return to the childhood illusion that for us time knows no bounds, form the very atmosphere that love breathes? When a man is expecting his beloved, when he holds her in his arms, covers her with kisses, or surrenders to the ecstasy of possessing her, are these not the supreme moments in which time, and the need to grow old, are really forgotten? That is why every lover swears eternal love" (Bonaparte, 1940, p. 434).

TIME MODES IN MIDADOLESCENCE

The Past and the Present

The past and the present begin to be viewed quite differently by the midadolescent. These new attitudes reflect the profound psychic reorganization that is taking place and foreshadow the emergence of more mature thinking in late adolescence.

"In his actual separateness and independence he experiences an intoxicating sense of triumph over his past and slowly becomes addicted to his state of apparent liberation" (Blos, 1967, p. 167). This shift is made possible by regression and the gradual decathexis of the infantile objects. "Regression under these auspices seeks not simply to reestablish the past but to reach the new, the future, via the detour along familiar pathways. A sentence by John Dewey comes to mind here. 'The present,' he says, 'is not just something which comes from the past. . . . It is what life is in leaving the past behind'" (Blos, 1967, p. 184).

Exhilaration is not the only feeling experienced in leaving the past. The process is also contaminated by the pain, suffering, and loss inevitably experienced during the decathexis from the infantile objects. Although he increasingly views the past as a time of physical and psychological limitation and immaturity, the midadolescent also begins to realize that the maturation process has burned bridges behind him. His dilemma is similar to that of the oedipal child, but in reverse. Just as physical immaturity eliminated the possibility that the young child could win the oedipal object, so does the presence of an adult body shatter any chance of again enjoying the simple, naïve, physical and psychological intimacy between parent and child that characterized the infantile past and childhood. The analyst's awareness of this process can have considerable clinical value, furthering an understanding of transference phenomena and providing a framework for interpretation (Rees, 1978).

The Future and the Ego Ideal

Piaget (1969) sees adolescence as a time of profound intellectual change which results in "the possibility of manipulating ideas in themselves . . . the adolescent is an individual who is capable (and this is where he reaches the level of the adult) of building or understanding ideal or abstract theories and concepts. The child does not build theories. . . . He is content to live in the present. . . . However, the adolescent is capable of projects for the future . . . of nonpresent interests, and of a passion for ideas, ideals or ideologies" (p. 105).

This cognitive development enhances and to a degree makes possible the equally significant change that is occurring simultaneously in the superego-ego ideal. The temporal developmental task is the integration in these evolving psychic structures of the ideal use of time in the adolescent and adult future. This is just one aspect of the extremely complex elaboration of all ideal expectations in regard to standards and behavior. Through identification, experience with parents and other significant objects in regard to their use or misuse of time is intermeshed with the representations of Mother and Father Time that were elaborated during preceding phases of development. Together these representations constitute the core around which the adolescent's expectations and use of time are formed. As with all other developmental progression, this change grows out of conflict. In midadolescence the keenly felt struggle between the urge to use time for instinctual gratification or for work, study, and other forms of instinctual delay is intensified because of the emergent readiness (physical and psychological) for sexual and other independent action.

Another temporal attitude that is integrated in the superego and the ego ideal stems from the adolescent's observation of the manner in which his parents and grandparents face middle and old age. Watching those two generations engage the developmental tasks of middle and late adulthood imprints on the evolving ego ideal a plan, an example, to be emulated or avoided, for living these future phases of life.

MOMENTS OF TRUTH: THE REVOLT AGAINST MOTHER AND FATHER TIME

As indicated, revolutionary intrapsychic work is occurring as real external battles are being fought over the use of time. As they separate and individuate healthy adolescents demand greater control of their time. In *The Race against Time* (1985), Robert Nemiroff and I, using an analogy to the point in the corrida when the matador is about to kill the bull, described those powerful organizing incidents, "moments of truth," in the lives of adolescents and parents when both come to realize that the adolescent is physically dominant, able to overpower the parent *for the first time in their relationship.* The issue precipitating the confrontation is often the control of time; the inevitable result, greater control of his own time by the adolescent.

Consider the following example, told with a mixture of pride and nostalgia by a young adult analytic patient:

> I was 16, I think. I stayed out late one night, 'til about 2 A.M., drinking and looking for girls. When I got home my dad was waiting for me; we were supposed to bale hay at 6 A.M. that morning. He just glared at me and said to be ready at 6 o'clock, like I couldn't because I'd stayed up late. I don't know why it happened then, I just knew I had to stand up to him. I stayed up all night, rattling around the house so he could hear me. I woke him up at 5:30, and we were in the field by 6:00. He tried all morning to break me. By 10 o'clock it was hot, and he was starting to wilt. I didn't say a word, I just kept baling. About noon he said he guessed he'd taught me enough of a lesson. I just looked at him and smiled. We both knew who had won. From then on I did what I wanted, when I wanted.

By late adolescence, when many individuals leave home to live on their own, their assumption of control over their own time is nearly complete. The need to be secretive about time, to hide its use from the parents, began in the oedipal phase and latency and reached a peak in early and middle adolescence. As the intrapsychic separation from Mother and Father Time continues and is complemented by moves out of the parental home, the late adolescent/young adult is finally able to control his time as he sees fit.

TIME SENSE IN LATE ADOLESCENCE

According to Seaton (1974), the late adolescent is "a present being assaulted and beckoned by an all-too-close past, assaulted and beckoned by an all-too-urgent future" (p. 796). The late adolescent's attempt to make sense of his temporal experience, which Seaton sees as quite distinct from earlier and later efforts, is called *psychotemporal adaptation.* This lifelong developmental process "requires that in infancy and early childhood there has been a continuity of experience and constancy of object, and that in late adolescence there has been adequate resolution of superego problems of guilt and ego problems of autonomy" (p. 796f.).

COMING TO TERMS WITH THE CHILDHOOD PAST

A major developmental task of late adolescence is a redefinition of the childhood past. For the first time, an entire phase of life must be consigned to the past. This process, which is gradual and painful, brings closure to an epoch of life and forces a further redefinition of aspects of psychic structure, particularly the superego and ego ideal, and the self. The late adolescent can no longer think of himself as a child and so must continue the comprehensive intrapsychic reorganization that will lead to his redefinition as a young adult.

This process is as inevitable as the onset of the oedipus complex in the 3-year-old or puberty in the young adolescent and is precipitated by relative mastery of the following adolescent developmental tasks:

1. Acceptance of a physically and sexually mature body, leading to the primacy of the genitals. One is no longer a child in appearance or action; the maturation process is irreversible.

2. Decathexis from the infantile objects. The second individuation brings a recognition that the dependent position of childhood, the *need* of parental figures for emotional and physical survival, is no longer tenable.

3. Engagement in adult work or the preparation for a career. The realistic and psychological need to work, to use time in adult ways, continually sharpens the distinction between the childhood past and the late adolescent present.

In those instances in which the late adolescent physically leaves home, the intrapsychic process is stimulated by the constant equations *home = childhood past* and *present location = late adolescent present,* be it the workplace, the military, or college.

These psychotemporal struggles often occupy a central position in clinical work and are readily available for study. Blos (1968) noted that "adolescent development can be carried forward only if the adolescent ego succeeds in establishing a historical continuity within its realm. . . . One adolescent spoke for many in saying that one cannot have a future without having a past" (p. 256f.).

Even as the past emerges as a distinct, sharply defined block, it must be connected to the present and still ill-defined future. Because the past is experienced with such clarity and force, a special effort is required to facilitate the ongoing process of duration, i.e., continuation in time. A similar situation existed at the beginning of latency when the newly crystallized superego precipitated a repression of infantile experience and produced a sense of estrangement from the oedipal and preoedipal past.

Aided by cognitive maturation (Piaget, 1969), this adolescent recognition that the childhood past can slip away, never to be retrieved, leads to a consideration that the present and indeed the future are limited as well. The cognitive and emotional understanding of temporal loss is the contribution of adolescence to the emerging acceptance of time limitation and personal death which becomes a psychic reality in young adulthood and a central, normative preoccupation in midlife (Colarusso and Nemiroff, 1981).

The consolidation of the childhood past is a significant intrapsychic force propelling the late adolescent to transform other important aspects of the self that are vital to healthy functioning in young adulthood.[1] Among the most important is the establishment of an adult work identity. The late adolescent is in the process of crossing a bridge from one phase of life to another. As a young adult his super-ego-ego ideal will expect him to work, to hold a job, to make money, to postpone pleasure, and, in temporal terms, *to give up much of his freedom to use time as he wishes* (for childhood and adolescent play) and willingly relinquish control to a boss or self-imposed structure. In many occupations and training situations, such as medical school, blocks of time that before were set aside for play, such as evenings, nights, and weekends, are invaded and coopted by the demands of work.

HEALTHY FUTURE ADAPTATION: THE SUPEREGO AND THE EGO IDEAL

Restructuring of the childhood past is a prerequisite for consideration of the future by the late adolescent and young adult. As the childhood past recedes, accompanied by the loss of gratifying, protective dependency upon the infantile objects, the late adolescent is propelled into highly cathected conscious and unconscious considerations of the future. This work continues into the 20s and is one of the temporal bridges between the developmental stages of adolescence and young adulthood.

Seaton (1974) sums up the absorption of the late adolescent in this temporal psychic restructuring:

> The issue of the future is a cardinal one for the college student as it has not previously been in his psychological development and as it is not again until the late middle life with the approach of the end of life. In the late adolescent, the future is dominatingly active as a reality in the

1. As Arlow (1986) pointed out, the self is a time-bound concept, one in which "identity implies that a self . . . is the same entity at different points in time, no matter what changes or transformations may have taken place in the intervening years" (p. 521).

objective present . . . he should be particularly concerned with the choices that will determine his career, marriage, life style, the person that he is and will become. . . . Through this very concern, the past dims in significance and time seems to begin anew. . . . The more the late adolescent is focused on where he is going, the less he is immediately concerned with where he comes from, providing things back there have been dealt with sufficiently well [p. 807].

If the superego and ego ideal are basically sound and the adolescent structuring and restructuring of both fairly well completed, these psychic agencies are in a position to steer the ego's attention to an integrative consideration of the future. If the late adolescent superego-ego ideal views the childhood past as a time of physical and intellectual accomplishment, sexual maturation and integration leading to genital primacy, and transformation of object ties to infantile objects and peers, then he is unlikely to experience wrenching shame or guilt from these transformed psychic agencies, although he may experience considerable realistic anxiety about the future, a feeling based on the recognition that no matter how well prepared he may be, no matter how intact, he cannot know what the future holds. In the next five to ten young adult years he will make vital decisions about work, spouse, children, a place to live, which will determine the course of his adult life.

The following clinical material from the last year of the analysis of a 21-year-old college senior illustrates these developmental issues and themes, stated so well by Seaton (1974): "It is the ego ideal, and later the superego, that states the future, that is the inner mental configuration of the kind of person the individual aspires to become, feels he must and should become, and it is that inner future against which he measures his inner present" (p. 804).

As he entered the second semester of his senior year of college, Jack became increasingly preoccupied with the adult future. He *had* to find a job. Where? When? He joked that he was being slapped in the face by reality and was ready to retire. "I've sponged off my parents long enough. I'll just jump to 65 and let Uncle Sam take care of me." Such regressive thoughts were momentary and did not diminish his relentless preoccupation with the future. Money, *his* money, which he would earn would *first* have to go for rent, car insurance, health insurance, and *then* for "booze, dates, and cars." Grades were viewed strictly in terms of the effect they would have on getting a job, no longer as a means of gaining the approval of parents or teachers. The normative conflict between urges to progress and to regress was always evident: "If I flunked, I could have another year in this loafer's paradise, but then I'd have to go through this again next year. It's not worth it." Women were still viewed in terms of "how many and how fast," but the young adult quest for intimacy was beginning to emerge: "I better start changing that tune. I'll probably meet my wife in the next five years." Jack summed up his temporal preoccupations nicely, "I'm living too much in the future. I'm not paying enough attention to now."

As an aside, this patient also demonstrated an interesting change in attitude toward day and night. "I can do it now [have sex] in the daytime. I mean I sometimes prefer it. Watching myself and my girl is fun." I understood this change, which did not grow out of a focused analytic consideration of the issue, as evidence of normal psychotemporal developmental progression. During the oedipal phase the dark was a time to be feared because of the phobias and nightmares associated with the infantile neurosis (Colarusso, 1987). During early and middle adolescence the night became a time of instinctual gratification, for dating and drinking. The dark hid the unintegrated sexual actions from others, including parents and partners, and the self. Late adolescence and young adult mastery of these childhood attitudes may sometimes be found in the individual's comfort, or lack thereof, with engaging in sexual activity in daylight.

Conversely, infantile temporal attitudes may be hidden in inhibitions and rituals. One 35-year-old analytic patient casually described, without any sense of embarrassment or recognition of inhibition, his preintercourse ritual of closing the blinds, turning out the lights, and climbing under the covers. My inquiry into the need for such rituals opened the door to a series of voyeuristic-exhibitionistic conflicts that had within them infantile temporal attitudes toward nighttime and the dark.

PROBLEMATIC FUTURE ADAPTATION

While preoccupation with the future can be a consuming mental activity for the healthier, well-functioning adolescent, it may be actively avoided by the disturbed or culturally deprived individual with few prospects. If the childhood past was a time of major disappointment or deprivation and the present is a time of disorganization and disarray, then a significant psychotemporal regression may occur in the form of either abandonment of realistic and intrapsychic preparation for the future or a pseudomature posturing, acting as though an adult integration had already occurred.

Nineteen and in his senior year of high school, Brad did everything possible to avoid thinking about his future. Ungainly in appearance, at the bottom of his class, ignored by his peers, he had achieved little success in his life. Significant perceptual problems, a parental divorce, and constant criticism from his father were among the factors contributing to his dismal position. Unlike Jack, who constantly brought his thoughts about the future into our analytic work, Brad volunteered nothing, ignoring the fact that graduation and a significant transition of some kind were just months away. When I broached the subject, he either ignored my comment or angrily told me to mind my own business. As these defensive postures were interpreted, we were able from time to time to speak about the future. "I don't know what I'm going to do tomorrow, let alone next year. Maybe I'll go to college or join the army." Although he was deeply interested in women, everyone he asked out refused him. This made a consideration of the future exquisitely painful. "Four girls have turned me down for the senior prom. I don't think I'll ever find somebody to marry. Too bad. I think I'd be a good husband and father, better than my father was."

While Brad handled his insurmountable feelings about his past and future through denial and withdrawal, other troubled late adolescents go to the opposite extreme and rush headlong into impulsive activity. The temporal issue for them, indeed for all late adolescents, is the relationship between impulse gratification and future sense. "If the gratification of an impulse can be relegated to the future, its discharge is more easily delayed and its energy susceptible to displacement or transformation. But if this gratification is incompatible with the future self, or if indeed there is no conviction of future, postponement may be very much more difficult. The fading of futurity in reality weakens aspects of superego function and prompts living as if there were no tomorrow" (Seaton, 1974, p. 809).

Joan was an exceptionally bright, promiscuous college senior. Although her promiscuity was multidetermined, she related her behavior to future concerns. "Why shouldn't I? Everyone, including me, sees me as an ugly egghead who'll end up unmarried, teaching philosophy at some jerkwater college. At least now I've got a pretty nice body and guys want me. In a few years when I get old, nobody will. And don't try and tell me the right guy for me will come along. I can't believe that anymore. I'm going to take what I can get *now*."

PSYCHOTEMPORAL ADAPTATION VERSUS SUSPENSION

The pressures of dealing with the past and future, real and imagined, impinge on the way the late adolescent present is viewed and lived. I am suggesting a normative intrapsychic conflict between the work of psychotemporal adaptation and attempts to suspend this painful process. This psychic suspension may take various forms and serve adaptive or regressive aims. During it "the adolescent defers both the issue and the consequences of attempting to measure up to his ego ideal. While the suspension of psychic time may serve the same developmental purposes as Erikson's (1968) psychosocial moratorium, which also removes the pressure of time, the two are not the same. The suspension of psychic time is a self-granted delay, a defensive maneuver, which is not sanctioned by the society, even though it may be in part culturally determined, whereas the psychosocial moratorium is an institutionalized delay which grants time for development through an extension of the adolescent phase, a sanctioned deferring of adult commitments" (Settlage, 1972, p. 83).

The normative aspects of temporal suspension are related to the uncertainty of facing the young adult future and the decathexis of the childhood past. By living impulsively in the present, seemingly disconnected from the past and the future, the late adolescent delays the process of decathexis from infantile objects and the reorganization of the past to include all of childhood and avoids facing the demands of the superego and the ego ideal in regard to ongoing preparations for the future. The process may range from a momentary daydream or a night of drunkenness to a semester of indolence. All are episodes of revolt against a superego weakened by the withdrawal of parental cathexis and still in the process of psychic reorganization.

While Jack experienced only occasional moments of temporal suspension and Brad was overwhelmed by them, Hal's experience held elements of Erikson's psychosocial moratorium. He had not become pubertal until the end of his junior year in high school and was now in the second semester of his senior year. After months of therapeutic consideration, he decided on the following. "I don't think I'm going anywhere after graduation. I think I need some more time at home. I haven't dated yet, and I don't know what I want to do with my life. I'm starting to look like a man, but I'm not there yet. If I grow as much [physically and mentally] in the next year as I have in the last one, I'll be ready."

BIBLIOGRAPHY

Arlow, J. A. (1986). Psychoanalysis and time. *J. Amer. Psychoanal. Assn.*, 34:507–528.
Blos, P. (1962). *On Adolescence.* New York: Free Press.

———— (1967). The second individuation process of adolescence. *Psychoanal. Study Child,* 22:162–187.

———— (1968). Character formation in adolescence. *Psychoanal. Study Child,* 23:245–263.

BONAPARTE, M. (1940). Time and the unconscious. *Int. J. Psychoanal.,* 21:427–468.

BRUNSWICK, R. M. (1940). The pre-oedipal phase of the libido development. *Psychoanal. Q.,* 9:293–319.

COLARUSSO, C. A. (1979). The development of time sense: from birth to object constancy. *Int. J. Psychoanal.,* 60:243–251.

———— (1987). The development of time sense: from object constancy to adolescence. *J. Amer. Psychoanal. Assn.,* 35:119–144.

———— & NEMIROFF, R. A. (1981). *Adult Development.* New York: Plenum.

ERIKSON, E. H. (1956). The problem of ego identity. *J. Amer. Psychoanal. Assn.,* 4:56–121.

———— (1968). *Identity, Youth and Crisis.* New York: Norton.

FENICHEL, O. (1945). *The Psychoanalytic Theory of Neurosis.* New York: Norton.

GIFFORD, S. (1960). Sleep, time and the early ego. *J. Amer. Psychoanal. Assn.,* 8:5–42.

LOEWALD, H. W. (1962). Superego and time. *Int. J. Psychoanal.,* 43:264–268.

MAHLER, M. S. (1975). Symbiosis and individuation. *Psychoanal. Study Child,* 29:89–106.

MEERLOO, J. A. (1948). Father time. *Psychoanal. Q.,* 22:587–608.

NEMIROFF, R. A. & COLARUSSO, C. A. (1985). *The Race against Time.* New York: Plenum.

PANEL (1972). On the experience of time. J. S. Kafka, reporter. *J. Amer. Psychoanal. Assn.,* 20:650–667.

PIAGET, J. (1969). The intellectual development of the adolescent. In *The Psychology of Adolescence,* ed. A. H. Esman. New York: Int. Univ. Press, 1975, pp. 104–108.

REES, K. (1978). The child's understanding of his past. *Psychoanal. Study Child,* 33:237–260.

SEATON, P. H. (1974). The psychotemporal adaptation of late adolescence. *J. Amer. Psychoanal. Assn.,* 22:795–819.

SETTLAGE, C. F. (1972). Cultural values and the superego in late adolescence. *Psychoanal. Study Child,* 27:74–92.

SOLNIT, A. J. (1984). Preparing. *Psychoanal. Study Child,* 39:613–632.

TERR, L. C. (1984). Time and trauma. *Psychoanal. Study Child,* 39:633–665.

WINNICOTT, D. W. (1967). Adolescent process and the need for personal confrontation. *Pediatrics,* 44:752–756.

The Terminability of Adolescence and Psychoanalysis

H. SHMUEL ERLICH, PH.D.

THE SIGNIFICANCE OF TERMINATION—AS A PHASE, A STATE, AND A SPECIAL treatment goal—in every analysis is by now very well established. So is the crucial importance of the management of termination in adolescent analyses as well as the links between termination and the normative processes undergone by the adolescent. These include the central position and multiple implications of the need to separate from early and current, preoedipal and postoedipal parental objects, as well as aspects of body and self that are ridden with infantile significance and attachment value. There is also no doubt whatsoever that the issue of termination in adolescent analysis—the "whether," "when," "how," and "what" would constitute a "good" or "bad" termination as well as the role played by varying ways of relating to and handling termination—that all of these are indeed valid and difficult clinical and technical problems, demanding our attention and consideration.

It seems to me, however, that by addressing ourselves so exclusively to these issues we are possibly falling short of some of the implications contained in Freud's monumental paper (1937). Freud chose as his title the terminability of psychoanalysis, and not its termination, with all the difference in nuance and implication contained in this wording. Although he touched briefly on some technical aspects of termination, he was not concerned, in the main, with questions of "when" and "how." Indeed, his focus and attention were shifted and transformed through the clinical facts of termination to the much wider vistas of the values, ideals, and evaluation contained in *terminability* ("the quality of . . . being terminable, i.e., capable of being or liable to be termi-

Senior lecturer in clinical psychology, Hebrew University of Jerusalem; member, Israel Psychoanalytic Association; faculty, Israel Institute of Psychoanalysis.

An earlier version of this paper was presented at the Yale University Child Study Center, July 1987.

nated" (Oxford English Dictionary). He was especially concerned, it seems, with the implications of the dialectics of the facts and questions of termination and terminability for human growth and functioning. In so doing, Freud achieved a transposition in which technical issues (e.g., the length and duration of an analysis, the immunity for living it promises to impart in an "average expectable traumatogenic environment," etc.), issues that were themselves born out of theoretical advancements, now became the stuff and generators of new and further theorizing and exploration or, as Freud coyly referred to it, "phantasying" (1937, p. 225).

In addressing himself to the theme of terminability, Freud soon adopts a parental posture. In fact, he begins to sound in many ways like the parent of an adolescent. Are not the very questions he raises variants, perhaps at some points even duplicates, of the questions asked by a normally concerned or anxious parent about his soon-to-be-graduated or confirmed offspring: How well have I prepared him for the "real" life that awaits him out there? Have I truly done enough in order to "immunize" him against future strife, trauma, and conflict? Do I regard him as strong enough—constitutionally, psychologically, spiritually? Where and how do I think he stands in comparison to others, to the "norm"?

We would rightly regard such soul-searchings as the parent's working through of his or her overreactions to the offspring's termination of childhood. We understand this process as the parent's moral and psychological accounting for himself and the quality of his parenting as he is about to part from what has been such a central constituent of his ego, self representation, and self ideal for a good part of his adult life. Would it not be correct to regard the analyst as undergoing a similar or parallel process, in which he becomes concerned, involved, or immersed, as the case may be, with the terminability of his patient's analysis? It seems to me that his consideration of the terminability of an analysis makes the analyst assume a role and stance analogous indeed in many ways to that of the parent of an adolescent.

Termination and imminent loss may be regarded in this context as giving rise to the reverse of the usual mourning process. Rather than the incurred loss inaugurating the work of mourning (Freud, 1917), in both terminations under discussion—of normal adolescence and of psychoanalysis—it is the commencement of what I would propose to define as an "anticipatory mourning process." This anticipatory mourning process signals, precedes, and paves the way for the anticipated loss and separation. It finds expression in the worried questioning and efforts at evaluating the past and glimpsing the future that are so characteristic of both the parent of the adolescent and of the analyst at a particular phase of the analysis. I suggest that this process of anticipatory mourning makes the issue of terminability an indicator or signal as well as a necessary, though not sufficient, condition for termination to take place.

When in the course of a normally conducted analysis such self-searching questions and reflections concerning a patient's capacity for terminability begin to abound in the analyst's mind, they should not be dismissed too readily as exaggerated concern and loss of analytic neutrality. Naturally, they may represent such digressions, or, if not properly handled, lead into them. But properly noted and treated, such a concerned reflectiveness on the part of the analyst, when focused, constitutes a powerful signal. It would indicate that the issue of *terminability* has arisen in the analysis, and the analysand is grappling with issues that are both newly adolescent as well as revivals of particular infantile and childhood dilemmas, most likely centered around separation-individuation, now appearing in its second edition (Blos, 1967) and proper adolescent size and weight. From this point on, realistic questions of *termination* may well become focused issues for analysis— to be fought over, analyzed, used by the patient to provoke, to attempt to gain premature independence, or to prolong closeness, fusion, and merger, all of which would be worked through, resolved, and integrated.

CLINICAL ILLUSTRATION

I would like to present a clinical illustration which may serve to highlight some of these thoughts. Miss A., just short of 17 years of age, was referred to me in a fairly advanced and difficult state of anorexia nervosa, following two years of unsuccessful psychotherapy. A tall and strikingly beautiful girl in spite of her emaciation, she was ready and eager to begin work. The daughter of a wealthy businessman, she had lost her mother several years ago, after an early mastectomy followed by a prolonged struggle with cancer. Both the extent of family pathology and her own preference for isolation as a defense were evident in a history of incestuous play with her older siblings, which was related fairly straightforwardly and laconically. From an early age she was heavily involved in a series of promiscuous sexual relationships with both her contemporaries and older male figures. A very bright and verbal person, she was almost incapable of any emotional display or relatedness. Instead, she was extremely pragmatic in her instrumental and "realistic" approach to the therapeutic task, accepting in a surface manner the need to understand matters so as to "exorcise" her difficulties. That this was not a mere figure of speech became evident when a host of obsessive-compulsive mechanisms carried over from childhood—rituals, magical thinking, and practices—was related. Most significant among them, as well as by far the most dramatic, were "her demons," who governed her every moment cruelly and mercilessly, and who had to be pacified and obeyed. At best they could be evaded on occasion, to be followed by bouts of immense anxiety about what would happen when they discovered her treachery and disloyalty.

Our work soon centered around two issues. The first concerned her relationship with her father, which had a strong oedipal cast. She feared and loved him, revered and worshipped his power and knowledge, and saw herself as his half-willing, half-protesting, abject victim. At the same time, she was always deviously nurturing and extending her own power and hold over him, in reality seemingly manipulating him at her will. This struggle with the powerful and dominating father came through vividly in voyeuristic fantasies, primal scene contents, real or imagined, in the present, and dreams of overt rape by the father or the analyst, as the transference quickly intensified.

The second issue was an apparently more deeply set experiential difficulty. It was apparent early on, and capable of interpretation, that she felt phony and false, acting her own experience instead of feeling and living it. This was reflected in her choice of defenses—isolation, intellectualization, and to some extent reaction formation. More importantly, it meant that she was effectively cut off from her own experiencing self, in a way she came to term her "disability," implying a kind of crippledness. This disturbance of self experience was by far the more serious problem. It manifested itself in the transference in her flat insistence, both willfully and affectlessly, on having little or no feelings toward her analyst, with the exception of erotized fantasies and, later on, infrequent but strong outbursts of anger and negative affect, occasioned mainly by her running into some of the rules of the analytic situation.

Her more intense transference feelings were thus experienced and interpreted along oedipal lines—as powerful wishes to gain and be dominated by the father-analyst sexually, to possess the penis and incorporate it, etc. Despite such undercurrents of powerful drama and passion, and despite the fact that the interpretation of these elements proceeded in a systematic manner, followed by relief and considerable improvement, it nevertheless produced no amelioration in the area of self experience. She continued to experience herself, throughout her 4½ years of analysis, peculiarly estranged from both herself and the analyst. This was a fairly subtle experience, which came through in two essential ways: she often felt false, phony, and cut off in some way she could not fully describe or comprehend; and she consistently managed not to include the analyst in her real-life experiences, insisting that, after all, what counted in analysis was her inner life, and she could not see what difference it made if she related boring details about what she did in her real life. This was not only a way of emasculating the analyst, or of expressing her resistance. After a great deal of work it turned out to be the missing link to what had been most conspicuously absent in the analysis until then, namely, her relationship with her mother.

She had not been able to mourn her mother's death. For a long time, the mother that she could summon and remember in the analysis was the crippled, sickly emaciated, and dying mother. Very gradually and tentatively, another part of mother was introduced: a mother who was not ill yet, who appeared to be powerful and capable of opposing and even dominating the father, and who omnisciently knew everything in and about Miss A., but contained and withheld this knowledge in a way that only further underscored her power and potency, now also buttressed by Miss A.'s feelings of guilt. It became exceedingly important to the young girl to earn her mother's love and respect by being meticulously clean, not permitting herself the slightest deviance or messiness. Her loving and libidinal strivings for this mother, the need to contain these powerful feelings as against the wish to exhibit and demonstrate them, as well as the self-punitive aspects of being a messy little girl who, at the same time, could not allow herself the enjoyment of her messy impulses and wishes—all these came through vividly in her memory of a repetitive childhood pattern: she runs home from school, so excited by the thought that she will be home and with mother at last, that when she reaches the front door, she wets her pants. She feels terribly humiliated, unable to look mother in the face. Mother sees her, knows she has wet herself, but does not say anything. This vivid interaction had almost the quality of a screen memory. It certainly contained many of the elements that accounted for this girl's tremendous need for control and messing (vomiting), sexualizing her tender and loving feelings and being incapable of sublimating them, and her tremendous efforts to contain reality and withhold it from me, in effect identifying with the mother who does not acknowledge reality, while projecting onto the analyst the little girl left alone with her inner world.

The emergence of these (and other) memories not only reenlivened the mother and her relationship with Miss A., formerly repressed and denied. It enabled her to reexperience her longings for mother, and very tenuously begin to entertain feelings of loss, of missing someone she loved and longing for that person. Such feelings had previously been either totally denied, or severely isolated, or powerfully sexualized and transformed, to be acted out in an oedipallike fashion. Her inability to tolerate absence and therefore to long for the loved object (Green, 1975) were experienced in the transference as a potent need to idealize the object (father, analyst) while devaluating another representation of it.

As these issues were crystallized and worked through, significant changes followed. Her anorectic symptoms all disappeared, the last to go being the ritualized and compulsive need to vomit and resort to diarrhetics. The need for sexual acting out, as well as for idealization of the father and the analyst, greatly diminished. She was able, for the first time, to arrange and take part in a family Seder on Passover, and on that occasion (as well as a number of others) to miss and feel real sadness and grief over her mother's absence from the festive gathering. She also developed a solid relationship with a young man who was both tender and understanding, as well as firm and supportive of her various needs and difficulties.

I now come to the issue of termination and terminability in this analysis. It is still very important to describe the setting in the analysis and her real life which now served as background for this.

Several important developments took place during the last year of analysis. The most important by far was her deepening relationship with her boyfriend, which was marked by a growing ability to share and discuss her thoughts and feelings, and especially her difficulties, with him, and find mutuality, understanding, and support in this relationship. Despite this great step forward, the conflicted nature of the gain was apparent in her reluctance to allow the relationship to become real within the analysis. Thus, for instance, it took a long time before she was able to mention her friend's name or other identifying facts about him in the analysis. She made the decision to get married and carried it out, again almost as if it were despite the analysis. She let the analyst know the date of her wedding almost as an aside, and insisted on coming for analysis on that day, though she did cancel the following two appointments. Splitting her life's reality off from her analytic reality, and denying the interrelatedness of the two, served to protect her from losing her inner hold and control, as she felt she would if she allowed them gradually to merge. She could thus carry on with her deep need to feel in control, combating and setting back the more childish, weak, and regressive parts of herself (Erlich, 1986).

She brought up her wish to terminate in the context of reality changes in her life that were due to her husband's studies, which meant moving to another city in the following year. She also felt that her attainments in analysis had been considerable; although she did not think that there were no issues left to work on, perhaps enough was enough. Her manner, approach, and attitude were reasonable, mature, and realistic, and yet she experienced some difficulty in deciding on a termination date. After considerable work on the possible meanings of this difficulty, a termination date was suggested by her. Again there were clear signs of difficulty, since her first choice of a date was so arbitrary, without consulting a calendar, that it turned out to be an impossible date. This too overcome, a date was set, again quite arbitrarily, for three months hence.

Although termination soon became a frequently featured theme in Miss A.'s thoughts, dreams, and fantasies, a feeling of dryness started to characterize the analytic sessions. Miss A. was, as usual, cooperative and reasonably productive, but something was missing, yet she did not know what it was. She complained that she could not see the point or need for such a lengthy period of termination. At some point, she spoke of her fear of needing and missing the analyst after she would leave. She said she experienced this as a threat to her relationship with her husband, on the one hand, while on the other it felt like some void inside her, which she wanted the analyst to fill. She had a dream in which the analyst appeared in a miniaturized version. I felt a sudden alarm: it became crystal clear to me that Miss A. would not leave the analysis without becoming pregnant. In this way she would gratify her long-standing wish for a baby (penis) from the father, and fulfill her powerful fantasies of being orally impregnated by him. At the same time, she would not have to experience separation and loss in relation to me and the analysis, taking us, as it were, along with her. It immediately occurred to me that, while the oral pregnancy wishes had been interpreted and worked through, clearly this had not been done sufficiently, and Miss A. was letting me know, perhaps aggressively and cynically, that the analysis had not really changed anything at all as far as she was concerned.

These thoughts and feelings were a source for considerable self-reproach, but I also was led to think through and understand more of what she was communicating, and what might be taking place intrapsychically and in the transference. I realized that another source for my dilemma was that she was also asking what would be my response to her wishes to realize her womanhood and femininity in her new relationship. The most serious problem, however, was in her inability to experience the longings occasioned by the impending separation and loss, which revived not only her still unresolved difficulties in adequately mourning her mother, but primarily the tremendous difficulty in *being* with her mother, which were now so preeminent in the dryness she experienced in the analysis. Overriding and overshadowing all of these, however, was the concern that I now experienced because of her imminent departure. What would be the meaning of her actually becoming pregnant in order to leave the analysis? Could I let her go, if that turned out to be the case? Should she be warned about this possibility of acting out her unconscious wish and need? Would this not be regarded by her as my rejection of her womanhood—and worse, as a sign of my lack of faith in her taking an independent course?

The above is but a brief, highly condensed version of the thoughts, feelings, and dilemmas I experienced when I realized with such force and clarity the unconscious meaning of Miss A.'s communication. What should be stressed, however, is the role played in these reflections by the background processes of termination and issues of terminability. Termination was, in this case, met and negotiated at the various levels of reality considerations, rational expedience, as well as real treatment gains, improvement, and a number of signs of greatly increased maturity. It would probably be a brash and somewhat unwise statement to make, but I felt that on every account and test this girl had traveled a very long and positive way in analysis, and if she wished to terminate, her decision could not really be faulted. In fact, it even seemed to me that the existence of areas in which I was well aware of some remaining problems was a further indication of the general adequacy of the decision to terminate: it seemed to accord with the general feeling of Freud's (1937) position of "letting sleeping dogs lie," and to indicate a more realistic, rather than idealized, resolution, and hence a better basis for termination. I still believe that, at that level, all of these considerations hold true.

What was missing in this termination process was precisely the questions of terminability referred to above. It was as if I had been willing to let her go without going through this, probably painful and difficult, process. My sudden rise of anxiety and apprehension ushered in all of these questions in an equally uncomfortable way, but probably again in an unavoidable fashion. It had also served to make me aware of more subtle forms of this process of anticipatory mourning, which had indeed been present earlier but had not received their full or due attention. The realization of Miss A.'s powerful wish to leave the analysis while pregnant brought all my concerns about her, and especially the anticipatory questions about her future being in the world of reality, into sharp and sudden focus. Working through these questions and concerns, with all the issues stirred up, could then serve the process of termination and become integrated into it.

I will only briefly summarize the subsequent course. In fact, I chose cautiously to interpret Miss A.'s wish to leave the analysis pregnant. She dealt with it positively but very briefly. Several weeks later, and about 6 weeks before termination, she announced that she was indeed pregnant. This raised all the above issues forcefully again, this time introducing them squarely into the analysis. She insisted on seeing her pregnancy as a positive expression of her progress and an assertion of her own self. Gradually, however, it turned into the poignant issue of her still considerable difficulty in *being* with the analyst and in the analysis, and allowing a fuller, less controlled, and willfully governed experiential participation. A freer mode of participation presented her with two threats: stirring up the powerful conflict around sexual submission to the father-analyst, with all the desires, incestuous prohibitions, and humiliation entailed; and stressing her difficulty in *being* relatedness, experienced in relation to both mother and analyst, and the subsequent inability to experience absence, loss, and longing for the object. This difficulty in *being* relatedness made her unable to enjoy and admiringly incorporate and assimilate the father-analyst's strength and potency on the one hand, while on the other it did not allow her to relinquish the mother-analyst without a defensive recourse to doing relatedness (i.e., becoming pregnant). This sequence may be regarded as the recapitulation of her childhood solution for achieving separation from her mother, and as the genetic bedrock of her characterological defenses. This solution also represented the essential aspects of her evolving self system.

As many of these issues became clearer, termination took place, and Miss. A. parted from the analysis with an air of indecision and uncertainty. She realized some of the issues raised and acted out by her pregnancy, which incidentally she would not terminate, but felt silly and unsure about changing her decision regarding termination. She felt it was artificial, but should nevertheless be maintained. She contacted me with some mild symptoms of anxiety and depression one month later, expressing her wish to resume analysis in order to work through these issues, which we did for a limited duration.

DISCUSSION

Considering termination from a psychoanalytic point of view immediately suggests at least three conceptual levels of discourse: (1) the idealization of termination; (2) the issue of resistance; and (3) the role and place of death. I would like to examine briefly the significance of each in the context of adolescent psychoanalysis, and in light of the distinction between termination and terminability.

1. Termination of an analysis forces both analyst and patient to deal with the degree of preparedness, the extensiveness of change, and the overall effectiveness of all participants—analyst, patient, and analysis as a therapeutic method. This raises issues of standards and criteria on the one hand, and of perfection and perfectability on the other. Probably the most overriding and elusive among the idealized end states invoked is the concept of mental health.

"Whatever one's theoretical attitude to the question may be, the *termination* of an analysis is . . . a *practical* matter" (Freud, 1937, p. 249; my italics). In this statement Freud summarizes the issue as it pertains to what he referred to as the "natural end" of an analysis. It is instructive that this assertion comes immediately after another one, which pertains to the *ideal* proposed for the analyst himself, to seek analysis every five years. In this connection Freud states: "This would mean . . . that not only the therapeutic analysis of patients but his own analysis would change from a *terminable into an interminable* task" (p. 249; my italics).

It is quite clear that in referring to the natural end of an analysis, Freud uses the term "termination" and stresses its pragmatic aspects. In making a recommendation as to an ideal to be pursued by the analyst himself, as a developing and evolving professional, Freud switches to the terminology of "terminability." This distinction between the pragmatic and idealized aspects of termination can be elaborated in terms of my proposed division of the experiential realm of psychoanalysis between two experiential modalities: one of *being* and the other of *doing,* each possessing its own lawfulness, giving rise to parallel and complementary mental processes, or experiential universes (Erlich and Blatt, 1985). In the present context, the issues and considerations of *termination* are the pragmatic, technical and clinical ones that pertain to the *doing* modality. The questions we meet with in this dimension are those of when, how, how much, if-then-what, and the like. The issues and considerations that arise in the *being* dimension, on the other hand, are those qualitative questions met when we tackle the problem of *terminability:* what will he or she be like, or what life will be for him or her? *Being* considerations necessarily and intrinsically partake of ideals and idealization. It is the ego ideal and its component ideals that provide the guidelines, values, and aspirations which guide our efforts to assess questions of essence, of quality of being, and characterize any attempt to assess the basics of life and *being*, like Growth, Development, and Health. One is tempted to characterize the problems of termination as superego considerations of correctness, while terminability pertains to issues of goodness of quality, as measured against the yardstick of the ego ideal.

The adolescent, both in and out of analysis, is constantly faced with precisely these two issues and the problem of finding his own unique integration of them. He must find a rewarding pattern and outlet for his *doing* experience, in which his ego will make use of specific social roles and functions (Erikson, 1968), including and incorporating his drives, impulses, wishes, and their satisfaction. And he must simultaneously become capable of experiencing his own self as an integrative, continuous existence possessing value, quality, and worthwhileness, as the new and ongoing expression of his *being* experience. It is the integration of both modalities and attendant experiences that finds expression in identity formation (Erikson, 1956; Erlich and Blatt, 1985).

The analyst in the course of an adolescent analysis is faced with an overwhelming array of pressing issues and difficulties, including sexual and aggressive conflicts and impulses, shifting characterological and defensive constellations, tendencies toward or gross displays of acting-out behavior, and acute transference and countertransference challenges. He has his hands full, so to speak, and for the longest time is concerned with keeping his head above the stormy waters. I believe the clinical material presented supports my contention that there comes a point in the course of an adolescent analysis when the analyst finds himself preoccupied, concerned, or even worried about some variety of the question of what his patient is going to be like. He is then concerned with the idealized aspects of his patient's image as a person and an adult. His own hopes and aspirations for the patient may then become a decisive factor in the terminability of the analysis and the success of its eventual outcome.

2. Termination is a fulcrum of resistance, in that it serves as a source, target, and modality for it. It stirs up anxieties and conflicts related to object relations and ego, self and ego-ideal definition, function, and status, while simultaneously acting as a lightning rod for these problem areas. As a content area, as well as a potential course of action, termination may be used to act out and resist further change and understanding. For the adolescent, so keen upon gaining distance from childish dependency and so fearful of its abrogation, this is a particularly heavy burden. For him, the very fact or situation of being in treatment is often a concrete reminder of his dependence and immaturity, without

the ameliorating distance that cushions this experience for the adult patient and allows him to experience it symbolically. This makes it more difficult to draw the line between the adolescent's recourse to termination as an area of conflict and resistance and his legitimate need to leave treatment as part of his growing up. I believe that, at least to some extent, the distinction between termination and terminability may be of help in this. In the first place, the analyst's own concern with the *terminability* of the analysis may serve as an indicator of readiness, providing a watershed between the relative weight of purely resistant issues and legitimate growth needs. Secondly, the contents and style of the analysand will provide a clue, if understood in terms of the relative dominance of *being* vs. *doing* in his associations and communication. The analyst will then have to assess the extent of lack of resolution and need for further work *in either* track, and make a determination about the analysand's position on *both* termination and terminability.

3. Termination, in the aforesaid, was considered chiefly as an active process. There is yet another side to it, however, more apparent when regarded from a passive vantage point. Here it signifies the state or experience of being terminated, ended or finished. Terminability, in this context, would mean one's potential finiteness, or the end of one's being, and hence death. Interminability, on the other hand, would suggest one's endless or infinite being, hence one's immortality. In either case, it brings to the fore the perennial struggle with inertia and death.

Adolescence is probably the most conspicuous and crucially important developmental stage in which this aspect of terminability is hammered out. Although the struggle with death, mortality, and finiteness is present throughout and accompanies all of development, the centrality as well as the reverberations of its resolution in adolescence deserve to be claimed as definitive and formative in several critical ways.

The major link is to the area of narcissism, in which we may distinguish two important subareas: First, the fiber and strength of the ego ideal, now receiving its final cast, depends vitally on the capacity for incorporating in it the notion of its own terminability. This notion, available truly for the first time due to cognitive developments, puts to the test the extent to which the adolescent is capable of relinquishing narcissistic investments in himself, including childish grandiosity and omnipotence, in favor of integrating more libidinal and realistic object relations. In the terms I have employed above, the question is to what extent he can integrate his *being* relatedness with currently pressing *doing* relatedness.

A second, related and equally important issue is the degree to which the adolescent can forego and separate himself from the pull of early merger experiences and *being* object relations, characterized by fusion and oneness, and his longings for them. Such longings, coupled with cognitive mishandling of death as an infinite (interminable) state, rather than a finite one, greatly increase the risk of turning to suicide as a solution during adolescence (Erlich, 1978).

Lastly, I would like to assert the existence of a linkage between the resolution of these aspects of terminability as it relates to death and three cardinal disorders of adolescence: asceticism, anorexia nervosa, and schizophrenia. It is clearly beyond the scope of this paper, but in each we may discern the struggle with the issue of terminability of the self, and the ego's incapacity for achieving a good enough integration of its *being* and *doing* experiential domains, of its aspirations to interminability with its adaptive responsivity to termination.

BIBLIOGRAPHY

Blos, P. (1967). The second individuation process of adolescence. *Psychoanal. Study Child,* 22:162–186.

_____ (1980). The life cycle as indicated by the nature of the transference in the psychoanalysis of adolescents. *Int. J. Psychoanal.,* 61:145–151.

Erikson, E. H. (1956). The concept of ego identity. *J. Amer. Psychoanal. Assn.,* 4:56–121.

_____ (1968). *Identity, Youth, and Crisis.* New York: Norton.

Erlich, H. S. (1978). Adolescent suicide. *Psychoanal. Study Child,* 33:261–277.

_____ (1986). Denial in adolescence. *Psychoanal. Study Child,* 41:315–336.

_____ & Blatt, S. J. (1985). Narcissism and object love. *Psychoanal. Study Child,* 40:57–79.

Freud, S. (1917). Mourning and melancholia. *S.E.,* 14:237–260.

_____ (1937). Analysis terminable and interminable. *S.E.,* 23:209–253.

Green, A. (1975). The analyst, symbolization and absence in the analytic setting. *Int. J. Psychoanal.,* 56:1–22.

Inner Themes and Outer Behaviors in Early Childhood Development

A Longitudinal Study

HENRY N. MASSIE, M.D., ABBOT BRONSTEIN, Ph.D., JOSEPH AFTERMAN, M.D., and B. KAY CAMPBELL, Ph.D.

SEVERAL YEARS AGO WE BEGAN A PROSPECTIVE LONGITUDINAL STUDY OF key elements of early personality development. The study sought especially to describe how a mother's personality is reflected in her behavior with her infant, and how these maternal behaviors become transfigured (if they do at all) into the child's own emerging character.

Our study focuses on how the mother responds to her infant in moments of mild to moderate stress. The responses that we look at are specific actions: How does she gaze, vocalize, touch, hold, show affect, and maintain closeness to the upset baby? Equally important to these external responses is what lies beneath the surface: Why does the mother minister the way she does? Her overt responses are instinctive

Henry Massie is director, child psychiatry residency training, St. Mary's Hospital, San Francisco; Abbot Bronstein is director of psychology, psychiatric services, Children's Hospital, San Francisco; Joseph Afterman is on the faculty of St. Mary's Hospital, and supervising analyst, San Francisco Psychoanalytic Institute; and Kay Campbell is in private practice in Southfield, Michigan.

We are very grateful to several colleagues who have instrumentally assisted in different stages of the project: Martha Harris, Toni Heineman, Naomi Low, Debra Melman, Riva Nelson, Candace Pierce, Judith Rosenthal, Gabrielle Thomson, Ruth Weatherford, Eleanor Willemsen, and Myla Young. In addition, we are most appreciative of the generous support of the Morris Stulsaft Foundation, Children's Hospital, and St. Mary's Hospital, San Francisco.

as well as shaped by conscious beliefs she has about raising children; these in turn are further shaped by ideas of which she has little or no conscious awareness. These instinctive responses and conscious and unconscious action-determining ideas may be said to compose the mother's personality, which influences her capacities to mother her infant.

We simultaneously examined the child's response to the mother. How did the baby gaze, vocalize, touch, hold on, show expression, and seek closeness or distance? The baby's response is mediated by his degree of distress and also by his temperament and perhaps genetic or neurodevelopmental proclivity toward a certain modality, such as a preference for visual rather than tactile receptivity. As a precis of our findings, we observed that very quickly mother and infant create a style of interaction with each other which the baby gradually transforms into his own particular style of adjusting to events in his life. Likewise, as time passes and language arrives in the second and third years, the child's mode of adaptation gains meaning for him; this becomes his own belief system, which like his mother's will have its own unconscious dimensions.

The concepts we are describing did not spring full grown into research methodology. Rather, this study evolved from our own earlier research (Massie, 1975; Massie and Rosenthal, 1984) in which a series of family-made home movies of the infancies of autistic and pre-psychotic children demonstrated disturbances in mother-infant interaction prior to the actual appearance of symptoms of illness toward the end of the first year and early in the second year. More specifically, we had found how the above-mentioned parameters of mother-infant gaze, vocalizing, touching, holding, affect, and proximity were different in index families prior to actual illness compared to control families. Therefore, we designed the current study to examine prospectively these same behaviors and interactions over time.

This research exists in the broader context of the work of Bowlby (1969) and Ainsworth et al. (1978), who also draw our attention to the phenomena of attachment; and in the context of Tinbergen's (1973, 1983) ethological descriptions of newborn animals imprinting upon contact with their mothers. Likewise, Winnicott's discussions (1965) of the maternal holding environment—literally how the mother holds the child and figuratively how well she is tuned into her baby—emphasize its critical importance in the child's healthy ego development. Also providing the theoretical backdrop for the current study have been psychoanalytic researchers such as Bibring et al. (1961), whose focus has been the maternal psychology of pregnancy; Brody and Axelrad

(1970), who amplify the meaning of nurturance; the Yale group (Ritvo and Solnit, 1953), and Escalona (1968), who have followed groups of children over time with in-depth descriptions of their developing personality; and Anna Freud (1965) and Mahler et al. (1975), who have outlined the psychic structure of early childhood.

In addition, our work has developed in the more recent climate of microkinesic and frame-by-frame analyses of mother-infant interaction pioneered by Brazelton et al. (1974), who glimpsed the origins of reciprocity; Tronick et al. (1978), who recognized the infant's response to entrapment between contradictory maternal messages in face-to-face interaction; and Stern (1971), who visualized the structure of mother-infant play.

However, in reviewing the preexisting research, we recognized that in the late 1970s important theoretical and methodological links between mother and child had not yet been addressed. Research that had carefully studied the mother's personality, or alternatively childhood personality, had not had available the newer microkinesic methodologies to document mother-infant behavior. On the other hand, microkinesic investigators were not doing long-term follow-up to assess the developmental significance of their documentation of dyadic behavior in infancy. Finally, we were able to find no studies that attempted to link maternal personality to microanalysis of mother-infant behavior and to subsequent child personality. Our own project therefore designed a methodology to redress these gaps in existing research.

Within the general plan of looking at maternal personality, mother-infant behavior, and childhood personality, we distilled three questions:

1. Do particular patterns of behavior characterize very early mother-infant interaction and become embedded in the mother-infant relationship so that they continue throughout childhood? Alternatively, if they exist in early life, do they become obsolete, merely leaving behind fossilized traces in the child's personality?

2. Are there areas of unconscious conflict and adaptation within the mother that she transmits to the child by means of her behavior?

3. Can we discern patterns of behavior in the infant and toddler that prefigure early character, defenses, and even psychopathology if that is to be the youngster's fate?

We selected for our study a group of 20 primapara couples in the third trimester of pregnancy. We filmed, tested, and observed mother and child (and at times the fathers) intensely for 3 years. Then when the children reached early grammar school, we made contact with the families again to do our follow-up study.

METHODOLOGY

Twenty primapara families volunteered, having been told that we were interested in "studying how families grow together." The mother-infant unit was to be the focus of the study, we explained, even though we were also interested in the father, but would not study him as closely as the mother and child. Approximately three-quarters of the families responded to an announcement of the project in the obstetrics clinic of Children's Hospital in San Francisco. The other families were referred by the parents' psychotherapists who recognized that parental psychopathology placed the to-be-born child at risk and felt that the project might offer additional support for these families. Thus the study population was anticipated from the outset to include both normally functioning and impaired families. All socioeconomic and several ethnic groups are represented, although the population is largely white and middle class.

Research operations included maternal psychological testing, developmental assessment of the child, an adaptation of the Ainsworth Strange Situation (1978), sequential family interviews, and structured and unstructured films at home and during well-baby clinic visits for the first 3 years, and a follow-up in grade school. The Massie-Campbell Scale of Mother-Infant Attachment Indicators During Stress (ADS scale, 1983) was used by "blind" raters to document mother-child reciprocal affect, touching, vocalizing, gazing, holding, and proximity in the films in the 3 minutes immediately *after* the pediatric well-baby examinations during infancy. We term this the "reunion episode" when mother comforts the child, who in turn responds.

FINDINGS

The wealth of data in the study defies easy reporting and requires much selecting and ordering. We found that in many ways the data teach us more when we describe them as a series of case studies, actually biographies in the process of becoming as our children grow. Therefore, in this section we will present two families in depth—one in which the child appears at emotional risk from infancy and the other in which there was no obvious risk to the child. For each family in the study there emerged one or two major themes or organizing myths particular to the family, which captured their adaptational style and major conflicts, around which we were able to structure their biography.[1]

1. Ziegler and Musliner (1977) also recognized the salience of persistent family themes in their pilot 15-year follow-up of Sander's (1964) mother-infant interaction data.

FAMILY 1. CHARLES T.

For the T. family the theme was the parents' conflict over having a dependent child versus a grown child, which they expressed through their physical closeness to their child. From Charles's birth the mother had a clear idea that she wanted her boy to grow up strong and independent. This led her consciously to deemphasize aspects of holding and nurturing of the baby. The father was closely aligned with the mother in this attitude, although mother was the primary caretaker. A second theme derived from the main one. The parents, both successful business people, felt that their primary task was to teach the child rules of proper behavior, to "help Charles become a good citizen," and to provide him a good education. With these fundamentals the parents believed their son would have the necessary tools to succeed.

Mrs. T. was one of 8 children in a hard-working family where there was little opportunity for relaxation and close contact with the parents. The mother had pushed herself through college and successfully into a business career where she exercised considerable authority over people. There was no past psychiatric history. She and her husband volunteered for the project because they thought they would learn from it how to be especially effective parents. During pregnancy, Mrs. T. was depressed. She remembered her own rigorous childhood, especially her feeling that her parents had been too hard on her. There was a longing and sense of identification with an aunt with whom she had spent much time and upon whom she wanted to model herself. Nonetheless she respected her parents' control and concern for her, especially since she felt she had not been a very likable child—stubborn, ungainly, and unattractive. Mrs. T. planned to breast-feed her baby as her own mother had done with her children. "My mother breast-fed us and we were healthy." Mrs. T. did not enjoy the physical discomforts of pregnancy and planned this to be her only child.

When Charles was born his mother cared for him until she returned to work full time at 5 months and placed him in daycare with a neighborhood woman. At 1 year the child had his first separation from his mother. His parents sent him out-of-town with his maternal aunt for two weeks for their summer vacation, a pattern that has become a yearly tradition. Developmental milestones have been normal, but noteworthy was mother's unsuccessful attempt to toilet train the boy just prior to his stay with his aunt at 1 year.

Mother's Psychological Testing. Mrs. T.'s Draw-a-Mother-and-Child projective test in the third trimester of pregnancy (fig. 1, p. 222) and her Rorschach when Charles was 1 year showed depression and anger indicative of interferences during the oral phase of development.

Mother-Infant Films and Interviews. In the very first film at 9 days of life, we noted that during breast-feeding the mother docked the child's mouth to her nipple without cradling his body to hers. The infant lay in the bed nursing like a small boat tethered to a buoy. The baby was not lying on the mother or in her arms, and there was little skin-to-skin contact. Mother and child were in close proximity but not fully physically close in terms of body contact. "You're so greedy," the mother said to the child, while at the same time affectionately gazing at his face while he nursed.

We interpreted this behavior as indicative of the mother's love for her child admixed with her sense of personal neediness, which she had denied and compensated for with her strength and independence. It made her wary of allowing her newborn too great a dependence on her. She appeared to fear allowing herself to regress into what Mahler et al. (1975) have termed a mutual symbiosis with the baby, for it might make them both weak and vulnerable. Furthermore, we wondered if the mother doubted her ability to meet her baby's voracious needs.

This pattern continued throughout the 18-month filming period. Physical closeness in the form of chest-chest holding was not prominent. By contrast, the mother emphasized distal interaction via talking to and looking at Charles. In addition, the films captured other moments: the mother prematurely pushing Charles's gross physical accomplishments such as crawling; the mother engaging in vigorous teasing play which embodied her specific ambivalence over physical intimacy and in which she loomed close to his face and retreated. When Charles was overstimulated at moments such as these, he frequently broke eye contact, which he then reestablished moments later. Mother and child did get in touch with each other, so to speak, but the mother seemed not to prefer what we can term low-intensity moments of alert inactivity, mutual quietness, nurturance, and dependency.

A scene at 6 months, 14 days was especially instructive. It repeated the kind of interaction seen earlier and continued the main theme of this couple, while it also illustrated another aspect of development. Mother and child were seated face to face at home. The mother with an animated face drew the child into a game of pat-a-cake. Charles became excited, got closer to mother, salivated,[2] then tried to put both his

2. Charles's actions highlight how salivation is a "psychosomatic" response to excitement in the pure or nonpathologic sense of the word. That is, in a moment of heightened interaction with the mother, the 6-month-old seemed to fuse his and mother's hand into a "joint mother-child hand" and incorporate it by taking it into his mouth. At a moment like this, Charles's pleasurable arousal had little use for ego boundaries. We have also observed similar psychosomatic responses at moments of strong dysphoric

and mother's hands in his mouth. But mother pulled away at this point. Charles became irritable, then cried, then slowly quieted. Thus there had been no consummation of the excitement between mother and child.

Finally, at the very end of the scene Charles was still irritable after his mother had cut off his excitement. He then reached for his mother, who did pick him up and drew him close, but after an instant she turned him outward and wiped his nose. In this manner her concern with cleanliness reasserted itself over quiet closeness. However, these instances in which the mother did not join in excitement or turned Charles away were not the full "preverbal double bind" we observed at this age in a child who subsequently developed autism. There the mother physically turned away from the child at the height of mother-child play rather than just dampen the excitement (Massie, 1975). Mrs. T.'s need to dampen the excitement (stopping the full seductive eye, voice, kinesthetic pat-a-cake stimulation) is a direct outgrowth of her own stern upbringing which instilled in her the sense of deprivation that was evident on her psychological tests.

Similarly, throughout Charles's infancy we observed in other micro-interactions how the mother cracked the symbiosis between her and the baby. Unaware of this microprocess, the mother cracks the symbiosis to ward off her sense of Charles's voraciousness and her anger. More obviously, she breaks the connection with her child when she and her husband vacation away from Charles beginning at 1 year. At those times she is aware that she is trying to train the boy toward independence. Thus the mother nurtures, but within limits. She fosters appetitive behavior and cuts it off. It was these momentary and larger events during the first year of Charles's life that made us feel he was at psychological risk. Affectively both mother and child were somber, though as Charles gained ability for locomotion as an early toddler his face brightened considerably. Therapeutically, supportive and educational comments to the mother did not alter her behavior.

The Attachment During Stress Scale (ADS scale) ratings generally supported clinical impressions. Charles and/or his mother were often below the median for all families in the study for holding, affect, vocalizing, and proximity. They were typically at the median for touching. Only for gazing did mother and infant reach or exceed the median consistently in the first 18 months.

---

interaction. At these moments, Charles and other infants may put their own hand in their mouth and ruminate upon it or flap their hand or fist in a transient stereotypy (Massie et al., 1983).

At 24 and 36 months, the Block Task took place in which the dyad was asked to make something with blocks. Both times the mother controlled Charles's play and the fantasy. For example, at 2 years Charles wanted to build a train. He put some blocks together, pushed them, and went, "Choo-choo." Mother, out of synchrony with her boy's developing fantasy life, derailed it by not seeing what he was doing and instead suggested that they build a house. The task became relatively rigidly structured rather than an opportunity for discovery. Toward the end of the Block Task at 2 years, and especially at 3 years, Charles was better able to focus on building with blocks. However, there was a sense that he was concentrating compliantly and playing parallel to his mother rather than playing with her or being allowed to take the lead himself.

Follow-up at 7 Years. After 36 months we said good-bye to the family for 4 years, wondering how they would look when we greeted them again and what surprises they held in store for us. Two unexpected things were apparent when we met the family at 7 years. The first was that the mother no longer showed signs of depression. She was fashionably, colorfully dressed, lively and assertive. The second was that a baby brother had been born 3 years earlier, a welcome addition to the family where the parents had once planned to have but one child. Now in a much happier frame of mind than 7 years earlier, the mother no longer held grudges about her childhood. "Love was just understood in our family. Even though my parents weren't openly affectionate, weekends were fun loving." In comparison to their childhood families, Charles's parents felt they were more openly affectionate and cuddling in their home. They spoke of themselves as satisfied.

Nonetheless, the 7-year follow-up did not augur well for Charles. In the *family session,* Charles was restless and reserved. Though not disruptive, he tended to tease. In response the parents quickly enforced good behavior. The father especially was stern and somber. When sitting, Charles was next to his mother. He drifted away when not asked by his parents to stay with them. In this manner, the theme of closeness but not close continued from infancy. When the interviewer asked about family modes of discipline, both parents acknowledged their concern about their son's stubbornness which the mother likened to her own stubborn streak. There were only rare spankings, but when Charles had gone through a period of masturbation between 2 and 3 years, the parents had told him that it was bad and had yelled at him, "You have to behave yourself."

Charles's *classroom teacher's report* gave us the gloomy news that in his competitive school he was not keeping up and required considerable one-to-one instruction to which he would respond. The teacher characterized him as sweet but lacking in self-esteem, unhappy, something of a crybaby, and disruptive in a silly way to get attention, sometimes by wandering and procrastinating. This made him the occasional butt of jokes. There had been some petty stealing from other kids. If the class were going on an outing, Charles was one of the children who liked to hold the teacher's hand.

In the *unstructured play interview,* Charles was subdued if not inhibited, finally choosing airplanes and missiles to play with. A theme of resignation crept into his voice when he spoke of toys at home that would not work. His attention then drifted to other toys. He gave an overall sense that there were things he wanted to accomplish or try, ways in which he wanted to show the interviewer how competent he was, but something kept interfering.

The filmed mother-child *Block Task at 7 years* showed the mother bright and no longer suffering an angry depression. Now in the supportive presence of his mother, Charles flourished, as his teacher had also noted him to do when she was able to give him personal encouragement. The mother sat on the floor with the blocks between her legs and Charles opposite, so that the blocks were between them. At first, the mother took the initiative—similar to the 2- and 3-year Block Tasks—and suggested they build a castle. Quickly the boy became intensely involved and active in building. The mother smiled, pleased, and allowed Charles to build upward while she worked on the foundation. They enjoyed working together, cooperatively taking turns. Her assistance was happily facilitating, and overall they shared a castle fantasy successfully, although when Charles placed a car in the castle, the mother was unwilling to allow this truly fantastic inconsistency and said, "They didn't have cars then."

The last follow-up data were Charles's *psychological testing.* The WISC-R showed him to have an overall IQ of 110 with performance considerably higher than verbal. Fund of knowledge was low, while comprehension was adequate. His ability for abstract reasoning was weak. Projective drawings of a boy and a girl (fig. 2) suggested the possibility of mild interferences secondary to neurodevelopmental maturational imbalances because of distortions in the size, shape, and organization of the drawings; while the absent hands, short limbs, and large feet on the boy suggested concerns with controlling aggressive impulses. Drawings of females were peculiar in having spear and swordlike phallic protuberances in their dress which gave them a more powerful quality than males. There was a general lack of bodily detail and differentiation for a 7-year-old, an immaturity that recalled the

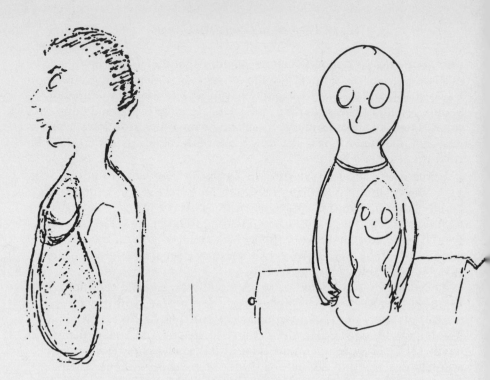

Figure 1. Drawings of Family 1 (Charles). Mrs. T.'s Draw-a-Mother-and-Child in third trimester and at 12 months

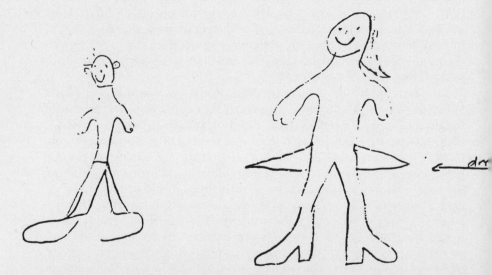

Figure 2. Drawings of Family 1 (Charles). Charles at 7 years: Draw-a-Person and Draw-a-Person-of-the-Opposite-Sex

mother's ghostlike mother and child drawings during the third trimester of pregnancy and at 1 year (fig. 1). The emptiness and lack of development in the mother's drawings and in the child's at 7 years expressed depression.

On the Rorschach, Charles's specific anxieties were fears of separation and fears of body damage, especially castration anxiety.

In sum, at 7 years Charles is a child whose development has been affected by his parents' earlier ambivalence over nurturing him. Their ambivalence stems in part from their childhood experiences remembered as not having enough access to their own parents as children. Charles is thus reproducing disturbances that have been handed down from generation to generation. He is somewhat sad and frustrated with attempting to suppress his longings. To get attention, he overreaches and becomes confused or makes himself helpless. His character, though still in formation, tends to include a reliance on action, a making himself vulnerable to elicit attention, stubbornness, and withholding. Paradoxically, the conscious major goal of Charles's parents, which was to raise a highly independent and assertive boy, seems to be handicapped now by an underlying separation anxiety that Charles experiences.

FAMILY 2. MOLLY P.

In contrast to family 1, there were few concerns during gestation and infancy that the child was at risk. The parents self-referred themselves to the project when they saw the notice in the obstetrics clinic. Both junior college graduates in their late 20s, the father was a career army officer with a permanent assignment in the San Francisco computer center. The mother worked as a secretary. Both parents came from intact middle-income families with two siblings, and recalled their childhoods with contentment. Both parents wanted 2 to 3 children. Pregnancy was happy for the couple who anticipated a rewarding relationship with their child.

The P. family lived close to the grandparents with whom they did not feel conflicts and whom they planned to use for support in child rearing. The mother expected to be a full-time housewife. The parents were congenial yet serious in demeanor, eager to participate in the project. A handsome, plainly dressed couple, they were at the same time somewhat stiff and deferential. Their attentiveness to the project team's instructions was also consistent with a strong respect for authority. Although there was a traditional division of roles, and the mother said that the father would have to make final decisions, she was at the same time more active in making day-to-day family arrangements. As with family 1, the parents were in agreement about their ideas about child rearing.

The theme which characterized this family made its appearance in the initial weeks of Molly's life. It was the parents' conflict between their desire to indulge and gratify their child and their fear of spoiling her. They feared that discipline might be hurtful—a concern never voiced by Charles's parents—yet disliked the idea of being ruled by a bratty child. Thus where closeness and independence were the central concerns in family 1, setting limits and controlling aggression came to the fore in the P. family, although it was only gradually over the years that we fully recognized their centrality to the emotional life of the family, in contrast to Charles's family where the motif of parental closeness to the child was quickly apparent.

The P. family's concern with limit setting versus gratification appeared in the first weeks when the parents were somewhat perplexed because Molly cried more and had more difficulty establishing nighttime sleep than they had expected. They made more use of the project team than other families for help with problems such as these and voiced guilt that they were not paying us for our time. They were uncertain how long to let the child cry, not wanting to be punitive while also wanting to allow the baby the chance to develop the capacity to soothe herself. The child's night wakefulness continued well into the third year, so that periodically the parents would wonder with us whether to bring Molly into their own bed to comfort her, which they did on occasion.

Mother's Psychological Testing. The Draw-a-Mother-and-Child during pregnancy and at 1 year (fig. 3, p. 230) and the Rorschach at 1 year both indicated a self-assured woman who nonetheless felt conflicted over aggressive and sexual impulses, tended to control affects, and avoided percepts that disturbed her.

Mother-Infant Films and Interviews. This was a happy family which took great pleasure in their child. Molly's developmental milestones through toddlerhood were normal except for the nighttime wakefulness, slightly slow walking at 16 months, and also a mild speech delay. Her language comprehension and vocabulary were always normal, but articulation was slow, for which she received therapy in her fourth year. Molly was at home with her mother until she went to nursery school without difficulty in her fourth year. The mother also breastfed Molly into her third year. Bottle-feedings had also been provided from the fifth month. Molly was toilet trained at 2 years.

Separating from their child was anxiety-provoking for these very conscientious parents. Their first evening away from Molly was at 6 months after they had discussed it with the project team. Their first overnight separation did not occur until the second year, and there have been no separations longer than a weekend to this date. The family did not use babysitters, but relied mostly on the maternal grandmother in whose house Molly slept in her own mother's childhood bed.

Like her parents, Molly was a serious baby who was very attentive to people and events about her. As she gained locomotion toward the end of her first year, she became bubbly and animated. Still she remained self-contained and well behaved. This quality appeared to be in response to the mother's emphasizing politeness, which she enforced by regularly citing rules, telling Molly to be a "good girl," and giving her time-outs alone in her room. The mother's concern with good behavior was a reflection of her previously noted fear and sense of danger in being dominated by an unruly child. Likewise we felt that it grew out of the mother's need for Molly to reflect well upon her as an extension of herself. The father was less active in controlling his daughter. Molly herself was able to say no, but her rebellions were brief and tantrums rare.

The mother's intense investment in her daughter made her very tied to her child, as indicated also by the long breast-feeding. "I wanted her always to have my milk . . . but wish she could also have taken it from a bottle. . . . I wish I could have gone away for an hour or two in the first 6 months, but I couldn't." When the mother pondered weaning at 2½ years, she said, "If I stopped nursing, Molly would scream; but if I take a firm stand, we would get through it . . . she looks for you to weaken. That's the only area where I do weaken."

For her part Molly was equally tied to the mother. For example, for several weeks beginning at 3 months, Molly had an early phase of stranger anxiety in which she cried whenever her mother left the room. This stranger anxiety included the father, so that he went through a period of feeling excluded by the mother-child bond. In actuality he accompanied the mother to the child's well-baby visits more frequently than any of the other fathers in the project.

In addition, Molly's intermittent sleep disturbance may have been related to her own strong dependence on, submission to, and love for mother, in whose presence she was manifestly secure and gratified. The mother conveyed to the project team and to her child that only she could ultimately comfort her daughter; Molly too seemed to indicate that only mother would do during the pretoddler months. The sense of Molly's attachment to her and her effectiveness with her daughter thus seemed to contribute further to the mother's sense of her own power, which caused her a measure of anxiety.

An interaction observed during a home visit at 2½ years illustrates still another dimension of the family theme, the control of unruly behavior. The interviewer, mother, father, and Molly had been chatting. Molly was sitting on mother's lap and began to put her fingers in her mouth. The mother asked her to take her fingers out, "You're a big girl now. Do you have your finger in your mouth because you're hungry?" The father responded, "Do you want some milk?" He appeared to be softening mother's firmness about the fingers in the mouth and her calling Molly first a big girl and then a little girl. Molly replied that she would like some milk, and the father got it for her. Molly was briefly subdued by mother's injunction, and after a few moments cuddled close to mother again. This led to a group discussion of defiance. The mother was proud that her daughter had shown "no terrible twos. She's a delight . . . sometimes she says 'no' to requests and is sent to her room; but she comes out quickly, smiling and cooperative, and gets a big hug." In fact, this did occur later in the interview; Molly did not clean up some toys when asked by her mother. In this manner, Molly already is adept at controlling her behavior so as to limit the wedges she drives between herself and her parents.

Analysis of the films of mother-child behavior adds further to the picture of this family. In the initial newborn film at 1 day, the mother was breast-feeding lying on her side and cradling the baby almost to her side. Although she appeared a little uncomfortable, she asserted determinedly with a smile that she was in fact comfortable. The baby sucked contentedly. Here and later the mother preferred holding and watching her baby to other modes of interaction. She did not emphasize talking, touching, patting, or grooming.

In subsequent films in the first 6 months, the child was also a strong gazer, responding with curiosity to stimuli. When Molly became apprehensive, she compared faces in the room and locked into mutual gaze with her mother. This calmed her. She became unusually tense in the presence of doctors and nurses between 3 and 6 months (her early stranger anxiety) and mirrored her parents' serious attentiveness.

During well-baby examinations, the mother never stopped monitoring her child; but, seemingly in deference to the authority of the female pediatrician, the mother stepped to the other side of the room to allow the doctor more room. Typically, at the end of well-baby examinations Molly cried lustily and her mother quickly came forward. The mother would pick her baby up and easily soothe the child in her own self-contained, slightly awkward manner. The parents would quickly lose their tension and beam when Molly relaxed in her mother's arms.

In a well-baby visit at 4 months the mother was talking face to face with her child, heightening her excitement and playful anticipation of being picked up. The child reached toward her mother, but the mother did not follow through and pick Molly up. This was an example of appetitive behavior not being consummated, similar to the more regular occurrence of such instances described in family 1. In response to the frustration, Molly's fingers started flapping briefly and fanning.[3] Then a few seconds later the child sobered and after a few more seconds became sociable again, smiling and imitating mother's restrained but happy voice.

The ADS scale ratings indicated that Molly and her mother did not establish an obvious pattern, unless the pattern lay in the shifting about of their interactions. That is, for a time the mother might score above the median in a behavior and the child below; in the next month this might reverse; and at times both mother and baby were together in scoring above or below the median in a particular modality.

The Block Tasks at 24 and 36 months were similar to each other. In both there was an initial tendency for the mother to overcontrol and lead the child to build at a level that was too cognitively advanced. However, the mother was able to correct herself quickly and then allow the child to lead while offering her reassuring support and autonomy to build separately if she wanted. Thus the child exercised intermittent leadership, while the mother organized the overall space. On both tasks, Molly created symbolic representations of things. This was a dyad that was clearly comfortable with each other and even, on the 3-year task, high spirited.

Follow-up at 7 Years. When seen again at 7, Molly was a lithe, attractive schoolgirl with long hair, smiling, and an eager friendly demeanor. She and her parents were proud of the baby son who had been born 3 years earlier, although Molly interspersed caring for her brother with big sister bossiness and hurt feelings and protest when he took some of her toys. The family itself was otherwise little changed. They were more economically secure, the father was progressing professionally, the mother was the full-time caretaker for the baby brother who in fact had not yet been left overnight with the grandparents. The principal emotional theme immediately recurred when the parents asked for guidance in how to deal with the children's rivalrous aggression toward

---

3. This hand-and-finger mannerism seems to be part of the motor schema of grasping (Piaget, 1945). Likewise it may represent a motor memory of a pleasurable interaction of kneading at the mother's breast during nursing. This may be mediated through the hypothalamus and basal ganglia, and reproduced here in the absence of full gratification of appetitive behavior by a mechanism similar to the psychosomatic response of Charles (Massie et al., 1983).

each other. This concern over good behavior had now been emphatically internalized by Molly who volunteered that she enjoyed second grade very much, "Especially the kids who behave in class."

Molly's *schoolteacher reported* that her work was average to above average. Only in mathematics did Molly have trouble, and the teacher suspected that this was secondary to a minor learning interference since the child's intelligence was above average by all other indications. This perception on the teacher's part was consistent with the 7-year psychological testing, which like Charles's showed signs of a minor neurodevelopmental imbalance on the WISC-R. Likewise this finding was consistent with Molly's earlier speech articulation difficulty and slightly slow walking at 1½ years. Further, both parents added that they too had difficulty with numbers, for which the father had compensated by developing an interest in computers. Molly's teacher reported that socially the child was very outgoing, aware of friends' feelings, and ready to help and care for others to a greater degree than most children. As a measure of her independence, Molly's teacher reported that the child would try tasks first on her own and then ask for help if she had trouble. She was more cheerful and understanding of what was going on than typical children. There was no difficulty with reading and spelling.

In her *unstructured play interview,* the mother once again had some trouble separating from Molly, solicitously coming back into the room to remind her daughter that she had wanted to go to the bathroom. Molly's initial shyness passed, and she then went to the art materials, drawing a very colorful house with many doors and windows. While she drew, she spontaneously talked about her fondness for a teacher who had moved away, how she was glad there was only one mean kid in class, and how her brother sometimes pulled her hair and got into trouble with Mom. Her thoughts then went to the night her brother was born. Molly was at her grandparents, but she got an earache so they took her to the hospital, and "Guess what?" she said. "Mommy was there in her nightgown, and Dad brought both of us flowers." This is an interesting commentary on Molly's sibling rivalry and normative oedipal rivalry and identification with her mother for father's attention.

On the *Block Task* at 7 years, mother and child continued their now predictable pattern. The mother organized like a teacher until Molly asserted herself, and then her mother retreated to the role of facilitator. They built a castle where a king lived who sometimes became angry when people spray-painted his walls. The kids lived in another house. Mother and child were able to play with Molly's rebellious spray-paint fantasy, although the mother finally affirmed that spray-painters are bad.

On *psychological testing* Molly achieved a full scale IQ of 108. Actual IQ is probably significantly higher if one discounts her performance on the digit span subtest. For example, her capacity for intellectual abstraction is in the 130 IQ range. In addition to the mild visual-motor and memory-organization interferences, mild performance anxiety also depressed her scores. Molly's nervousness over doing well, of course, is remindful of the parents' own concern over doing a good job with their daughter. In her drawings (fig. 4), Molly demonstrated an adequate and solidly organized body image, although there were slight distortions of shapes and an unusual placing of the figures so that they were askew, tilting to one side. Strong male-female differentiation showed in the drawings, which were accentuated with jewelry and clothes, demonstrating Molly's strong wish to be feminine and grown like Mom combined with an age-appropriate pull to still be a little girl. The family drawing showed the members as joined together and happy, suggesting also defensive elements of reaction formation and denial of any disruptive affect. This is similar to mother's adaptive style; and these defenses likewise came across on Molly's other projective test responses. There Molly denied angry and jealous feelings in CAT stories and on the Rorschach. This led to some constriction of her imagination as she was careful not to reveal anything bad, in spite of breakthroughs of her rivalrous feelings toward her little brother in her stories.

The tests showed a normal girl in early latency with early indication of a personality style characterized by some avoidances of affect, attention to body details, and perception of herself as potentially vulnerable to both masculine and feminine deprivation and control. This is similar to mother's style. Technically, for lack of a better term, we speak of it as a hysterical style. To find her way she feels she must inhibit aggression, which nonetheless gets expressed from time to time in moments of frustration. The tester concluded that Molly was a delightful girl on her way to healthy development, moving through latency well, with appropriate resolution of sexual identification and struggles around phallic and oral concerns.

To summarize, we see Molly as a successful schoolgirl who has adjusted well developmentally to her parents' expectations that she be well mannered. It seems that the child has accomplished this nicely through getting in tune with her mother by identifying with her mother's particular need that Molly be a good, big girl. Molly clearly sees pride in her mother's face and knows she has to follow rules. For her

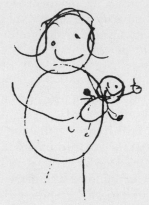
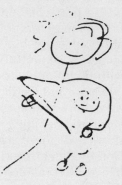

Figure 3.   Drawings of Family 2 (Molly). Mrs. P.'s Draw-a-Mother-and-Child in third trimester and at 12 months

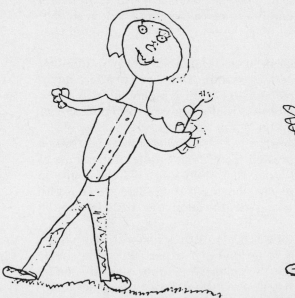
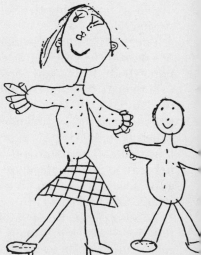

Figure 4.   Drawings of Family 2 (Molly). Molly at 7 years: Draw-a-Person and Draw-a-Mother ("They are happy. It's my mother and brother.")

part, the mother has been able to adjust to her daughter. When she gradually perceived that Molly could regulate herself and was able to sleep, feed, and curb her aggressiveness, the mother could relax her fears of being either too forceful or too passive with her child.

These particular fears were observed in a more microfashion in the films which showed the mother to be ever-vigilant but at the same time reserved and cautious in physically making contact with her baby. The mother successfully balanced her reserve and emphasis on socialization with her attentiveness and the generosity of the extended breast-feeding she offered Molly until 3 years of age.

The evolution of this case contrasts to that of Charles, where parents and child have not so successfully adjusted to each other. Molly's mother has charted a steady course in her emotional life, changing very little if at all. By contrast, Charles's mother has gradually overcome a significant depression which had strongly marked her during the pregnancy and well into Charles's toddlerhood. The parents' wish to foster independence in their boy through early separations—reflected also in the mother's microbehaviors of regularly disrupting or avoiding moments that would consummate a closeness between them—has taken its toll on Charles. Table 1 summarizes the longitudinal course of the two families.

DISCUSSION

Tolstoy wrote in *Anna Karenina,* "Happy families are all alike; every unhappy family is unhappy in its own way." Our beginning understanding of the families in our project would have us modify Tolstoy's famous opening line to "Every happy family also tells a different story." Molly's and Charles's families—both intact, in agreement over their child rearing, and avowedly secure and content—organize their emotional and physical lives around central themes which are quite personal. Likewise we are teasing out specific central themes from the other families in the project.

In this section we review the principal issues that the two case studies highlight, and amplify certain ideas with illustrations from other families. The question of continuities in development provides one of the most intriguing issues in research. Some workers such as Kagan (1984) tend to downplay continuities, emphasizing instead the steady appearance of cognitive and social functions. Similarly, Thomas and Chess (1977) found that in the New York longitudinal study the only variable that was predictable over time was that of infant temperament.

Nonetheless, psychoanalytic theory postulates continuities as the

Table 1. Summary of Longitudinal Findings, Infancy to 7 Years

Child's name	Family theme	Maternal conflict	Mother-infant behavior	ADS scale ratings (0–18 mos.)	Strange situation (18 mos.)	Child in latency	Mother at 7 yrs. follow-up
CHARLES (Family 1)	You can get close but not too close	Mother denies own & child's dependency needs	Baby's appetitive behaviors unconsummated; early separations; mother's affect gloomy	Mother & child largely below median except gazing	Unclassifiable. Child does not show clear distress	Restless, clinging, below average in school, sense of impotence	No longer depressed, happy, second child
MOLLY (Family 2)	Be a good girl	Mother worries about being too strong with child; neither does she want to be ruled by child	Mother responsive, watchful, slightly stiff; breast-feeding for 3 years	No clear pattern	Secure attachment. Child upset on separation; uses mother for comfort on return	Joyful, independent, sociable; above average in school	Unchanged, content, competent, second child

cornerstone of its developmental and epigenetic points of view (Anna Freud, 1963), in which one layer of psychological attainment leads stepwise to the next; one faulty step leaves a weakness in the structure. Likewise, research in attachment theory suggests something similar. Recently Erickson et al. (1985) and Main et al. (1985) have shown that aspects of preschoolers' and grammar schoolers' behavior could be predicted from the findings of the Strange Situation response of the child at 1 year. Secure attachment at 1 year presaged greater flexibility of response and adjustment in school. Charles in our study illustrated how a lack of a rating of secure attachment at 18 months foreshadowed his dependent behavior in school at 7 years. Molly similarly demonstrated continuity but with a different outcome: secure attachment correlated with better school adaptation.

But the issues are much more complex than this. Infant, toddler, and schoolchild have very different internal worlds to go along with their vastly changing external world. The healthy schoolchild has an inner structure that includes the constancy of libidinal objects, a good degree of self and object differentiation, a sense of competency and efficacy, an increasing autonomy from inner drives and pressures for instant action and gratification, as well as a working style of defenses and characterologic adaptations. The child has arrived there by internalizing the pattern of the mother-infant interactions which create in the baby the capacities to contain both inner and outer stimuli. Mahler et al. (1975) speak of the early months in which the child is scarcely psychologically separate from the mother; and the mother herself undergoes a process of psychological dedifferentiation—or regression as Bibring et al. (1961) have termed it—which facilitates her attunement to the relatively undifferentiated baby.

Our study showed how regularly mothers gave what appeared to be psychologically regressive responses on projective testing at 1 year, while at the same time they were functioning competently from a clinical point of view. The psychological testing apparently picked up the normal loosening of the maternal personality which may be a prerequisite for the empathic transcending of one's own ego boundaries so as to be able to project oneself into the baby's inchoate states. This makes possible maternal "attunement" to the baby (Stern, 1985), a more precise description of Winnicott's (1965) holding environment, which helps the infant gradually achieve self-regulation of his own states.

After this earliest period of life, there occur the child's processes of separation and individuation in the latter half of the first year and through the second and third years. For the mother it is also a time of psychic restructuralization. Many of the mothers in the study, of which Charles's was one, came out of this time happier and more effective than before pregnancy. For them, raising their first baby had permitted a reindividuation and reseparation from their own mothers, so that they felt in less conflict with the ways in which they still identified with or resembled their mothers. Other mothers such as Molly's did not show this kind of change. She remained emotionally on an even keel throughout, even while undergoing the normative dedifferentiation of ego boundaries that imitates psychopathology during her child's infancy. Another mother, Peter's, exemplified still another maternal course that we observed. She escaped from a feared identification with her somewhat helpless, passive mother via the excitement and activity of raising her baby. After Peter's infancy, however, this mother became confused by the reemerging threat of being too much like her own mother.

Erikson (1950) wrote that the creation of a sense of trust, autonomy, and industry was the psychosocial task of these early years. Still earlier psychoanalysts had described the fantasies that characterized an oral, anal, and phallic time during these first three years, with potentiality for interference with psychological growth if they were not well attended to by the parent. Now we attempt to invoke the complexities of the process by calling it a dance between mother and infant. And if mutual reciprocity and contingent responsiveness are the rhythm of the dance which the current generation of baby watchers has discovered, affective states are the melodies. Together they create the dyad's or family's theme, of which we have spoken, with ample room for a unique choreography as well as missteps.

Thus, what we found especially rewarding in working up project families was following the melody which, in this metaphor, corresponds to the affective component of the family theme. In the outline of normal development, empathy (Basch, 1983), which is critical for effective parental responsiveness, involves the capacity of the mother to recognize and *project* herself *into* her baby's mood. The mother recognizes what the baby's affect would be like in herself and identifies with it. To do this, she must be attuned to the infant's rhythm and state. If the baby is fatigued, distressed, bored, eager, adventurous, or cautious, for example, the parent feels what it is like, almost automatically, and enters into that world. Once there, the parent sometimes takes the lead, but often it is otherwise and she allows the baby to do the regulating of himself and mother. Even if this sometimes means suffering at the whim and cry of the baby (Brody, 1970), the mother must be able to accommodate to him. Her ability to recognize her baby's mood and be influenced by her baby is of critical importance.

There are elements that support or interfere with this, for parental projection is hardly ever pure. Molly's and Charles's families showed the individuality of the process. What Charles's mother seemed to *project onto* her son, out of her fear of personal weakness and neediness, was a conscious image of him as stronger than he really was. The mother was in fact unconsciously repudiating her own sense of neediness by force of denial and accomplishment, although it nonetheless was the root of her depression during the first 3 or so years of Charles's life. By warding off her perception of her baby's needs, she was not able to empathize effectively with his own needs for closeness. Thus, we recognize two projection mechanisms at play in child rearing— parental *projection into* a baby's mood of one's self to identify with the child, and parental *projection onto* the baby of one's own image of him. These two processes are linked in the parent, affect the parent's overt behavior response, and finally affect the child's own emerging ego functions and self image.

Remindful of Lewin's (1950) description of the normative oral triad of the wish to eat, be eaten, and sleep were Charles's mother's anxieties about her baby's nursing and her fantasies that this would deplete her. This led her to behaviors we described. Recall her docking of the infant at her breast without body contact like a dirigible at a pylon; her comment that "he's so greedy"; the abrupt weaning at 6 months and shift to full-time daycare; the regular vacation separations beginning at 1 year; the Attachment During Stress (ADS) scale ratings for the first 18 months, which registered mother-infant distance in all parameters except touch and eye gaze. In fact, it was this gaze that communicated the mother's obvious love for her child, along with the pride, humor, and affection in her voice when she talked about Charles.

Even with gaze there were examples of how the mother had to break the mutual lock—cracking the symbiosis, we have called it—in the service of a relationship that was close but not too close. Play and enveloping holding were rare. It seemed that the mother could get in touch with her son as she saw the image of him which pleased her: an active, sturdy, moving, and pliant boy. At these times both connected. On the other hand, when in the grip of oppressive depressive feelings she could ill "tune in." Perhaps Charles's loss of emerging ego functions begins here in the abrupt breaks in the mutuality of the pair, in the difficulty the mother had allowing low-intensity moments to occur between her and her son and also the difficulty in allowing her son to consummate high-intensity appetitive behaviors he directed to her. This may have laid the ground for disruption of nascent homeostatic and regulatory functions (Greenspan, 1981) in the child that are the precursors of early ego functions. Likewise the breaks in mutuality may have prevented the mother from providing Charles the auxiliary ego assistance that promotes the unfolding of self-regulation.

We saw derivatives of the interferences with self-regulation in subsequent phases. For example, in the Strange Situation at 18 months, Charles ran to and fro the length of the room after his mother left. We took this as a motoric sign of attempts at restitutive activity to forestall an increasing sense of disorganization. Likewise this form of restitutive activity may have the meaning for Charles of complying with his mother's wishes for him to be active. By acting in this way he can invoke an image (a self-object image) of himself and mother that re-creates pleasing experiences and defends against the separation from mother. In this way the to-and-fro action can defend against separation anxiety and simultaneously be a motoric regression to ward off disorganization.

Charles's behavior on the Strange Situation, though not classifiable by Ainsworth et al.'s (1978) original categories, fits Main et al.'s (1985) description of their new category Insecure-disorganized/disoriented. In their study, children rated this way at 12 months were followed up at 6 years. They showed less balance and fluidity in speech with their mothers, and less optimal social and emotional functioning and task orientation with an examiner than children who had been earlier rated as Securely Attached. When shown a picture of a child undergoing a separation from his parent and asked what they would feel and do themselves in such a situation, the 6-year-old children who had formerly been rated Insecure-disorganized/disoriented were more likely to be reticent, depressed, passive, or disorganized.

We also saw signs of Charles's particular motor response to stress on the Block Task at 2 years. Although his mother was present, she and Charles were unable to connect around the task, creating in effect a psychological distance. Charles responded by a passive-to-active reversal in which he ran away from his mother's field and the blocks. It appeared that early interactions had a significant templating effect, so that the core underlying dynamics stayed consistent while the external form evolved and activities changed. This also appeared to be the case in Charles's follow-up at 7 years. We found him somewhat dependent and clinging to his teacher and ill at ease in competitiveness with peers. His teacher labels him as somewhat needy, sad, and anxious, which are precisely the same types of behavior that have threatened his mother.

In this manner we can see a transmission of parental conflict which is beginning to pervade Charles's own individual experience. The boy's mother has been able to repress relatively successfully her depression and longings to be cared for via denial; her son is unable to do it. He is becoming clinging and discouraged by second grade. This is a variation of what Freud (1896) described as "the return of the repressed." However, here it recurs not in the original person but in the next generation.

Further, in our 7-year follow-up, psychological testing raised the possibility of a minor, central nervous system, developmental, integrative imbalance reflected in the boy's awkward spatial orientation of representations and visual-motor rendering of representations. Therefore, Charles's 7-year-old capacities and incapacities may be the final common pathway of an interference with emerging ego functions whose work is to synthesize and integrate affective, cognitive, and motoric activity. In its magnified form, we are now familiar with how gross psychological disorder can accompany physical defect in the young child. For example, Fraiberg (1977) described how an autistic syndrome can result in blind infants from the emotional and physical isolation that is the fate of these children unless they are given highly nurturing care. Similarly Engel (1979) and Dowling (1977) found that children with congenital esophageal atresia that requires tube feedings until surgical correction after infancy, and who miss the experience of a feeding cycle, grow up with a blunting of their affective and fantasy life. And earlier, Spitz (1945) and Provence and Ritvo (1961) recognized the anaclitic depressions of children bereft of even surrogate parenting in inadequate foundling institutions. It is possible that a family such as Charles's illustrates the more temperate effects of moderate ongoing mother-child dyssynchrony and organic vulnerability on psychic development. Yet another factor in Charles's equation was the father's relative emotional distance. He was in concert with the mother and therefore could not be an ameliorating force.

We now turn to Molly's family. With Charles we focused on how the mother had to repudiate the dependent part of herself leading to a premature projection onto her baby of a view of him as independent, which in turn promoted his own later difficulty with independent functioning. Molly's mother also was not comfortable with aspects of herself which she likewise projected onto her baby, seeing her as unbridled. But for Molly at 7 years the outcome seems much more auspicious.

The key seems to lie in the intensity of the parental need to disavow unacceptable wishes and aspects of the self. The more pressing the need, the more likely it is that the parent will have to resort to a massive defense to get rid of what is reprehensible in the self, usually by making it—and the defense as well—unconscious. Johnson and Szurek (1952) recognized an aspect of this in their delineation of superego lacunae in which a parent does not recognize antisocial impulses in himself through projecting them onto (and into) his child, who then acts out for him. Kohut (1972) also viewed the phenomenon of narcissistic rage as an individual's attempt to obliterate what offends in one's self.

If a part of the self is intensely disavowed, it cannot effectively be used to empathize with a young child, which leaves the child in limbo when caught in the grip of the state that the mother avoids. We have seen how this affected Charles's development. What Molly's mother did not want was for her child to be unruly, especially if this meant that the child dominated her. However, this mother had no need massively to disavow strength and control; rather, these issues made her uncomfortable within a range she could tolerate. She viewed herself as competent and forceful, and used reaction formations to mitigate guilt associated with her abilities. She did not need to so deny her assertiveness as to become clinging and give up her forthrightness. Aware of her ability, she also feared being too powerful in a way that might crush Molly's movement toward autonomy.

What distinguished Molly's mother's conflicts from Charles's was that they were less intense and they remained largely conscious. She was able to recognize that the issue of control was an area of conflict for her and was able to entertain it in consciousness, which gave her more flexibility than Charles's mother. Molly's mother's behavior with her infant followed consciously held beliefs about the importance of order and moderation on the part of parent and child alike that were not incongruent with repressed affects. Thus Molly's mother was conscientiously vigilant for aspects of herself that might crop up in her daughter and lead to willful or unbridled behavior. They had to be controlled, not denied, so that the mother countered them with her firm sense of "the right way to behave." Likewise she countered her limit setting by balancing it thoughtfully with extended breast-feeding. In infancy, the mother cradled the child to her side and to her breast. The child responded with a good suck, and over the next 3 years shared with the mother the pleasure of the breast-feeding. Had Molly's mother been more conflicted over either her own power or her daughter's assertiveness, unconscious projections might have interfered. In such a scenario the mother might have seen her daughter as aggressive when she was only upset, or crushed by maternal rules when

Molly was only daunted. Either view would have disrupted maternal empathy and mother-infant mutuality.

As it was, both mother and child had to work at being comfortable with each other. They both were distressed at times at this process. Paradoxically, Charles and his mother enjoyed greater surface tranquillity (and a more stable pattern of interaction on ADS scale ratings). Molly, by contrast, slept restlessly throughout infancy, a phenomenon which Paret (1983) found correlated with extended breast-feeding, and went through an early prolonged period of stranger anxiety and separation protest. The mother periodically doubted her daughter's ability to establish self-regulation of her crying, sleeping, eating, and fears. Able to consider her hesitations and conflicts, the mother occasionally asked for assistance from the project team and pediatricians in order fully to trust in her daughter's excellent development. She did not need to ward off advice as Charles's parents did.

The ADS scale ratings seemed to capture Molly and her mother's on-going working at adjustment to each other's reciprocal influences. No stable pattern appeared. Sometimes one or the other ranked higher on one or the other parameter of initiation, avoidance, and response, yet ultimately they seemed successfully to work out their relationship.

This is in agreement with Main et al.'s (1985, p. 101) finding in their examination of mother-child speech patterns at the 6 years of age follow-up of children who had been rated secure or insecure in the Strange Situation in infancy: "the very secure dyads were the dyads most free of predictable, 'rule-like' regularities and patternings in discourse." Apparently where the internal representation of the mother is more stable, the child is able to function more autonomously, and mother and child are less governed by rules that guide their behavior. Consistent with this, at follow-up at age 7, both Molly and her mother showed a similar sense of confidence in their effectiveness as individuals and clear signs of mutual identification, which contrasted with Charles's sense of impotence.

The prevailing background of Molly's breast-feeding may have given reassurance to both that all would go well.[4] Another factor that had exerted a steadying influence in this child's development was the strong involvement of the father from birth. Attitudinally he was in agreement with his wife on issues of child rearing; behaviorally he sometimes offered nurturing to Molly to soften his wife's limit setting.

---

4. A side note to this is the possibility that the prolonged oral gratification in the feeding may have contributed to the delay in the emergence of speech articulation.

To begin to broaden our findings, what this research accents is the strong effect of the prevailing mother-child interaction (and the supporting role of the father[5] in influencing this dyad) on the young child's emerging ego functions and self-differentiation. It was striking to us that we could see traces of the mother-infant interactions in the child's subsequent development. What we identified as family themes seem to be organizers of the family at all levels of feeling and behavior, which shape development from conception. It is not that this process rigidly fixes growth, but it is likely that these themes channel the wide boundaries of development.

SUMMARY

A principal reason that we conducted much of the early observation and filming in a naturalistic setting like the pediatric well-baby clinic was to learn the kinds of parent-infant phenomena predictive of later development that can be recognized there. This site is one of the very few places that child care professionals routinely meet young families. With the project findings in mind, we now have a better understanding of the importance of what can be seen in infancy so that we can begin to refine therapeutic interventions in order to prevent severe distortions of development in the child.

At the beginning of this report we described how we designed this study to redress some of the gaps existing in developmental research. Specifically, we wanted to correlate a careful understanding of the mother's personality with the actual behaviors she brought to her interactions with her baby, and we wanted to correlate close observation of patterns of mother-infant interaction with the child's subsequent emotional growth. Doing this has provided an eyeful of visual impressions and an earful of ideas. Together they create an array of meanings. Perhaps none of these is more important than recognizing that preverbal experiences that occur in mother-baby interactions form enduring patterns that can be discerned early in life, and viewed years later in an altered derivative but equivalent shape when the youngster can also express them in relation to other people, and in language, fantasy, and activity. Likewise, as part of this evolution, we have been able to see how parents do transmit their conflicts to their children by expressing them, at the most primitive level, in their actions with their

5. Main et al. (1985) also found in their study of secure attachment in infancy and childhood that individual difference in the infancy relationship to mother, but not to father, predicted the 6-year-old's responses.

babies. The child adjusts to the parents' world in this process, with the possibility of a relatively broad band of adaptation. Nonetheless, the adaptations the children in our study make are at different functional levels.

BIBLIOGRAPHY

AINSWORTH, M., BLEHAR, M., WATERS, E., & WALLS, S. (1978). *Patterns of Attachment*. Hillsdale, N.J.: Lawrence Erlbaum.

BASCH, M. (1983). Empathic understanding. *J. Amer. Psychoanal. Assn.*, 31:101–126.

BIBRING, G. L., DWYER, T. F., HUNTINGTON, D. S., & VALENSTEIN, A. F. (1961). A study of psychological processes in pregnancy and of the earliest mother-child relation. *Psychoanal. Study Child*, 16:64–91.

BOWLBY, J. (1969). *Attachment and Loss,* vol. 1. New York: Basic Books.

BRAZELTON, T. B., KOSLOWSKI, B., & MAIN, M. (1974). The origins of reciprocity. In *The Effect of the Infant on Its Caregiver,* ed. M. Lewis & L. A. Rosenblum. New York: Wiley, pp. 49–76.

BRODY, S. (1970). A mother is being beaten. In *Parenthood,* ed. E. J. Anthony & T. Benedek. Boston: Little, Brown, pp. 427–447.

––––––– & AXELRAD, S. (1970). *Anxiety and Ego Formation in Infancy.* New York: Int. Univ. Press.

DOWLING, S. (1977). Seven infants with esophageal atresia. *Psychoanal. Study Child*, 32:215–256.

ENGEL, G. (1979). Monica. *J. Amer. Psychoanal. Assn.*, 27:107–126.

ERICKSON, M., SROUFE, L. A., & EGELAND, B. (1985). The relationship between quality of attachment and behavior problems in preschool in a high-risk sample. In *Growing Points of Attachment Theory and Research,* ed. I. Bretherton & E. Waters. Monogr. Soc. Res. Child Develpm., serial no. 209, vol. 50, nos. 1–2, pp. 147–166.

ERIKSON, E. H. (1950). *Childhood and Society.* New York: Norton.

ESCALONA, S. K. (1968). *The Roots of Individuality.* Chicago: Aldine.

FRAIBERG, S. (1977). *Insights from the Blind.* New York: Basic Books.

FREUD, A. (1963). The concept of developmental lines. *Psychoanal. Study Child*, 18:245–265.

––––––– (1965). Normality and pathology in childhood. *W.,* 6.

FREUD, S. (1896). The etiology of hysteria. *S.E.,* 3:189–221.

GREENSPAN, S. (1981). *Psychopathology and Adaptation in Infancy and Early Childhood.* New York: Int. Univ. Press.

JOHNSON, A. & SZUREK, S. (1952). The genesis of antisocial acting out in children and adults. *Psychoanal. Q.,* 21:323–343.

KAGAN, J. (1984). *The Nature of the Child.* New York: Basic Books.

KOHUT, H. (1972). Thoughts on narcissism and narcissistic rage. *Psychoanal. Study Child*, 27:360–400.

Lewin, B. D. (1950). *The Psychoanalysis of Elation*. New York: Norton.

Mahler, M. S., Pine, F., & Bergman, T. (1975). *The Psychological Birth of the Infant*. New York: Basic Books.

Main, M., Kaplan, N., & Cassidy, J. (1985). Security in infancy, childhood, and adulthood. In *Growing Points of Attachment Theory and Research*, ed. I. Bretherton & E. Waters. Monogr. Soc. Res. Child Develpm., serial no. 209, vol. 50, nos. 1–2, pp. 66–104.

Massie, H. (1975). The early natural history of childhood psychosis. *J. Amer. Acad. Child Psychiat.*, 14:683–707.

——— Bronstein, A., & Afterman, J. (1983). A report of neuropsychological differentiation and de-differentiation in very young children in conflict, with special reference to autism. Presented at the annual meeting of the American Academy Child Psychiatry, San Francisco.

——— & Campbell, B. K. (1983). The Massie-Campbell scale of mother-infant attachment indicators during stress. In *Frontiers of Infant Psychiatry*, ed. J. Call, E. Galenson, & R. Tyson. New York: Basic Books, pp. 394–412.

——— & Rosenthal, J. (1984). *Childhood Psychosis in the First 4 Years of Life*. New York: McGraw-Hill.

Paret, I. (1983). Night waking and its relation to mother-infant interaction in 9 month olds. In *Frontiers of Infant Psychiatry*, ed. J. Call, E. Galenson, & R. Tyson. New York: Basic Books, pp. 171–177.

Piaget, J. (1945). *Play, Dreams, and Imitation in Childhood*. New York: Norton, 1962.

Provence, S. & Ritvo, S. (1961). Effects of deprivation on institutionalized infants. *Psychoanal. Study Child*, 16:189–205.

Ritvo, S. & Solnit, A. J. (1953). Influences of early mother and child interaction on identification processes. *Psychoanal. Study Child*, 13:64–91.

Sander, L. (1964). Adaptive relationships in early mother-child interaction. *J. Amer. Acad. Child Psychiat.*, 3:231–265.

Spitz, R. A. (1945). Hospitalism. *Psychoanal. Study Child*, 1:53–72.

Stern, D. N. (1971). A micro-analysis of mother-infant interaction. *J. Amer. Acad. Child Psychiat.*, 10:501–517.

——— (1985). *The Interpersonal World of the Infant*. New York: Basic Books.

Thomas, A. & Chess, S. (1977). *Temperament and Development*. New York: Brunner/Mazel.

Tinbergen, N. (1973). *The Animal in Its World*, 2 vols. London: Allen & Unwin.

——— & Tinbergen, E. A. (1983). *Autistic Children*. London: Allen & Unwin.

Tronick, E., Als, H., Adamson, L., Wise, S., & Brazelton, T. B. (1978). The infant's response to entrapment between contradictory messages in face-to-face interaction. *J. Amer. Acad. Child Psychiat.*, 7:1–13.

Winnicott, D. W. (1965). *The Maturational Processes and the Facilitating Environment*. New York: Int. Univ. Press.

Ziegler, R. & Musliner, P. (1977). Persistent themes. *Family Process*, 16:293–305.

CLINICAL CONTRIBUTIONS

The Psychoanalytic Process in Adults and Children

SAMUEL ABRAMS, M.D.

I FIND IT USEFUL TO CONCEPTUALIZE THE PSYCHOANALYTIC PROCESS AS that sequence of steps which proceeds within the mind of the patient as the treatment moves forward. The process begins with the patient's character and ends with new integrations. The goal of analysis is achieved when pathogens are uprooted from an earlier psychological organization and freshly placed into a more mature one where they can be transformed. While I believe that the overall process is similar in patients of all ages, the impetus for therapeutic action and the steps in the sequence are somewhat more complex in children. By focusing on the similarities and differences I hope to illustrate the usefulness of these points of view about process.

I shall describe two cases, one an adult woman, the second a little boy. They share a clinical curiosity. Each developed a relationship to a stuffed animal in the course of the work. I hope to demonstrate what that relationship meant to them and how it expressed features of the emerging treatment process within each.

RHINO AND THE LADY

Jessica was 11 years old when she came upon a small stuffed rhinoceros at a country fair in Grand Rapids, Michigan. He was one of a sibling

---

Clinical professor, The Psychoanalytic Institute, New York University Medical Center.

The Freud Lecture, Psychoanalytic Association of New York, April 27, 1987. Many ideas in this paper were developed within two discussion groups: the Child Analysis Faculty Seminar of The Psychoanalytic Institute at the New York University Medical Center, chaired by Roy K. Lilleskov, M.D., and "The Many Meanings of Play in Childhood," sponsored by the Psychoanalytic Research and Development Fund, chaired by Albert J. Solnit, M.D. I am especially grateful to Peter B. Neubauer, M.D., a member of both discussion groups, for his stimulating ideas about developmental phases and treatment processes. Dr. Neubauer and Dr. Edward Weinshel offered valuable suggestions while I modified earlier drafts of this paper.

group of very similar rhinoceroses. However, because he was black with red paws and beady eyes, he was regarded as less attractive than the others and the least likely to be sold. Jessica felt sorry for him and bought him. She named him Rhino. Rhino joined her stuffed animal collection, comprised by then of some 25 other creatures.

He evoked little interest for several years. When it was time for Jessica to go to college, however, she chose him to accompany her. He sat idly on the dorm shelf as she made her way through school. Upon completing her studies she moved East to get a job. Rhino was packed along with her books and once again settled peacefully among them in her New York City apartment.

Jessica found work in the creative arts and soon became seriously involved with a young man. But neither the work nor the involvement seemed gratifying. She felt constrained at her job, and she saw the young man as overly demanding. When she became ill for a while, he seemed too distant; and when she became well, there were times when he was a bit brusque and even rude. She was a self-demeaning young woman and partly as a consequence of this feature of her character had cultivated particular kinds of relationships—caring women, protective men. She very much wanted to be a more independent and assertive person, but she feared that this would alienate her from her beau and from her many friends who were accustomed to her retiring behavior. Her unhappiness intensified; she began to have nightmares and often found herself weeping uncontrollably. A close relative had experienced a successful outcome from analysis many years earlier; so when Jessica's situation became sufficiently painful, she too decided to try it. She was 23 years old when she began.

Jessica was the second of three children; there had been a girl before her, a boy after. She recalled her mother as an enthusiastic home-maker, a creative person, sly in her dealings with the children. The father was an acknowledged success in business, a model of independent enterprise and moral virtues. Jessica's older sister had followed her father into the world of commerce, but Jessica always perceived herself as more artsy, like her mother. She had been very close to her 15-month younger brother in spite of her envy born of the belief that he was the preferred child because he was a boy. The three had been cesarian births. Jessica had always known this and carried the image of her abdominally scarred mother in her mind from her earliest days. Even with this picture of females as physically flawed and less valued than males she had always wanted to be a "lady."

In her first dream in analysis, she found herself studying for a difficult history exam while desperately trying to make her room look pretty; and, in her second, she was repudiated by her sister and a childhood girlfriend. Around these two brief dreams there soon consolidated themes of feeling unattractive and condemned. As a child she believed she was ugly; her knees were knobby and her legs too thin. There were times when she thought that she looked more like a little boy than a girl. Despite this impression or perhaps on account of it, even at the age of 3 she was fond of donning one of her mother's dresses and prancing about with one strap hanging suggestively off the shoulder. She wanted very much to be a pretty, grown-up lady.

Almost from the moment the analysis began, she reacted to my comments as if they were reproaches. Sometimes she felt demeaned, sometimes condemned. Often she burst into tears. These responses reflected how she processed the ambiguity of the treatment setting. She conveyed the impression that she was a fragile and easily wounded person who might fall apart were I not overly solicitous and overly supportive. It offered me the opportunity to activate the analytic process. I focused on the form, paying less attention to the content of the exchanges for quite a while. It required considerable effort on my part to maintain what she regarded as such a cool and remote stance because her cowering was so intimidating. The cowering soon blended into another surfacing phenomenon: she frequently imagined voices in her head—voices that often sounded like her father. The voices would describe her as "bad," sometimes matter-of-factly, sometimes in an accusatory manner. "Bad" encompassed a variety of subcategories: bad was weak, bad was female, bad was dirty, and bad was immoral. The effect of the cowering and the voices was to keep her uncompromisingly good almost all of the time. Analysis was a genuine danger: it threatened to call forth all her wickedness and all her ugliness were she to be stripped of the approaches that had seemed so effective until now.

Whatever their real and imagined advantages, the traits of cowering and self-condemnation also proved burdensome. She lived in a universe that was continually dangerous and depressing. However, as she dramatized these views of herself within the analytic setting, she felt their influence wane a bit outside of it. After a few months, she was able to act upon her own interest on matters that affected her career and her personal life in ways quite uncharacteristic for her.

The tension created by the difference between her expectations and my actual behavior provided me with another opportunity. I used it to demonstrate just how much her life was influenced by what she envisioned about people and situations as contrasted with what people and situations really were. This brought her to the topic of her imagination, which had always been quite vivid. When she was little, walks in ordinary open fields were recalled as experiences of exploratory adventures, while evenings at home were dominated by menacing monsters. She always needed someone to guard her from the monsters. Her mother was the preferred protector, but sometimes the family dog or her stuffed animals would do. The stuffed animals proved most reliable (her mother was not always around at bedtime, and the family dog finally died), so the teddies and the rabbits became her regular companions and not only at night. They also were assigned roles in the dramas she loved to make up during the daytime.

Until she was 4 years old, Jessica's father was probably her preferred partner in the stuffed animal adventures, but a mysterious barrier developed between the two of them—it seemed quite sharply demarcated in retrospect—and her younger brother became her co-star. The stuffed animals were her babies; she and her brother were wife and husband, exchanging evening kisses amidst giggles. For two years or so she played out a day-by-day grown lady existence as mother and wife.

The earlier years with her father had been so filled with pleasurable memories and excitement that it seemed imperative to trace the events that had led to the rift between them. Initially in the analysis, Jessica remembered that she had told her mother that she wanted to marry her father; her mother had reacted with mock earnestness at the news and wondered what would become of *her*? Reflecting on that recalled exchange, Jessica concluded that she had created the barrier to her father herself in order to protect her mother. Much later in the treatment a different account surfaced. Jessica had assertively proposed marriage to her father, frankly without much regard for her mother. However, he turned her down, explaining that he already had a wife. The rebuff left her angered and vengeful. From that point forward, she saw her father as cruel and autocratic, excessively moralistic and demanding. At the same time she continually measured herself against his real and envisioned severe standards and usually concluded that she was wanting. The lost father was retained as a set of unachievable demands; her own fury fueled those demands and her failures sustained them, guaranteeing continuing despondency. The original bond of loving playfulness was transformed into a bond of cruel reproach and surfaced in the traits of cowering and self-condemnation. This was increasingly evident as the traits were rolled back in analysis and the childhood relationships that had given rise to them revived. The activation of Rhino signaled that revival.

I first became aware of the little stuffed rhinoceros in the seventh month of the treatment, although another half year would pass before

I would meet him personally. One day Jessica reported that he had quite unexpectedly jumped from the book shelf to her bed the evening before; she told me who he was and when she had acquired him. At the time he came forward, Jessica was involved with what she labeled as homosexual ideas, recollections of her interest in the bodies of other young girls during her teen-age years. Such an interest during adolescence had alarmed her and made it even more imperative that she hurry up and become a grown-up lady. The anxieties and the shame about being "queer" were revived in the treatment; the renewal of a supportive relationship with a stuffed animal facilitated the recall of these humiliating memories and made many forbidden thoughts thinkable. She told me of thumbing through issues of *Playboy* even before her adolescence, always arrested by the striking centerfolds. Sometimes she was aroused by the pictures, while at other times she hoped to become such an alluring lady herself someday. The teen years became a time of mixed and apparently irreconcilable aims. What kind of lady did she want to be? An irresistible licentious one? A damaged mother? A lady who loved other ladies? Or a continuously indicted sinful lady?

After some months occupied with descriptions of such experiences, she issued a warning: something of crisis proportion was intruding upon our relationship and it might very well disrupt the analysis. Since I had persevered in spite of her declarations of ugliness and wickedness, she was becoming concerned that I looked upon her as an attractive and desirable young woman rather than a dirty little girl. The idea horrified her.

She actively consulted with Rhino at home about the wisdom of continuing the treatment. He tried to reassure her that I was a reputable physician. I had come well recommended and my credentials were in order. My behavior had always been proper and respectful. However, if she thought it would be useful, he would make a personal inspection. So, in the thirteenth month of the analysis, within this crisis precipitated by heightened transference danger and excitement, Rhino came and attended sessions regularly for the next seven months.

At first Jessica was uncertain what role to assign Rhino in this new drama. Sometimes he sat perched on her shoulder staring at me, clearly a sentry on guard; sometimes she placed him supine on her stomach as if he too were free associating. The sessions became affectively explosive with hitherto unexplored personal matters. She spoke of orgasm for the first time, of the experience of evil, dirty fluids oozing forth from her, of the variety of holes "down there" and her uncertainties about her ability competently to control them all. The poorly differentiated perineum of her childhood was recalled. She also remembered an early distinction she had made between boys and girls, a distinction allegedly reflecting the difference between having "outside" or "inside" genitals. Men were more streamlined, more honest, but also more vulnerable; women were less sleek, more secretive, and better protected. Women faked orgasms; men couldn't. She described this very matter-of-factly, as if such broad inferences from anatomy were self-evident. Rhino supported her perspective.

Rhino's presence in the sessions, a solution to one crisis, soon provoked another. Jessica's mother insisted that bringing a stuffed rhinoceros to an analyst's office was quite a strange thing to do; and if, somehow, it were being encouraged in any way by her doctor, the treatment would best be broken up. Her father responded differently. Clipped and abrupt during phone calls until now, he began to inquire about the little fellow; he wondered about Rhino's health (his nose had been injured in the subway) and asked about his explorations of the Big Apple. Jessica recognized with pleasure that the earlier stuffed animal dramas between the two of them had been revived. She also wondered if her mother's warnings about impropriety within the therapeutic interaction mirrored a long-forgotten reproach of her play with her father. Jessica's insights into the group reenactment brought an end to the newest threat to the treatment.

The insights also emboldened her. She openly wondered what an affair between us would *really* be like. Visions of our imagined sexual encounters became graphic. Fantasies of oral impregnation surfaced along with desires secretly to witness sexual scenes or seductively exhibit herself. How delightfully filthy it would be to do a striptease right there in the office. And wasn't all this revealing of fantasies tantamount to a striptease anyway? Without controls she could become a woman with voracious perverse desires. Rhino sat quietly by as she offered these ideas, now a sentry, now our baby, now an expression of an aspect of herself, now a feature of me. Whatever other roles he played, however, he remained concretely the link to the earlier dramas created with her father when she was little and the unrecognized sexual desires embedded within them. The entrapment of that tabooed relationship within an earlier psychological organization constituted the pathogenic core of her disorder.

Seven months after Rhino had begun attending sessions, he announced to her that an important step was at hand. He would have to return to his world of stuffed animals and she would have to reside thoroughly in the world of real people. He urged her to go it alone in the analysis. The next day she arrived without him and reported this dream:

I am with a huge teddy bear, my "buddy." We go every place together and it's wonderful. Then I discover that I don't own him at all; that he's only a rented teddy bear and what's worse that there's a real man inside of him. I feel betrayed. I had a similar feeling of betrayal the other day. I closed my eyes and imagined that Rhino wanted to have sex with me; he took out his thing and peed on me. When I opened my eyes, I was so relieved to see good old Rhino as always. But then I had an image of you taking advantage of me, violating me physically. In the image my mother sat by smoking a cigarette, saying I deserved it.

A further movement forward was at hand for Jessica, a movement that would require another reach backward to a still earlier relationship with her mother.

So much for an illustration of the sequence of the empirical expressions of the underlying psychoanalytic process in adults. What is demonstrable is the revival of pathogenic experiences that were bound in another time and another place and the tracking of these experiences through character, the transference, and the past, so that they might be unbound and then freshly transformed by the mature personality. What is also demonstrable is the implicit operational aspects of the process, i.e., what she did and what I did to facilitate and sustain the sequence.

Mr. Beary and the Little Boy

Next I describe aspects of the treatment of a little boy named Leslie in order to illustrate some of the conceptual similarities and differences between adults and children and how that conceptualization influences my view of the therapeutic interaction. As with the adult case, I tried to help Leslie reach backward to understand how he got into all his troubles, but you will also hear me trying to facilitate the pull forward toward necessary new experiences so that his ways of knowing the past would be expanded and so that the foundation for his future might be more securely laid.

Leslie was not yet 4 when he was brought for treatment because he insisted he was a girl. His parents had prepared the two of us for our first meeting. They told me of the many concerns they had about his development and they told him that I was a doctor who helped people who had worries.

Leslie was the child of enterprising parents who seemed buoyant with energy and bursting with inventive business ventures. He was the second of two children, named for a man with great strength known to both parents. It was not until I brought it to their attention that either one realized that Leslie was as much a girl's name as it was a boy's. His sister, 4 years older, had always been an active child but was never a source of concern. Leslie appeared entirely normal in his first year of life—at least when measured against the conventional yardsticks— except for some food idiosyncrasies that were destined to persist for a while. Because of his finickiness, when Leslie joined the family at the table his mother elected to serve everyone what he tolerated best so that he would not feel stigmatized by his food restrictions. She reacted in a like way during the period of his toilet training. She instructed every- one to behave with considerable indulgence to his "accidents" so that he would not feel ashamed of them. In his second year, his mother sensed that something was seriously wrong with her son, but he was still unable to express himself in ways that would permit her to define the fault. By the time he was 3, however, his words were loud enough and clear enough. "You see that picture of a girl in the magazine?" he would say, "she's like me. I'm a girl." He began to behave like a female; he walked with a lilt and with his hands slightly extended, and he even asked that he be called by a girl's name at times. He made surprisingly sophisticated comments about coordinating shades of color in clothing or home decor and openly admired selective features of his mother's wardrobe. He loved wearing bracelets and necklaces, which he often lifted from the local five-and-dime; and he also swiped his sister's earrings and her nightgowns, which he wore to bed. She, like her mother, preferred to indulge him in his idiosyncrasies rather than be confrontative, because the screaming that followed any thwarting was unbearable to her. Leslie especially loved to prance about in his moth- er's high heels. He would often insist he had breasts, although he was confused about whether breasts were different from "boobs" and what nipples should be called; he also insisted that he had a vagina and frequently declared that he had no penis. His behavior in public was an embarrassment. His parents stopped taking him to restaurants, and his sister stopped having sleep-over dates. What all of this achieved was difficult for anyone about him to understand.

The consultant the parents finally visited confirmed that their alarms were valid, but they dragged their feet about going ahead with treatment. They had what they considered to be an enlightened view about individual development and contemporary society. They knew that gender confusions happened and that such matters often ap- peared quite early in life; if this meant that Leslie was destined to be a homosexual, they hoped that at least he would not be too humiliated about it. They were worried that an analyst would insist upon Leslie asserting his masculinity and thereby create conflict and low self-es- teem. They also feared that treatment might encumber his talents, which they properly assessed as considerable. He was curious, attentive, good-looking, clever, witty, and, at least when he did not feel threatened, sunny in mood and disposition. Some other features of his personality irked them far more than the high heels and the earrings and it was probably these that won the day for treatment. He had difficulty defining the limits of his own territory; when he went into homes or stores or met new people, he had to be restrained from poking about in areas that most children would have immediately recognized as restricted. He was terribly possessive; everything was his, once he said so. If a dispute about an item seemed likely to be settled against him, he would hide it somewhere to guarantee ownership. He was intolerant about the setting of limits; he watched what he wanted on TV, and he watched it when he wanted to. This was especially true at bedtime when he would become thoroughly autocratic. And as one might expect, he was having serious difficulty acclimatizing himself to nursery school.

In our first meeting Leslie's curiosity about my office was boundless and bordered on the intrusive. No drawer was left unopened, although, mercifully, he accepted restrictions about how closely he could examine the various components of my computer. The items he inspected were placed into two categories: things were either broken or they were not broken. He toyed with some Scotch tape and the tape got tangled; he tossed it away saying that it too was now broken. I sensed an opportunity. I realigned the tape in the dispenser and declared that it was fixed. I further commented, somewhat casually, that I was a doctor who also fixed broken feelings. He seemed quite unimpressed and went on with his dogged inspection of the office.

In our second meeting he resumed the pattern of inspecting, but he also introduced the gender issue. I made the assumption that this was a preferred adaptive strategy now being applied to the threatening ambiguity of the treatment situation. He playfully painted his face so that he looked like a clown—or was it a clownish woman?—and he modeled the new fashionable shoulder bag he had insisted on his mother buying him on the way to the session. There was a certain imperious quality to his manner even as he modeled, but I also recognized he was confused and frightened. I further assumed that being autocratic and being female made him feel safe, although I was not at all sure what the dangers were.

The attitudes intensified. He appeared at sessions with bracelets, necklaces, or earrings. He played at applying makeup. Sometimes he strode about in a "swish" walk, as if he were mocking a woman's gait. He displayed his color sense; his capacity to differentiate subtle shades of color impressed me, especially since he was so blurry in other areas. For a while he chose to spend much of his time dusting, polishing, and vacuuming my office. If, in the course of his activities, he injured himself ever so slightly, he would burst into uncontrollable tears. Once he fell on his chin and screamed that his face was "ruined"; the hour was aborted and he was taken home in anguish.

He took a liking to me quickly. Both the rapidity and the intensity were a bit unsettling. I counted it as a minus in my assessments. He often told his mother how much he missed me on weekends. The interruptions were becoming more and more unbearable. However, he avoided discussing his feelings about me during his sessions and concentrated instead on objects in my office. Since Leslie was accustomed to making things his own, he quickly laid claim to whatever aroused his interest, relinquishing each succeeding claim with ever more reluctance. We had a real showdown over the rubber stamp I use to endorse my checks. He insisted that it was his. The fact that it had my name on it was not evidence to the contrary. His voice climbed in intensity once my firm opposition asserted itself. His insistence was followed by crying, crying by howling, and howling by the pounding of feet. The din was such that I wondered if the conditions of my office lease were being violated. I said to him that the stamp was so important because he did not like leaving *me* and he wanted something of mine to take with him. The interpretation, which I thought was accurate, well timed, and emphatically delivered merely had the effect of his raising the intensity of the howling and the pounding. I needed another approach to help him "know" what I was trying to have him understand, so I said that he could not take what was mine, but that we could draw a picture of what he wanted and he could take the drawing home with him. The tantrum aborted suddenly. As we drew the picture of the rubber stamp, I commented that he got a "take home feeling" a lot of times and we would have to try to figure out why. Once I learned of his interest in singing, that phrase was put to music, and sung repeatedly. If Leslie became demanding, which almost always happened at the ends of sessions, he or I would break out into "The Take Home Feeling," and the crisis would be over. The song would soon become more elaborate as more differentiated verses were added. I was pleased that he was able to accept the picture as a substitute for the stamp and even more pleased that our singing together further helped him deal with the threatening separation. These seemed like necessary steps forward from the all-encompassing introjection that had been his preferred strategy until then.

Despite the drawing and the singing, Leslie was still unable to talk about me directly, even though I was clearly the most desired object in the room. It was in the context of my recognition of the intensity of these feelings and how helpless he felt about them that he came upon a teddy bear hand puppet in my toy chest and named him Mr. Beary. The puppet was one of a variety of play items that I had collected some 20 years earlier, when I believed such objects were necessary for doing child analysis. Every now and then a child would spend some time with this puppet, but none fancied him as much as Leslie. From the moment of his naming and for almost two years thereafter, Leslie's visits were not to me but to his friend, Mr. Beary. He would enter the office, instruct me to don the hand puppet, and he and Mr. Beary would proceed with the session. I created a voice that seemed appropriate for a 6-inch-tall teddy bear and at first only spoke in my own voice when I was addressed directly or to announce an administrative detail, the end of the hour, or an anticipated missed session, for example. Leslie was openly affectionate to Mr. Beary. He hugged him on entering and hugged him on leaving. When Mr. Beary had trouble holding on to some blocks and dropped them, Leslie calmly assured him that everyone made mistakes now and then and kissed him affectionately.

He told Mr. Beary about terrifying dreams—ghosts, monsters, witches, Dracula, Frankenstein. This seemed to account for the tyranny around bedtime; he was substituting imperiousness for anxiety. On one occasion, while reporting the dreams, Leslie assaulted Mr. Beary; he beat him, stabbed him, soiled him. Speaking in my own voice I suggested that he preferred feeling mean to feeling scared. The words reached him. The beatings waned; Mr. Beary thanked me for the timely interpretation.

Tales of horror surfaced. He and Mr. Beary went on hunting expeditions to gun down menacing creatures who were fond of eating people. Initially, the imagined hunt was devoid of any story line—it was simply the struggle of good guys against bad guys. Invariably the good guys triumphed and the monsters were driven back. And as all these new ways of dealing with loss and danger were being developed, the bracelets, necklaces, and earrings ceased to be prominent adornments and the "swish" walk disappeared. Leslie became more congenial in nursery school and more actively involved with other children. He spoke of his new boy's jacket with some pride and visited Dad at his office.

One day he discovered that it was possible to pass a piece of paper through a slot on my desk and have it fall unnoticed into an underlying file drawer. He called it the disappearing paper trick. He told Mr. Beary that he was a magician and while Mr. Beary stared in astonishment, Leslie worked his magic. He elaborated the fantasy: the papers were Mr. Beary's precious documents and as one after the other vanished, Mr. Beary was required to plead for them to be spared. Leslie responded with sadistic glee. After numerous repetitions of actively intimidating poor Beary, Leslie announced, in a way that was almost a non sequitur, that even though he was just a little boy, he was no longer afraid of anything. He was especially not afraid of having his penis chopped off. With hardly a break in the action, he invented a card game making up the rules as he went along so as to be sure he would win. At one point he accused Mr. Beary of trying to steal some of his cards. I spoke in my own voice, admonishing Mr. Beary lightly. "Those cards belong to him, you cannot take what's his." And Leslie added, thoroughly tuned in to the displacement, "And you cannot have my penis either." I took this view of what was transpiring: the earlier threat of losing people and the defensive strategies adopted to deal with that danger were in the process of being reassembled on a new level of organization.

For a while the theme of the penis that might be taken overlapped with the theme of lost persons. Leslie attacked Mr. Beary bodily after almost every weekend separation, pulling his eyes out or punching his face in. Leslie also tried to address the feeling of sadness more directly, and it was a more differentiated feeling than it had been earlier. Words were added to the "take home feeling" that stressed the missing of people, the anger at parting, the threat of the feelings of anger, and the preference for anger over sadness. In expectation of weekend separations, Leslie soon became accustomed to stroking Mr. Beary fondly at the farewell, while the two of them bravely threw kisses toward one another. Sometimes, he required that I draw a picture of a smiling Mr. Beary to take home with him. It would act as a reminder that Beary could tolerate the interruption without destructive wishes.

The scenes of anger and sadness over loss interwove with his drawings of naked people. He became confused and irritated and either scribbled over or tore up his drawings. At first his naked women all had penises, his naked men had vaginas and boobs. Everyone had everything; no one had lost anything. In describing himself, however, he no longer claimed to have a vagina. He talked openly about his penis and his little balls. He told me he had nipples and that only women have boobs.

A year or so into the treatment, his play took on a different shape. The struggle between good and evil was pulled into a three-character drama. A weak or dependent woman was being stalked by a monster, often an alligator or a shark or a whale intent on voraciously swallowing

her up. At the eleventh hour she would be rescued by a hero, sometimes sword-laden, sometimes merely two-fisted. At first, Leslie tried
on the role of the stalked woman and invited me to be the attacking
shark while Mr. Beary was the heroic rescuer. As the woman, he was
clearly excited as he anticipated the assault with a sly smile of pleasure.
Then he cast Mr. Beary as the hapless lady, while he became a super-
hero, leaping over furniture, surprisingly indifferent to scrapes and
bruises. More rarely he was the voracious shark. He sustained the play
for some months, elaborating, embellishing, and extending while continually switching roles. Once as hero, he brandished a stick, and wondered if he should be a rescuing witch with a wand or Robin Hood with
a sword. It was a crossroads metaphor: the stick could stand for the
illusory magical phallus of a woman or symbolize the extension of the
powerful phallus of a man. What would lead him to the one choice or
the other?

As the treatment moved along, Beary could transiently be put aside
as an intermediary in favor of one of my books. A nightmare would
often inspire this more sophisticated play, a play which even Leslie
recognized was closer to the expected model of analytic interaction. "I
had a dream," he said. "I am with two of my friends and my father and
we are fishing. And there are sharks. And I am afraid of the sharks."
Leslie asked me to consult one of my books to find out what the dream
meant. He had become phobic about kidnappers and robbers in recent
days and was left downright clingy by it all. I opened a book that he
chose and pretended to read, "If a boy tells a scary dream about a
shark, ask him what he thinks about." Leslie answered that he was
afraid his body would be hurt. I read on. "If a boy says he's worried that
his body will be hurt, ask him what part." "My penis," Leslie said to me
and to the book and went right on with "Sometimes it's soft and sometimes it sticks up. But nobody can take it away because it's attached to
your body. Except with a knife they could take it away. I like to sleep in
my sister's nightgown." "Tell the boy," continued the book, "that he
sleeps in his sister's nightgowns so that it looks as if he's a girl who
doesn't have a penis." "Then a kidnapper won't take me," Leslie added, "and a robber won't rob my penis," thus summing up his recently
developed fear of kidnappers and robbers rather succinctly, I thought.
He launched into a description of a vagina, explaining that it was like a
fold but that there was a hole some place in there; only one had to cut
through the fold to get at it. Then he spoke about all the teeth that a
shark had and how careful one had to be to avoid being bitten by a
shark. I read again from the book: "If a boy talks about a vagina and at
the same time also talks about being bitten, tell him he's worried that

the hole in the vagina could bite his penis." Leslie corrected the book. He said the vagina had no teeth, but that maybe it was a sucking hole and could suck the penis into it.

He was almost 6 now. There had been many features of his growth that were worrisome initially and some of them were still worrisome. A fluidity persisted, but it was no longer the global fluidity that characterized his self and object representations at the beginning of his treatment. The organizing fantasies necessary to actualize the inherent maturational pull forward were paying off in a more advanced developmental organization. The earlier annihilation of self was now experienced as a threat to his penis, the earlier thoroughgoing introjective stance replaced with a more organized set of identifications involving males and females, the initial gender disorder transformed into a conflict about sexual role. The new organization was also giving him a fresh vantage point to examine the antecedent pathogens just as it was proving felicitous for his future growth.

Discussion

The illustrations demonstrate the similarities and differences in the psychoanalytic process of adults and children.

In the case of the adult woman, I tried to show how aspects of her character were initially mobilized in the analytic situation and, after a time, regressively changed back into components of the original childhood fantasies, events, and object relationships from which they were derived. Features of form and content of that revived past were channeled through her stuffed animal and consolidated in the transference. I described her reenacting as well as her recalling portions of childhood, inside and outside of the treatment setting, and getting to know about the pathogenic influences of those portions. Because of the process that led to her knowing, elements hitherto kept out of development by conflict and defense could be newly acted upon, integrated into the existing adult structures and transformed. The inherent need for synthesis provided the impetus for the resultant therapeutic action. The first presentation should have captured the overlapping and interweaving steps in the sequence of the treatment process in adults: (1) character; (2) transference; (3) the revived past; and (4) the effects of insight.

In the second case a little boy used a stuffed animal as a vehicle for a set of emerging experiences with his doctor, experiences which seemed too much for him to manage at first. The emergence was partly shaped by the past; the stuffed animal channeled and buffered the antecedents akin to the transference consolidation of the adult. Within that consolidation, the upsets of a past world surfaced, and he got to know about them in an effective way, even though his knowing was only a child's way and not an adult's. For the little boy, the stuffed animal also became a center for a set of *new* experiences, which provided some of the ingredients needed to actualize an emerging developmental organization. As a result of the reorganization, the upsets of the past world were engaged with new words, new cognitive states, new affects, new qualities of relationships, and new ways of knowing. Maturation and the resulting developmental pull forward gave additional impetus toward change, enhancing the complexity of the steps in the sequence. The second presentation should have highlighted those steps: (1) characteristic modes of relating; (2) the finding of both an old and a new object in the therapeutic interaction; (3) the revived past as pictured from different organizational perspectives; and (4) the changes resulting from the pull forward and the new cognitive position.

The clinical descriptions also illustrate how responsibilities for promoting and sustaining the treatment are allocated between patient and doctor and how that allocation is shaped by the concept of the process.

The doctor-patient relationship is the foundation upon which all else rests. The patient introduces the *potential* for the process. He acts upon the ambiguity of the treatment situation in a distinctively individual way, even when his response appears merely commonplace. This is the seed of resistance. The analyst reacts to the distinctiveness, assuming that an adaptive strategy lies embedded within it. This is the seed of interpretation. Action and reaction, resistance and interpretation, the operational dialectic in psychoanalysis, *activate* the process and *sustain* it through the anticipated sequence. An adult has the task of reviving and consolidating the infantile neurotic constellation within the transference, while affectively recalling or reenacting the pathogenic past. A child patient does this as well but has an additional task: he searches for ingredients within the setting that will promote whatever developmental phase is being clocked in by maturation. The analyst is the *guardian* of the psychoanalytic process. It is moved along with adults when he is mindful of the unresolved antecedent conflicts; and, being so mindful, concentrates on approaches that permit the transference to consolidate, because the transference, a central step in the emerging sequence, is the embodiment of the decisive pathogenic past. The treatment is facilitated with children when the analyst is *also* mindful of the requirements of development, so that he may attend to the concomitant task of facilitating phase progression. The child analyst's task can sometimes be a bit more complex, since the evolving developmental process pulls the patient forward, while the analytic process tends to pull him backward. Finding one's way within these cross-currents without violating the requirements of either process can be more than routinely taxing, but it is also often more challenging and exciting.

A simple but not entirely accurate way of looking at the differences between adults and children is to say that adults use the experiences of the analysis to revive the past, while children *also* use the experiences of the analysis to establish structures that will prepare them for the future and enable them to deal with the pathogenic past more effectively.

SUMMARY

In describing aspects of the analyses of an adult and a child, I focused on the clinically demonstrable observations, suggesting with annotated comments how the psychoanalytic process, the infrastructure of the treatment situation, informed the empirical data. I tried to show that Jessica used Rhino to cultivate experiences that took her back to her past, whereas Leslie *also* used Mr. Beary to actualize experiences which served as the nidus for a newly emerging developmental organization. The case descriptions do, of course, lend themselves to other theoretical discussions, e.g., the study of character development, or the origins of the sense of gender, or the meanings of transitional phenomena. It has taken some effort to avoid the temptation vigorously to pursue these areas. But the effort seems justified. The customary clamor about technique or dynamics or structure too often interferes with the focus upon the silent shaping process; and, after all, what distinguishes psychoanalysis from other therapies resides within the view of that process.

These are the main points of the summary:

1. It is useful to distinguish between the conceptualization of the psychoanalytic process and the operations necessary to introduce and sustain it. The process itself belongs to the conceptual realm of psychoanalysis, not its empirical realm.

2. The psychoanalytic process may be viewed as that sequence of steps which appears within the mind of the patient as the treatment proceeds. The steps are more often overlapping or interweaving than they are sharply delineated.

3. For adults and children the steps include characteristic modes of relating, a transference consolidation, the revival of earlier pathogens, and the effects of knowing. Children also use the setting for new experiences in the service of emerging developmental organizations. This

causes what is at times bewildering cross-currents, forward and backward.

4. The psychoanalytic process is the vehicle for therapeutic action.

5. The impetus for such action arises from the ego's integrative capacities in adults and children and is further fueled in children by the pull forward of developmental organizations.

6. All patients also use the analytic situation to experiment with new identifications, to mourn lost objects, and to overcome areas of inhibited development. While these are valuable and often necessary treatment actions, they are not specific to psychoanalysis.

7. These views of the process are useful for clinical work since they underscore the tasks of both participants in the setting. The patient introduces the potential for the treatment by being who he is. The analyst, the guardian of the process, confronts the distinctiveness of that presentation so that the process may be activated. As the sequence evolves, both share in the responsibility for sustaining its direction by committing themselves to the essential dialectic—resistance and interpretation.

From the Analysis of a 5-Year-Old Boy with Pathological Narcissism

EVA BERBERICH, M.D.

IN 1984 EGAN AND KERNBERG POINTED OUT THAT THERE WERE FEW clinical reports on children who suffered from intense narcissism and an ego disorder. This comment encouraged me to report the initial stages of the analysis of a 5-year-old boy, whose disturbance appears to fall into this type of disorder. Apart from questions discussed in the literature with regard to the genesis and underlying factors of such disorders—for example, the contribution of family dynamics to their development and maintenance, which were also evident in my patient—I wish to describe and consider, as a special feature of the case, the difficult start in life which this child had. He was born prematurely (4 weeks early, birth weight 2,200 gm), suffered from severe respiratory distress, and had to be treated for some time in the intensive care unit of a pediatric clinic, where he was kept alive in an incubator.

In considering how to assess the significance of this postnatal trauma, associated as it was with many painful interventions and the deficit in contact between mother and child, I found Greenacre's paper "Predisposition to Anxiety" (1941) to be helpful. Greenacre attempted to relate early life-threatening situations—she explicitly mentions postnatal illness—and the resulting tension states at an organismic level, which gave rise to a raised basic level of anxiety or its organic components, to increased infantile narcissism, especially in the case of severe neurosis. "I believe this organic stamp of suffering to consist of a genuine physiological sensitivity, a kind of increased indelibility of reaction to experience which heightens the anxiety potential of later life" (p. 54). "It seems to me quite evident that an increased early infantile anxiety can be expected to be associated with a complemen-

Associate member, German Psychoanalytical Association; Institutes of Heidelberg/Karlsruhe and Freiburg.

tary increase in the infantile narcissism . . . ; that, in fact, excess narcissism develops as part of the organism's overcoming of the excess anxiety before it can function even slightly as an independent unit in the environment" (p. 48). She also states that these patients have a strong tendency to exhibitionism, which is used unconsciously as an expression of anxiety and fear, not only to gain sympathy but also to control the situation by engendering anxiety and fear in the analyst.

Weil (1977) refers in a similar connection to a primitive linking of anxiety and anger which, in stress situations, can lead to affectomotor discharges and which reflects a kind of amalgamation of panic and rage.

In this report I should like to demonstrate how "endogenous physical distress" (Greenacre, 1966), combined with an early contact deficiency between mother and child, and certain pathological features of the parents, interacted with one another to give rise to a severe form of pathological narcissism and an ego disorder in such a young child. I would also like to describe how in the course of a year the pathological narcissistic structure could be replaced by more normal infantile narcissism, in keeping with the boy's age, thus enabling him to make a successful start at school. That so much could be achieved can be ascribed to the fact that the boy was able to cope with his blind or, as Greenacre and Weil term it, his amorphous rage/anxiety, because the attempt was repeatedly made to "reconstruct" these for him as results of his earliest experiences and thereby to bring them into an understandable connection with one another, even though he could not remember the experiences.

EARLY HISTORY

Max was 4 years and 11 months old at the start of the analysis, which lasted 2 years. He was brought to me because of his uncontrolled fits of rage, which made contact difficult for him in the kindergarten and also severely disturbed the family life at home. He was unpopular with other children of the same age because he tried to dominate them and order them about as if they were his underlings. He behaved in such a provocative and unpredictably aggressive way that dangerous injuries occurred, not just to himself but even more to other children. On one occasion, for example, he violently pushed a much smaller girl off a wall. Finally, the children in the kindergarten did not want to let him go on attending, especially since he completely destroyed other children's work if he found it particularly attractive. The weeping and protests of the other children did not seem to bother him in any way, or to make him either embarrassed or ashamed; on the contrary, he reacted in a cold and arrogant manner, quite without sympathy, so that even the adults were shocked by such callousness. More recently, the other children had begun to revenge themselves by making him increasingly into a scapegoat.

Max's mother also complained about his demanding behavior and the heartless manner in which he depreciated her and told her "to get lost" when she did not fulfill his expectations or anticipate his thoughts and wishes. He not only irritated his mother to exasperation, but also bullied his younger brother, especially in secret when no one was watching him. His relationship to his father was described as being less tense, but he had, nevertheless, recently threatened him with a plastic knife. When others rejected him, he usually thought that he was disliked and often withdrew completely. He would then be found sitting in a corner with an empty, lost look in his eyes and seemingly very wretched. He also once confessed to his father, "If things go on like this with the other kids, I don't want to live anymore."

The adults unanimously emphasized that Max seemed more relaxed when he accepted a special role or if he had someone's undivided attention. He liked to get to the kindergarten before 8 o'clock in the morning so that he could have the playleader to himself. He loved to converse with her in a completely adult way and became angry as soon as the other children appeared. He also made a habit, even before he was 5 years old, of not going directly home after the kindergarten. Instead he would wander around the downtown pedestrian zone. Apparently, the sales staff in the little boutiques were pleased to see him and greeted him in a friendly way. The fact that his absence was not noticed at home speaks for itself. His mother and younger brother would have a 2-hour nap after lunch and so, in any case, he could not get into the house. Later he was given his own latchkey.

His parents provided detailed information about Max's early history. However, they remained silent at first about their own personal difficulties, apparently being unable to see that their problems were connected with their child's disturbance. At the beginning of the analysis, therefore, I had only the following information: Max was the elder of two sons. His life had had a difficult beginning. Not only was he born 4 weeks prematurely, but he then developed respiratory distress which necessitated several weeks inpatient treatment and incubator care in a children's unit. The illness was followed by several bronchitic episodes during his first year of life. His father, who was a physician, himself administered the necessary injections and also, shortly before Max's first birthday, himself manually treated a paraphimosis the child had

developed. It is not hard to imagine that the life-threatening complications of the premature birth and immature lungs, which not only reduced the early contacts between mother and child but also resulted in
a series of painful experiences throughout the entire first year of life,
must have left their mark.

When Max was finally discharged to his mother's care she at first
found him "strange" and "difficult to feed." She described initial difficulties which were further exacerbated by the fact that Max's father
had been discharged from hospital at the same time, following a serious cardiac illness, and had also required nursing care. According to
the mother, however, the relationship with her first child soon became
"unbelievably close," and there followed a happy period for them both.
The mother carried Max around with her the whole day. She enjoyed
the way everyone reacted spontaneously to him because he was "beaming, interested, and lively." She did not, however, describe any play
activities which may have developed between her and the growing
baby.

As Max approached his second birthday, difficulties began to arise.
The mother was again pregnant at this time and herself observed how
she withdrew more and more from Max who, to her way of thinking,
was becoming independent much too early. She admitted preferring
small babies, whom one could mother and completely take care of. She
had on several occasions looked after someone else's baby around the
time that Max's analysis began.

The 18-month-old Max now began increasingly to emphasize his
independence. He not only rejected affection but often actually misin-
terpreted it as an attack. He developed sleep disturbances, which still
existed at the start of the analysis. He sat in his cot "howling like a
werewolf" (his mother's expression), was difficult to rouse, and only
calmed down in his parents' bed. Following a middle-ear infection
which he suffered about this time, he appeared to become hard of
hearing. During conversation at the dining table he often interrupted
with "What did you say?" and appeared actually to miss a lot of the
conversation. An operation which had been advised by an ear, nose
and throat specialist was canceled at the mother's request. She was
reluctant to believe that Max had an organic partial deafness, particularly as this could not be objectively confirmed. I also observed this
apparent hardness of hearing at the commencement of the analysis,
but interpreted it as a kind of "autistic withdrawal." Max often appeared unaware of my presence and behaved as if he were alone in the
room. As the treatment progressed, he was able to abandon this form
of withdrawal.

Initially Max reacted with interest to the birth of his brother—he was 2 years and 2 months old at the time. He was always present at breast-feeding times and occasionally was allowed a try at the breast. He wanted to know what had happened to him after his own birth, as compared to his brother. In the analytic sessions he was at first able to cope with the dangerous and frightening stories about his first weeks of life only by reinterpreting them, as though they conveyed an especial form of distinction, thus apparently making them favorable in his own eyes. In the weeks following the birth of his brother, Max became more aggressive and demanding, and hence more trying for those in his environment. One particular comment by Max's mother deserves mention. She emphasized that both her husband and her own mother believed Max to be "a special child"—a little genius. The grandmother considered him to be a kind of "brilliant first-born child," very much like the mother's 3-year-older brother, who had been similarly highly regarded, and in contrast to whom she herself had, from the beginning, been a failure at school. Max's mother herself was more reserved in her assessment of his abilities, but his father apparently believed and also hoped that his first-born child would accomplish all those things which he himself, despite his evident abilities, could no longer hope to achieve.

ASPECTS OF THE THERAPY

I wish to restrict my presentation to the first year of analysis, which took place four times a week. I would like to place particular emphasis on the relationship which developed between the child and myself, the ways and means he used to try to dominate and manipulate me, and the role into which I felt myself forced. I would further like to describe how, mainly with the help of the child himself, my original hypothesis regarding the early traumatization was supplemented by a growing awareness of the influence that the psychopathology of both parents was having on the child's disturbance. Each of these aspects had a decisive effect on my approach which, somewhat artificially, I will present step by step, according to the gradually developing change in the therapeutic atmosphere. Here I refer to the growing ability of the child to cope with the stresses of the analytic work, to allow interpretations, and to let his feelings surface without immediately having to get into a state of blind rage, anxiety, and tension in which he would no longer be accessible to intervention.

Max was a small, delicately built, restless boy with a sensitive face. He had large, dark eyes which could sometimes blaze incredibly with anger, but at other times he had a lost and empty gaze. From the very beginning I had two main difficulties to contend with. First of all, Max was apparently convinced that only one of us could be in charge and that it must be he. I had to defer to him, to submit to his tyrannical will, and to admire him whenever he so desired. It was always Max who possessed all available weapons with which he threatened me mercilessly, while I had to remain powerless and, indeed, to some extent actually felt myself to be so. He obviously expected only trouble, threats, and destructive acts from me, and for his part tried to forestall these by opening each session with dramatic attacks on me, even before he had entered my consulting room. He himself expressed this on one occasion by saying, "The robbers are wicked first, so that nobody can be wicked to them." Incidentally, he constantly addressed me with his mother's name and, in moments of great anger, also seemed to be somewhat confused as to who I actually was. Then there were other moments when I did not even exist for him, or at most only as a kind of slave. "You are my bear, since I haven't got another at the moment, and you've got to do what I say at once if you don't want your ears boxed." He also used to denigrate, in an unchildlike manner, everything I said or did. He succeeded in inducing in me a feeling of complete subjection, helplessness, and incompetence as well as powerless anger; it really seemed in such moments that there was nothing I could do. Everything happened so quickly that I hardly had time to understand, much less to interpret, what was going on. If I had not kept a careful record of each session, and received supervision[1] enabling me afterward to gain insight and, time after time, to come to cathect the child and the analysis positively once again, I should presumably have begun to want to break off the therapy. Indeed, I gradually came to fear the sessions with Max. However, I soon realized that it was not only a matter of his own feelings of helplessness and absolute subjection, experienced in the postnatal period, being transferred in that he was making me feel weak, dependent, and threatened, but I also began to suspect that he wanted, in addition, to make me understand how people were still behaving toward him and how he experienced this. Corresponding interpretations had no influence at this juncture; he simply covered his ears and said, "I am deaf."

The second difficulty was presented by his blind, undirected attacks of rage and panic, which threatened to overwhelm him completely and which were always provoked by his being confronted with his own limitations or else by other trivial, to me at first hardly perceptible,

1. I am greatly indebted to Dr. L. Schacht for the supervision of this case.

causes. Sometimes he arrived completely tensed up, and only the slightest frustration was needed to send him off the rails. If earlier I had been almost afraid of him, I now became afraid for him; he would go so completely wild that I could not help fearing he would "go to pieces." He himself seemed to fear his own rage and called it "frightening." My room often finished up in utter disorder; however, this rather seemed to have a calming effect on Max, as if he felt that this inner turmoil had been transferred to his surroundings.

Despite all the turbulence which reigned in the sessions, I was more and more led by the boy to pay increasing attention to his parents and their personal difficulties, as well as to his own early history. I was helped in this by Max who had quickly grasped how I was seeking associations since I had, from the beginning, shared my conjectures with him—however vague, tentative, or indeed misdirected they might be. He had a great ability to make statements about himself and to offer explanations or interpretations by using catchy metaphors, or in the guise of fairy tales which he had transformed in an entirely personal way. He did this indirectly and without immediately exposing himself. For the time being he was saved from confrontation with the underlying painful content.

I gradually became aware of three distinct themes, which crystallized during the therapy and which were also confirmed as important by his parents. The diverse forms he used to express his feeling of being threatened could not be explained simply by the actual threat to life in his early days, the projection of his own aggression, or the threatening quality of his normal infantile drives.

First, there was the theme of being threatened, not only by me during the sessions, where I had to be very careful that he did not injure himself, but also outside them, where he created situations dangerous to himself in a very concrete way. In doing so, he sometimes suffered quite serious injuries. He also liked to deal with his feelings of being in danger through stories about other small boys, who were either killed in bicycle accidents or who died from brain tumors (his father was an oncologist).

The fairy tale "Little Brother and Sister" ended in Max's version with the little brother, disguised as a reindeer, being poisoned by an old lady. He related that Robin Hood, too, died from eating poisoned soup given to him by an old woman. I understood this as evidence of a threat from the preoedipal mother. Moreover, it became clear in the transference that I too was being referred to here. With the following story about a little panda bear, on the other hand, Max thematized a conflict which existed between himself and his father: "Once upon a time there was a little panda bear, whose parents wanted him to be dead. But they didn't know that he had magical powers, and he changed his father into a stone."

The second theme, that of being "dropped," seemed to be linked with the idea, "I must become something very special, otherwise Daddy won't love me anymore." During the sessions, Max brought up the question of how safe the gutters under my window might be. More than once he tested my reaction by unexpectedly leaning right out of the window and calling out, "Help, help, I'm falling!" I soon noticed that despite the undoubtedly high esteem in which he was held by his parents, they showed little empathy or readiness to respond to his needs. The parents' own interests always took precedence, for example, with regard to the regularity of attendance at the sessions. It happened occasionally that Max was not brought to his hours for some trivial reasons, or even that I was given false explanations for his absence. Max was always infuriated on such occasions, not because he suffered from the separation, but because he was made so aware of having to adapt himself to the wishes of his parents. In his anger he then planned to destroy the whole world and build a series of armored cars during the sessions, using his coat as a windscreen. Max was therefore aware—this became clear to me—of being exposed to the contradiction of high expectations linked with the demands for extreme conformity. The high expectations, with which he had identified, were expressed in his ideas about hobbies. These were not at all typical for his age but rather reflected the interests his father wanted him to share. They included sailing, surfing, fencing, flying aeroplanes, and riding powerful motor bikes—all activities that actually aroused anxiety in him, that he could not yet learn to do, and that confronted him once again with his smallness and inferiority. He stated firmly that he would be "dropped" by his father if he were unable to do all these things.

He could not express, however, how he would feel if he tried to come up to these expectations on his own. This brings me to the third theme which he indicated to me, namely, his feeling of lifelessness. He would say, "I have a heart of stone," or "Do you know the story of the little boy who got lost in the snow and never found his way home?" Or, taken from Hans Christian Andersen's story of the Snow Queen: "Kai could only do evil after the Snow Queen had given him a heart of ice." Or, finally: "Have you ever seen a knight in prison uniform?" This last example seemed to me to be the most telling metaphor for his internal conflicts. Signs that something else was concealed—perhaps something positive—came only fleetingly and furtively: "There is something one can't see and I must keep it secret. No one knows my names."

Discussions with his parents gradually clarified certain questions which had posed themselves. Prominent among them was his sense of being existentially threatened. This feeling was apparently shared by the parents. The burglar alarm they had recently installed in their house showed that they also had projected internal feelings of threat to the external world. Furthermore, it became clear that the father—once a brilliant student—had become to some extent resigned, and had abandoned certain ambitions; for example, that of becoming a professor. Since Max's birth, coinciding with his own illness which he had experienced as life-threatening, he had lived with the fear of suddenly "dropping dead like father" as a result of heart failure. He reported increasingly frequent "heart attacks" at night. Max's mother, for her part, had declared in front of the children that if this happened, she would kill herself and the children. She had been struggling anyway with depression and thoughts of suicide ever since the death of her own father when she was 15 years old. "Since Max could speak, he has only talked about death," I was told.

Max had attached himself firmly to his father, who in turn had focused all his hopes on this promising son. But he had made it clear to Max that fatherly love would only be forthcoming under certain specific conditions. One had to be splendid and brilliant; vulnerability, sensitivity, and anxiety were not permitted since they would cause disappointment to the father. Similarly, Max had said to me, "You can only win me over if you pluck the sky down for me." At the same time, Max was aware that these opinions and expectations of him did not really correspond to his nature. He was treated as an "as-if child" or "model child" and not as the person he actually was. He had, therefore, to hide his true feelings of inferiority, smallness, and sensitivity, and protect himself with omnipotent and megalomanic fantasies. I mentioned earlier the callousness used by Max to cope with his environment. I understood this to be a reaction to what he probably experienced as coldness when his mother withdrew herself as she again became pregnant: a coldness which he appropriated for himself and used as his own defense.[2] It led, as Ferenczi (1931) said, to a narcissistic splitting of the self into a know-it-all, unfeeling part and a painfully feeling but brutally destroyed part. The condensation of vulnerability and callousness was expressed in his frequent use of snow and glass as metaphors.

Considering the ways I tried to bring my influence to bear, I would say that my first efforts were directed to reducing his attacks of blind anger that almost led to disintegration. Any interpretations of conflict

2. I am using here a suggestion from Mrs. H. Kennedy.

made at such times had, in any case, no chance of success. I attempted to adapt myself as far as possible to him and to accommodate to his needs, trying to fulfill his wishes where these seemed to me to be justified. For example, because his parents did not accompany Max up the two flights of stairs to my office, I came downstairs to collect him. I later managed to achieve a situation in which he was once again brought all the way up. This delighted him. I was made aware that he hardly knew how to channel outbreaks of great joy and tended to turn rather to aggressive behavior. I gradually attempted to comment on the steps of my therapeutic contributions or on my attitude. The fact that I was able to remain calm and did not become anxious when he had his outbursts had already succeeded in subduing him a little. I began cautiously to express my conjectures about how children probably felt when no one paid attention to them or listened to them, whether they perhaps felt lost or insecure. Some would probably feel anger that was so great they would not know how to dispose of it.

At first Max was only capable of listening for a short time. Since we were now talking about other children, he did not feel threatened. One could see that he briefly considered and compared how it was in his case. He admitted feeling anger and that it was "frightening," but he categorically rejected at this stage the words "insecure," "lost," or even "anxious" as applying to him. But he was always ready to hear how these things applied to other children whose friendship he certainly secretly longed for. This provided an opportunity to bring certain things home to him, even if only in very small steps. At first he misunderstood my attempt to draw comparisons with his own situation as an attack; later, however, it seemed to appeal to him that I was taking so much trouble with him. "Think about it, then," he would say occasionally, "and tell me tomorrow what comes out."

He certainly liked to feel my constant interest irrespective of whether he staged destructive scenes, was bored, or came with seemingly interesting ideas, which he was then unable to realize because they were too ambitious and unchildlike, and whose failure he angrily blamed on me. For my part, I had a great deal of trouble, at least in the early phase of the treatment, constantly to recharge my interest in him and the analytic process.

Gradually, longer intervals would occur in which he did not know what to do with himself. Although he complained bitterly about this and put the blame on me, he allowed himself to be reassured by my supportive comment that it was of course difficult to tolerate not knowing what to do. Only as he allowed himself to experiment a little, with my contribution consisting merely of relieving his despondency and keeping his interest alive, something would arise spontaneously that pleased him and excited his enthusiasm. He marched out after such sessions with the proud air of a person who has accomplished something important. When failures occurred—at the beginning a reason for giving everything up—he soon became curious when I simply started a new attempt with the remark, "Let's think what we have to do differently." This was often enough for him to take the situation into his own hands again. He rediscovered his pleasure in painting, which he had completely given up, with the remark, "My Daddy said I am no painter."

After one year his ways of coping with anger, fear, and tension states had changed, so that such outbursts no longer occurred. Step by step his reaction to everyday frustrations had modified; above all it was no longer necessary for him to turn immediately to physical action. He was capable of turning over in his mind the various possible ways of reacting, ways which indicated his increased autonomy, more stable self-esteem, or healthy infantile narcissism as well as an increased ability for relative dependence. "You might as well help me a bit" was a completely new type of comment from him. At this stage, outbursts of anger began to give way to the idea that one could retreat from everything and go to another planet. If, however, one wanted to remain on earth, he continued, one could kill everyone, but then one would be alone, would have nobody to look after one, and would have to leave home. A better idea would be if one had a "Meister Eder"—a reference to a children's game on German television—who helped one to get out of all predicaments. Up to this point the clinical picture had been dominated by total dependence, first on an environment which took care of oral needs and then on an object that was constantly available. At a time when he did not pass the numerous tests of courage set by his father and could feel the latter's disappointment, he made a remark that could serve as the motto for his life up to then: "The day was shit—awful from the beginning."

A wild session which followed soon afterward was described by the boy, at my insistence: "At first I was sad, then I became anxious, and then I went wild in your room." He accepted my response that "being bad seems to be connected with anxiety"; in fact, he had himself shortly before explained, "When I am anxious, the first thing I do is to start hitting people." Then he proposed, "We'll have a game: you are me and I am you; then you'll know what it is like and you'll act bad." It was also becoming possible to talk more about anxiety in the face of demands connected with growing up, for example (he was just about to start school), and in the face of the demands from his father, who was not supposed to know anything about the boy's anxieties. However clear the association had meanwhile become for him, he nevertheless had no great hopes or optimism at this stage that without continual support from outside, he would be able to cope with his anxiety in any other way than by becoming bad. On the other hand he still felt it was quite alright if he became aggressive and possibly injured others when he felt anxious. However, it was still not clear to him that this could also be the reason for his loneliness. He was by now able to bear someone taking an interest in him, without misinterpreting such behavior, as he had formerly done. But he was still scarcely capable of adjusting to others: "The wicked animal has to be wicked forever, the witches have seen to that. It can be good for a little while if someone treats it well, then it is bad forever," he declared, apparently without emotion. And the little Lego-spirit figure which he brought to the last session before my summer vacation was only able to shine if a torch was beamed on it for 10 minutes. "But it is a kind spirit, I will put it outside my bedroom door, it drives the bad spirits away."

The summer break was going to be unusually long as a result of inept planning on the part of his parents. Max was going away with them for four weeks, and then there would be only one week left before my vacation began. In fact, the break lasted even longer because the mother of Max's father had died suddenly. She, too, had "simply dropped dead," like the father's father. Max's father was very depressed and anxious. He told me he could not bring the boy because the whole family was staying for the time being in the grandmother's house in another town in order to dispose of the house contents.

When Max finally did come, he was full of resentment and ambivalence toward me. He showed clearly his jealousy of the other children who had been coming in the meantime. He wanted to borrow a long piece of string from me, and said he needed it for his grandmother's garden shed. This was the only, very indirect comment that he made at first about his grandmother's death. My remark that we could perhaps have remained in contact with such a long piece of string was rejected by him with the explanation that there was no electricity in the string. Otherwise, he behaved as though nothing much had happened, took up an old game again, and offered once more—as he had already done before the holidays—numerous examples in support of his belief that as a child one was not heard, that attention was just not paid to children. "Why on earth doesn't anybody listen?" he asked suddenly, and this question also seemed to relate to the fact that nobody had brought him for therapy after his grandmother's death, even though (as I subsequently learned) he had developed breathing difficulties similar to hers. Later he told me that he had had to be taken by ambulance, with flashing blue lights, to the children's hospital as an emergency. This was not true, but was invented by him in order to give me a bad conscience. In this session he eventually brought up the question as to which of us would survive the other: whether he would throw me out the window or I would throw him out.

The question of who survives whom also was unresolved between his father and himself, and had, in fact, been so from his birth onward. It had already been raised before the holidays as well, when Max related the story of the television film. This question of who survives whom, when only one can survive, was now brought up between the two of us. Max had been sitting on the radiator and without waiting for my answer, he suddenly said, "I'm a snowman and I'm melting." Then he jumped off the radiator and wanted to look at a folder in which all his paintings were collected. It was the first time for a long while that he had wanted to do this, since, at some stage, he had decided not to paint anymore: "I'm not a painter, only painters do pictures." Now we looked together at all the pictures, and Max wanted me to tell him what he had said at the time about each picture. Although he sometimes remembered himself, he seemed to want me "to participate in the memories" (Schacht, 1978). It took a long time to go through them all, Max listening to me carefully and sometimes adding comments. He now liked all the pictures, although before he had never been satisfied with them. He indicated humorously all the colored pieces of cardboard which he had covered with scribble so that no other child would be able to use them. "I'll paint a new, much better picture," he decided. However, as the session was now at an end, he had to postpone this and, on leaving, said emphatically to me, "Please keep them all carefully for me."

Concluding Comments

I have ended my report here since our relationship underwent a change at this point, in that Max no longer had to fight constantly with me and denigrate "me and my helper's helper," as he had once referred to me. Instead, he was much more capable of exploring, together with me, the negative aspects of himself which he had previously projected onto me. His attitude to himself grew more critical and realistic. His grandiose fantasies became modified into normal infantile narcissism and a normal phallic-narcissistically toned self-image, appropriate for his age, with a reduction in tension between his ideal and real selves, which he found increasingly tolerable. He remained extremely sensitive about himself and preoccupied with his own affairs in an egocentric way. He showed little capacity for empathy, had brittle emotional object relationships, and was still unable to make friends.

Interestingly enough, like Matt, the patient of Egan and Kernberg (1984), Max had been able, during the first long separation from the therapist, to develop new ideas about the possibility, and indeed the necessity, of maintaining the connection to another person—in this case the analyst—even in this person's absence. At first Max had "eaten" me with obvious enjoyment. "You tasted good," he said. Nevertheless the feeling had remained that I could only protect him within the analytic setting. He also spoke about having a telephone cable for emergencies. In a dream Matt ate somebody who wanted to leave him and who was then turned into a gingerbread man. In his case, too, there was at first the same awareness of the need for constant supplies from an external source: oxygen in the form of the analyst. Max needed a "kind spirit" as protection. This spirit always had to be recharged; that is, Max needed continuing narcissistic supplies in order to deal with the "bad spirits." The "bad animal" could only briefly be good in those moments when it was kindly treated. Both patients, however, were later able to permit a more constant interpretation of the narcissistic defense and its ego function.

This phase of Max's treatment ended when "the snowman melted." It was the moment when the murderous fantasies and real feelings, still unresolved between him and his father/brother, were consciously expressed for the first time in our relationship.

In pathogenic terms, the child's low tolerance of frustration and anxiety, deriving from his postnatal illness, had resulted in a negatively toned perception of his mother and had bestowed dangerous and threatening attributes on the introjected mother that did not correspond to her real nature. I assume that she had in fact used the child to obtain emotional warmth because of her own depressed state, and had herself then experienced separation anxiety when Max began to be more self-sufficient as he entered the anal stage. Nevertheless, she seemed to have taken trouble to compensate the child for the suffering he had had to bear right at the beginning of his life; for example, she had carried him around everywhere with her in his first year. Her subsequent withdrawal, however, as Max entered the rapprochement phase, must have been experienced by him as inconsistency and must have lessened his sense of security and feelings of self-esteem, especially because in any case his ability to bear frustration was not great.

Turning to his father brought him esteem only if he promised to be brilliant. He tried to adjust to the image that his father projected onto him. However, this meant that only those aspects of his nature which corresponded to this image could find expression. Under these circumstances he had to develop a feeling of self-esteem which was not supported and maintained from within himself—a false identity that required the continuing reinforcement from others or remained dependent on a hypercathexis of grandiose ideas and deeds.

It seems to me that my clinical material provides confirmation for the ideas of Egan and Kernberg on pathological narcissism in children, broadened by the additional aspect of the vital postnatal impairment with its interruption of early contact with the mother: an aspect which contributed to the severity of the clinical picture and also determined the technical procedure at the beginning of the therapy. The subsequently satisfactory development of this patient shows that the boy could make use of the emotional growth process of therapy and become able to face his conflicts.

BIBLIOGRAPHY

BENE, A. (1979). The question of narcissistic personality disorders. *Bull. Hampstead Clin.*, 2:209–218.

EGAN, J. & KERNBERG, P. F. (1984). Pathological narcissism in childhood. *J. Amer. Psychoanal. Assn.*, 32:39–62.

FERENCZI, S. (1931). Child-analysis in the analysis of adults. In *Final Contributions to the Problems & Methods of Psycho-Analysis*. London: Hogarth Press, 1955, pp. 126–142.

GREENACRE, P. (1941). The predisposition to anxiety. In *Trauma, Growth, and Personality*. New York: Int. Univ. Press, 1952, pp. 27–82.

—————— (1966). Problems of overidealization of the analyst and of analysis. In *Emotional Growth*. New York: Int. Univ. Press, 1971, 2:743–761.

—————— (1967). The influence of infantile trauma on genetic patterns. *Ibid.*, 1:260–299.

KERNBERG, O. F. (1974). Further contributions to the treatment of narcissistic personalities. *Int. J. Psychoanal.*, 55:215–240.

—————— (1975). Normal and pathological narcissism. In *Borderline Conditions and Pathological Narcissism*. New York: Aronson, pp. 315–343.

KOHUT, H. (1972). Thoughts on narcissism and narcissistic rage. *Psychoanal. Study Child*, 27:360–400.

MOORE, B. E. (1975). Toward a clarification on the concept of narcissism. *Psychoanal. Study Child*, 30:243–276.

REICH, A. (1954). Early identifications as archaic elements in the superego. *J. Amer. Psychoanal. Assn.*, 2:218–238.

———— (1960). Pathologic forms of self-esteem regulation. *Psychoanal. Study Child*, 15:215–232.

SCHACHT, L. (1978). Die Entdeckung der Lebensgeschichte. *Psyche*, 32:97– 110.

TYSON, P. & TYSON, R. L. (1984). Narcissism and superego development. *J. Amer. Psychoanal. Assn.*, 32:75–98.

WEIL, A. (1970). The basic core. *Psychoanal. Study Child*, 25:442–460.

———— (1977). Maturational variations and genetic-dynamic issues. *J. Amer. Psychoanal. Assn.*, 26:461–491.

The Disavowal of Authority in a Child of Divorce

T. WAYNE DOWNEY, M.D.

AS ANNA FREUD (1969) HAS CAUTIONED, PSYCHOANALYSIS PERFORMED ON a "battlefield" may be impossible. If not impossible, it is likely to be overburdened by a variety of contemporary crises and conflicts between the individual and his environment which will constantly and unpredictably interfere with the establishment or continuity of an analytic process. Day-to-day events erratically impinging on the reflective potentialities of analysis keep the analysand in a state of alertness to external danger which greatly hampers internal developments such as the transference neurosis and depth-psychological events such as reconstruction. Ultimately the "battlefield" quality of the treatment may come to doom the analysis itself either by logistically blocking the patient's access to analysis or by destroying his psychological potentials for analyzability. Then we may be left, like Freud (1905) in the Dora case, to console ourselves with the sad dictum that analysis may have to settle for confirming certain aspects of the human condition where it is unable to assist the patient in substantially remediating his condition.

The narrative I am about to present falls somewhere in between. While Sally's case may sound both dour and dire, and indeed it is to some extent, the process of selecting it for this particular type of presentation enhances and retrospectively reinforces the more negative aspects of the treatment. I will focus on what in the family milieu of divorce interfered with the psychoanalytic process rather than what propelled it. As I will describe later on, child analysis was essential to Sally's recovery from a severe depressive state. The manner of her

---

Training and supervising analyst at the Western New England Institute for Psychoanalysis; associate clinical professor of pediatrics and psychiatry, Child Study Center, New Haven.

Presented at the 35th Congress of the International Psychoanalytical Association, Montreal, Canada, July 30, 1987.

recovery may have dissipated her suicidal potential. The paradoxical effect of child analysis was that it freed up Sally as an individual and opened her eyes to more clearly viewing herself, her parents, and the world. The analysis at a certain point conspired with inaccessible aspects of her preoedipal development *and* ongoing external events to crystallize partially into the antiauthoritarian disavowing character adaptation.

Sally came to analysis as a frightened, passive, withdrawn child easily overwhelmed by depressive affect and self-injurious preoccupations. She departed her unfinished analysis more actively engaged with the world. She rejected her parents in reality, while consciously and unconsciously she utilized the regenerated positive parent and grandparent mental representations to maintain self-esteem and self-integrity in a world of unending crisis.

In child analysis we are increasingly confronted by this "battlefield" dilemma as parents bring us their troubled children suffering in the throes of family breakdown. In this context of separation and divorce we may encounter severely ill children or children at risk of major disturbance. We assess children whose resources are scanty. We see children who have already been marked in their prehistory by the relational stresses of the marital couple. For these children who are at such risk of permanent psychological injury (if it has not occurred already) child analysis asserts itself as potentially the most effective treatment. At best it would aim to arrest regressive trends in the child's personality and restore healthy developmental processes. In the worst case situations child analysis would function as the most efficient mode of assessing psychological damage and maintaining "damage control." The risks in such hazardous circumstances are obvious. Environmental pressures and internal vulnerabilities may not allow the child to remove himself sufficiently from the marital fray. To the extent that the divorce remains "unconsummated" it provides the parents with a "license to hate," and their child's analysis may then become yet another opportunity for injuring each other and their child in the guise of rescuing the child from the other parent. As with adults, it is the child in such dire circumstances who can convert the exigencies of their life into fantasy and the life of imagination and who stands the best chance of utilizing analysis for personal gain. Sally presented as such a child.

Sally was an extremely sad and distraught child in such a raw situation. She was in analysis for 35 months. I have presented other aspects of her analysis focusing on some of her more positive psychological potentials and other developmental and analytic dynamics (Downey, 1984). When first seen she was literally crying out for help. Her parents were in the process of a final separation leading to divorce. She was referred for analysis by her mother's analyst. Another child analyst had offered a similar recommendation. Prior to this crisis period, just before her eighth birthday, Sally had been characterized as a quiet, sensitive, eager-to-please child. As her parents' permanent rift became more obvious, she became profoundly depressed. She was one of the most depressed children of her age that I have encountered. She cried constantly at home and in school. She cried herself to sleep. She became unconsolable. There were unpredictable outbursts of temper. Both of her parents remarked on a change in their perception of Sally. Whereas previously they had characterized her as loving and lovable, they now perceived her as frustrating and unlovable. She rebuffed her mother's efforts to hold and comfort her. When her teacher approached her in school, she would slump onto the top of her desk and bury her head in her arms. Her legs were bruised and scratched. Always a clumsy child, in her distress she became even more uncoordinated. She was forever tripping, falling, and bumping into furniture. She picked compulsively at her wounds. Her father found her motor behavior particularly aggravating. Although he was hard pressed to deny Sally's obvious emotional disturbance, he tended to attribute it to some vague condition of neurological dysfunction. At the depths of her despair she often blurted out her wish that she would die and be spared her suffering.

Clinically Sally was obviously a deeply disturbed child whose ego organization and object relations were markedly impaired. There were wide swings from open-eyed friendly engagement during which she was an articulate, even precocious, conversationalist, to bleak depressive withdrawal of near-psychotic proportions. In this latter state she would huddle on my couch, unapproachable and unresponsive, sobbing and sucking her thumb. She would pull her jacket up over her head, hiding her body almost totally from view. In this act she dramatically re-created the sense of invisibility which is so often the experience of adults in the throes of depression.

PRECURSORS

Sally M.'s parents met in professional school. Mrs. M. described herself as having had a happy childhood in an upper-middle-class family. Mr. M. described an affluent upbringing in a family where members of several generations on both sides suffered from depression. His father was an alcoholic who died in old age of his disease. His mother killed herself suddenly when Mr. M. was a young child. Mrs. M. idolized her young husband and particularly his intelligence, intellect, and energy. Mr. M. was attracted as much by his wife's family as he was to her. He converted to her Protestant sect to marry her. He suffered in adult years from seasonal depressions which left him feeling "dead" for 3 to 4 months of the year.

After several years the marital stresses became severe as Mrs. M. was unable to live up to her husband's impossible expectations. By both their accounts he attacked, criticized, and belittled her constantly. Mrs. M. guiltily and masochistically redoubled her efforts to please him. She likewise became depressed. In this embattled context both parents sought treatment around the time of Sally's birth. She was their oldest child. Mrs. M. entered analysis when Sally was 6 months old. Shortly thereafter Mr. M. impulsively left the marriage. He did not return until Sally was well into her second year.

Sally was an easily satisfied infant who made few demands. Her mother described her infancy in ideal terms. Some years later Mrs. M.'s analyst reported that Sally would be brought to analysis during her first two years (particularly while her husband was separated from the young family). She would lie on the couch with her mother and occasionally pull her mother's hair or bite her quite strongly. In spite of her analyst's efforts to call attention to this disturbed behavior in the dyad, Mrs. M. was as helpless to counter these assaults by her daughter as she had been to protect herself from her husband's. This biting and hair-pulling behavior of the infant Sally suggest that these attacks on her mother were perhaps her attempt to break through her mother's depressive withdrawal and reestablish a lively contact. It also served as the prototype for the hostile behavior toward her parents in her incomplete recovery. Indeed, as time went on, the couple's exchanges became physical, too. Sally was exposed to interactions in which arguing led to light physical force and then to intercourse between her parents.

Mr. M. returned after 8 months. He proceeded to idealize Sally. He was convinced she was an infant prodigy who was destined to become a genius. He indicated during an interview early in Sally's analysis that his departure in Sally's infancy had been a protective measure initiated by homicidal impulses toward wife and child. He had been dimly aware of these impulses at the time. They had been confirmed in Mr. M.'s psychotherapy.

The other significant traumatic development in Sally's early childhood was the birth of her brother Jimmy during her fifth year. Up to Jimmy's birth her father had indulged Sally in his love as much as he had hated her mother. Mrs. M. likewise vied for Sally's affection. Following Jimmy's birth her father summarily declared that Sally was defective, like her mother. He shifted his energies to Jimmy as the new prodigy. Jimmy's endowment better conformed to his father's expectations. He became the "easy" child for both parents. Sally was pushed and pulled and also retreated back more into her mother's orbit. She began a slow, petulant slide into despair, which finally flared into depression with her parents' impending divorce.

CHILD ANALYSIS PROPER

The preanalytic period and the early phase of Sally's analysis necessarily included many contacts with Mr. and Mrs. M. together and separately to ascertain the degree of their support for her analysis. They entered into the process relatively dispassionately as one of many necessary arrangements for the dissolution of their marriage. Though we may surmise that all parties were unconsciously searching for an idealized reunion of the family bound by Sally at the center, overall, the extrusion dynamics were most prominent! They came to me at the end of an unsuccessful 3-month attempt at a rapprochement. This had been preceded by a 6-month separation during which Mr. M. devoted himself to his first love, travel. (Between the first separation when Sally was 6 months and this last one, there had been innumerable shorter ones.) Both parents initially wanted, even insisted, on Sally's analysis. The logistics involved in a 40-mile round trip to my office four times a week were worked out with apparent ease. While the parents freely exchanged criticisms of each other when together with me, they were emphatic in their understanding of Sally's critical need for help and support at that juncture.

Sally responded immediately to the provision of analysis for her and to her parents' cease-fire where she was concerned. Her depression started to resolve rapidly, and both parents reported with pleasure that they were recognizing the loving child they once knew as Sally. Sally related to me in an expectable manner as a helper and as a positive parental figure. Her play mainly involved card games which emphasized predictability and regular sequences. There were also marble games based on finding "lost" or hidden objects. Obviously in this early phase she was working on reordering her world, banishing interpersonal chaos, and reestablishing a lost equilibrium. The analytic process depleted the depressive and suicidal potentials which she had voiced earlier. The analyst "is on my side, right?" she queried.

About 6 months into Sally's analysis, war suddenly erupted anew between the parents. Divorce negotiations were entering their final phase. Mrs. M. was holding the line with her husband. For once, she was not aquiescing to his demands. This had never happened before. While he initially maintained with me that he supported his daughter's analysis as much as ever, he became quite fearful that his soon-to-be ex-wife was "taking" him through his participation in Sally's treatment. He fired off the following note to his wife: "Because I think there are unequal sacrifices involved in the therapy with Sally (I have to give up something I really love and you do not [Mr. M.'s travel plans]), I am not willing to drive her back and forth to Guilford. The extra inconvenience that this poses for you should come close to balancing out the sacrifices we make to see that she gets proper psychotherapy." Mr. M. also abruptly refused to talk with me. This began a tug-of-war over which parent was contributing or sacrificing more to their children's welfare, which was to go on for years, long past the interruption of Sally's analysis. And thus began an ultimately futile attempt on the part of Sally's mother to fill the gaps in the economic and transportational arrangements supporting her daughter's treatment by employing a patchwork of family loans and hired drivers bringing Sally to analysis.

Sally was once again devastated. Her associations were to Jimmy's birth and her parents' last separation. This time, however, she became angry with her father rather than blanketed with depression. Against all evidence she had maintained an idealized image of both her father and her mother. If her father, in an overdetermined incident the previous spring, had lost his temper and slapped her, he had good reason to. He was right. She had no right to stand up to him and protest. She had been wrong. She deserved what he inflicted upon her. It was her deserved punishment.

Over the next 2 years she used the analysis to put her father into clearer focus. She stopped looking for his love and rationalizing his unexpected absences. The disappointments of visitation when he did not come to pick up herself and Jimmy diminished. "My Dad's crazy." "I can't think of anything true right now that he tells." She could not count on his love, let alone his baby. She slowly relinquished her wishes on both accounts. As she did so, her hatred and envy of her brother Jimmy for displacing her with her father came into bold relief. This, coupled with Mr. M.'s increasingly explicit negative equation of Sally and her mother and his obvious preference for Jimmy ultimately interfered with a potentially important, supportive coalition for both siblings during these troubled times.

The climate of Sally's analysis was never the same after her father withdrew his support. In subtle ways she was never again as open and enthusiastic about the help she might get from me. Her analysis became as precarious and tentative as the rest of her life. In addition to the usual separation issues around weekends and vacations, her statements that "I was afraid I wouldn't see you again" took on new meaning and new reality. Her idealizing transference was *prematurely* called into question by life's events. Her father's departure alerted her too soon to the "mortal" nature of her analysis. I and her analysis might vanish just as unpredictably as he did! She became more conservative in what she played out or brought up. A protective constriction set in.

Somewhat paradoxically the analytic stance of addressing realities enhanced Sally's sense of being on her own and alone with no one ultimately that she could count on. She tried again and again to make me that reliable and stable object, but events always conspired to erode her sense of that constant caring other. (Favorite games in this regard had to do with searching for changes in my appearance or in the consulting room after absences. She played a card game called "I Doubt It" where the participants attempt to determine when the other is cheating.) She dismissed her mother as helpless and ineffectual and also depressed. Her mother was ultimately not loving enough with her. Analysis helped her to reverse her guilty, self-injurious, depressive trends into a more cynical, yet self-assertive, independent, and isolated orientation. As she reiterated many times, "Nobody's perfect. Not me. Not you." This is certainly a common outcome among children of divorce. In Sally's case it seemed that child analysis may have contributed to a speeding up of this more typically adolescent development of a sort of cynical, desperate, and adaptive autonomy among children of divorce.

As she addressed her suicidal and her parricidal wishes, she shook free from some of the more negative aspects of both parents which she had internalized while holding onto the positive imagos. "I wish he was dead. He's going to kill himself, you know, and then I'm going to kill myself. I'm going to grow up, drive a car, and go to Mississippi and kill myself. . . . I'm just like my father. It's in the family." That had been her prediction early in her analysis. As she disavowed her father and mother as beloved authorities in her life, she cast off some of these negative identifications.

Ongoing events continued to contribute to Sally's growing perception that her parents were becoming increasingly powerless as they wrangled over divorce, child support, and visitation arrangements. Every few months one or the other parent would take the former spouse to court. Mr. M. went to court on many occasions to get decreased child support or permission to see the children separately. He often sought elaborate visitation schedules to redress his perception that he was the soft, sacrificing parent. Mrs. M. would countersue her husband to get child support reinstituted, as he usually withheld it at court times. Sally would respond in kind to these power moves on the part of her parents. She would refuse to visit Mr. M., talk to him on the phone, or read his letters. While overtly "sweet" and compliant with Mrs. M., she would steal from mother's sweets or steal her money to buy them.

In Sally's mind, the judge became the ultimate authority with the power of life or death and anything in between over herself and her parents. She became phobic about the judge and court appearances. She filled session after session with her distorted fears about the court and judges. The judge came to symbolize the abdication by her parents of loving responsibility for her care and protection. She came more and more to view them as fighting for the sake of fighting. As she put it, "They look for any anniversary to fight. I meant opportunity." She incorporated this perception into her own armamentarium much later as she approached adolescence. She seemed to fight on these very same terms.

During the many court crises that occurred, Sally's motivation to analyze (already compromised as I have indicated earlier) sank to near zero. She insisted on play activities which had to be pleasurable, mindless, and unreflective; or she obsessed about the fantasied dangers of court action. Occasionally she would draw aim on me as yet another adult who had let her down. Yet the analysis of the negative transference often turned into an entry to her own self-hatred and neurotic guilt at creating such unhappy circumstances for herself and her parents. Jimmy, however, usually deserved what he got, in her mind.

As an aspect of shutting out the unpleasantness in her life and refusing to examine current realities, Sally would stop working in school. She would become adamant and obviously antiauthoritarian about this. She would not budge, no matter what the threat or reward! School performance had special relevance for both parents. Not working in school also differentiated her from Jimmy, her now academically talented brother. It also reflected a tendency which was increasingly obvious in the analysis to "stonewall" (her term) when she felt the demands of the outside world were too threatening, intense, or otherwise intolerable. Where she had shut out the world with her coat and thumb as an 8-year-old, as an almost 11-year-old she would sit mute, looking away into space, avoiding eye contact, apparently impervious to those around her.

In the third year of her analysis, Sally's mother began to date. Sally experienced this as an ultimate rejection and betrayal. It had been difficult enough the previous year when her mother had reverted to her maiden name, leaving Sally and Jimmy with her father's name. But, her mother's dating brought to the surface a host of previously hidden, actively defended against, but probably partially conscious fantasies about her role in the marriage and divorce. They emerged relatively easily. They had a conventional, but powerful, dynamic quality. She felt herself responsible for all the family's difficulties. Only she could change and bring the parents back together! Mrs. M.'s dating also brought a new behavioral pattern to the surface. For the first time, Sally's mother described her daughter as acting in a conscious, purposeful, negative, belligerent manner toward her. That is, stonewalling was now joined by lying as part of Sally's psychological armor. Sally, defensively and defiantly, acknowledged her lying and her manipulation of her mother. There was no guilt or remorse. She felt justified in this. However, she went on to outline her contrary feeling of guilt, that she had caused her parents many separations and finally the divorce. If she hadn't been born, they would have lived happily. Jimmy was her "good" replacement. If she had enough time, she would "get better" and bring them back together. She felt that she needed to do whatever she could to keep alive the possibility that her mother and father might reunite. This development flew in the face of the realities of Mr. M.'s life with its parade of lovers. It seemed more involved in maintaining a secret, exclusive, sadoerotic relationship with her mother, which I described early in the paper but which I had no knowledge of at this time in the analysis.

In its third year, time finally ran out on Sally's analysis. She had made significant gains overcoming her depression and negative self-image. The frequency of treatment seemed approximately to keep pace with the erosive effects of the parents' ongoing hostilities and Sally's active counterattacks on each of them. Sally continued to maintain a qualified interest in me and the analysis. However, a number of events conspired to make that impossible. Mrs. M. moved to better housing even further away from my office. Even with a moderate fee, funding for the analysis became questionable as resources in Mrs. M.'s family of origin dried up. Jimmy developed a sleep disturbance which urgently required treatment at a site even further from home. With increasing age the realities and horrors of the divorce were more than he could deny. With Mrs. M. working full time and Mr. M. refusing to participate (even though he was now once again consulting me about the children), the logistics of the analysis became impossible. Mrs. M. was also in the process of engagement to a man who looked dourly on what he took to be her overreliance on mental health professionals. After her analysis was interrupted, I continued to see Sally for a number of years on a less frequent and less regular basis—but that is another story.

DISCUSSION

Sally's plight might be paraphrased as follows: "Authority is not what it promises to be. It is to be distrusted. We must grow to disavow it; particularly when what should be parental strength hurts more than it helps. No one *really* cares for me. My parents don't seem to. They must hate me because they certainly don't help me! If I didn't need one or both of them so much—if I were older and could be on my own—I would reject them more openly just as they reject me. They have defaulted. They have disavowed me! In their own battle they have surrendered their parental rights to a judge. I fear a judge. I fear authorities. No authority will govern my life. I will take my life into my own hands. I will live it with choices, with calculating, self-absorbed hostility if need be. It is a war out there. No one can be depended on. Tell people what they want to hear. Do whatever you need to get what you want." Traumatic divorce without cessation of hostilities requires disavowal of authority!

While the impact of any life event must be understood in terms of the particular capacities and vulnerabilities of the individual, some events may be so powerful as to shape the individual's reaction in particular, overdetermined ways. Sally's use of disavowal is such an instance. Faced finally with the impossibility of her task of reuniting her fractured and fragmented family, she ambivalently, yet resignedly attempts her own version of psychological divorce. She attempts to capitalize on the split in her ego to draw a psychological line between herself and her parents whereby they will be punished for their inadequacies in raising her. No longer will she feel as guilty about not meeting their irrational needs. Through disavowal she attempts to turn her parents into "people" (albeit ineffective people) way before the time in late adolescence when this usually occurs as a function of normal development. While it goes beyond the scope of this brief paper, it is worth noting that these developments in Sally augur an antioedipal development. In the analyses of adults who experienced divorce as children we not infrequently encounter such an antioedipal transference state. For her parents to cede their parental rights and prerogatives to judges and to the legal system was for Sally, as it is for some other children, an ultimate abandonment, a parental disavowal of their child. Such a crime against childhood requires some children of divorce to react as Sally did to preserve through defiance, disavowal, and negation some semblance of sanity in a world where through the course of events and the reason of analysis madness becomes impossible to mislabel or avoid.

BIBLIOGRAPHY

DOWNEY, T. W. (1984). Within the pleasure principle. *Psychoanal. Study Child,* 39:101–136.
FREUD, A. (1969). Remarks at the New Haven, Ct. meeting of the Association for Child Analysis.
FREUD, S. (1905). Fragment of an analysis of a case of hysteria. *S.E.,* 7:7–122.

Some Reflections on the Inner Space and Its Contents

YEHOYAKIM STEIN, M.D.

THIS PAPER DEALS WITH INNER SPACE OF WOMEN AROUND THREE CENTRAL themes:

1. The dangerous content of the inside of the uterus, mainly the menstrual blood.
2. The dangerous space inside the uterus.
3. The symbolism of the pregnancy-abortion-pregnancy cycle.

The clinical material is based on the psychoanalytic treatment of a young woman.

Case History

A native Israeli of French origin and a student of the arts, Ella, 24 years old, complained of an increasing fear that something might happen to her parents, especially when she was not at home. She also worried about her short-term relationships with men and her unsatisfactory sex life. She was preoccupied with small wounds on her skin and with the idea that she was contaminated with all kinds of diseases. The skin affliction precipitated her decision to seek therapy.

Ella had been a difficult first child for her mother, and began suffering from allergies in babyhood. Her overprotective and overanxious mother overfed Ella and took her from one physician to another. When she was 3 years old, her sister was born. According to her mother, Ella had "no time" to envy her sister because she was thrust into kindergarten prematurely, an act which she interpreted as a sign of her mother's desire to be alone with the new baby. (Her sister had suffered an accident shortly before Ella began analysis.)

Visiting scholar at the Sigmund Freud Center, Hebrew University, Jerusalem; member, Israel Psychoanalytic Society.

At the age of 7, Ella became asthmatic after her mother unexpectedly introduced a puppy into the home and gave it the status of a baby by giving it a bottle, a little bed, and "all mother's love." At that time Ella started to excel at school in order to please her mother. Gradually, she developed the tendency of tormenting her mother; she insisted, for instance, on seeing her menstrual blood. Upon being refused, Ella told her girlfriends that her mother was pregnant, which was not true. Ella was then sent for treatment with a female therapist. She felt deeply offended to find out that it was only in therapy that she could get the care and warmth which she expected from her mother. Nevertheless, she recollected positive memories from the time she spent with the therapist.

Ella had her first period at 15½, only a few weeks before her sister, who was only 13. She had been terrified that her sister might pass her. For several years she suffered from menstrual irregularities, hemorrhoids, and subclinical hyperthyroidism. At the age of 19, she underwent plastic surgery on her nose, after which she felt even uglier and more inadequate.

Her sexual experience began at 19 with an encounter with two young men who took her to the seashore, stating that they would "open her up, with a knife if necessary." While all three were together, she had sex with both of them. She appeared to be amused when she told me the story. One of these men, with whom she continued the relationship for a while, was later killed in an accident.

In her later relationships with men, she preferred fellatio. During coitus, she was generally dry, experiencing pain that felt gratifying. She pretended orgasm, never knowing what she really felt. Simultaneous with her masochistically developing sex life, she began to be worried by the idea that her mother was getting old and that something might happen to her parents. At that time she suffered from a fungal skin disease on her legs, which she neglected until it appeared on her hands as well. "Now everybody can see my dirt," she thought. It is quite apparent that she felt like a criminal, but she had not the slightest idea what crime she had committed.

She described her father as a good-hearted, pleasant fellow, but superficial in his contacts. He preferred Ella to her sister, maybe even to her mother, and never failed to let her know this.

A suspicious, bitter, and impulsive woman, Ella's mother felt that the world was her enemy and she did not want to be disturbed by anybody. From time to time, she warned Ella that she would put her in an orphanage and that she herself would convert to Christianity and leave Israel. Sometimes her mother declared her intention to commit suicide, and rumor had it that she made an attempt when Ella was about 9 years old. Her mother hit Ella until she was 16.

From the beginning of the analytic process, one could trace Ella's compulsive urge toward and search for complete intactness and self-sufficiency with regard to her own body image and in her object relationships.

THE ANALYSIS

The first stage of Ella's analysis lasted about one year. It was characterized by a quick and intensive regression into the world of fantasy. My room was experienced as an arena of the primal scene. In the seventh month of analysis Ella verbalized her fear that she might become a "bad girl" and leave analysis. She then related a dream in which she observed a T-shaped blood clot on her leg. Associating she said, "A skin eruption on the leg is like a mental disease of the leg." I reminded her of the first letter of her family name, and of a crucifix as well. She feared that her skin would reveal her dirt and badness the moment that such a defect appeared on the surface. The crucifix reminded her of her bad mother, who threatened to leave her, as well as of the poor mother, who was sent to a convent school by her own neglecting parents and who was forced to leave home completely when she was 15. Ella spoke about the "primal scene." Christianity symbolized the guilt and punishment for her bad deeds. In her dream, she expressed the desperate temptation to preserve the intactness of her skin so that the primal scene could not make itself visible. On the other hand, she expressed the wish that the skin defect would protect her from becoming insane.

At about the same time that she had this dream, Ella was preoccupied in the analytic process with her thyroid. She associated the thyroid with a shutter (in Hebrew, the word shutter is also used for thyroid): "Shutter regulates the light. I'm frightened to be seen in strong light. I want my problems to regulate the thyroid toward the phlegmatic direction, but the thyroid pulls toward nervousness. The eyes will be expelled." Ella wished to see in her thyroid a regulator that would facilitate her staying in a static, protected state; but the thyroid, like her mother, expelled her into the cold world and demanded a hyperactive position from her. She was forced to leave the womb. In this context, the expelling eyes symbolized the forced delivery, the refusal of her mother to let her stay inside her. In her analysis, Ella was "hyperactive" in her associations in order to get well quickly, in order to please me. She was afraid that I, like her mother, wanted to get rid of her as fast as possible and push her into the outside world. She saw it as her duty to cooperate with that wish of mine.

The analysis proceeded; associative productions flew endlessly. This was a reflection of her hyperactive attitude and a defense against the fear of abandonment. In my consulting room, Ella tried to hide from the light, asking me to draw the curtains. She wanted to be protected from overstimulation by the outer world. But, alas, after a while my room, and especially the curtains which she faced, became a source of many fears. She perceived my room as a dark cellar, an inquisition room. The curtains were full of dark, terrifying circles, "twistings of the soul," monsters emerging out of a nightmare—some of them were red like blood. She heard terrifying noises; it seemed that there were wailings, as if cats were hiding there. Maybe these were her parents. The curtains reminded her of murderous crimes. My room became a frightening space and she, inside it, endured a drama of torture. She desired to find in my room a dusky, protective, and pleasant milieu, but most of the time she was forced to live in this terrible, dark, and bloody inner space. She produced many associations connected with falling inside a space or into dark holes. The analysis was like "an open wound in the air, a process of digging." Sometimes it felt like bleeding. This drama which she produced inside my room was partly a projection of the drama that she imagined had happened inside her mother, and partly a recapitulation of the primal scene with early acoustic stimulations as well as oral and anal-sadistic elements.

After one year of analysis, Ella entered a new phase. The hyperactivity stopped. She felt like a sleeping baby, like someone in hibernation: "The soul is undergoing a process while I stand aside." She was frigid. She no longer was obliged to prove her independence to me, feeling free to seek my protection. Sometimes she felt as if she was hiding under her mother's skin or under mine. She demanded body touch and care from me. She asked herself if her mother would accept her in this state. She was hiding in the protective milieu of my room, avoiding stimulation from both outside and inside. Then she began to be annoyed by the notion that I would not accept her as she was, and that she must stick to me like a leech in order not to be thrown out. The skin became the image of a womb in which she was hiding. We then began to observe oscillations in the image of the womb: between the good, warm, protecting, and the bad, frightening, and expelling organ. Sometimes she would express depressive feelings which she had tried to avoid all her life and during the first phase of psychoanalysis. On the other hand, the hibernation reflected a way of not feeling anything and avoiding her growing fear of being thrown out by me, especially now that her real intentions—to stick to me—became obvious. The hibernation also was a way of avoiding aggressive feelings which she had earlier projected onto others, especially me.

In the middle of the second year of analysis, Ella came out of hibernation and ventured toward the unknown. Her oral needs diminished and she was no longer frigid. I, as a transference figure, was perceived as much more earthy, "blood and flesh," and she herself was also more willing to be in contact with her own blood and flesh. She looked inside her body in order to find out what dangers might emerge from it. In terms of defense mechanisms, this stage was a breakthrough after the projective stage and the following hibernation stage with the repression of aggressive fantasies. At that time, her mother unexpectedly underwent a uterine myomectomy. Ella relived in her analysis frightening images related to the womb. She recollected her mother's refusal to show her the menstrual blood. "Mother preferred dying to showing me her blood. Father and mother copulated and the punishment is blood. Menstruation is like dying." As a child, Ella saw in her mother's menstrual blood the evidence of her tendency to commit suicide, which had been concealed from her. Mother brought death upon herself by copulating with father. Her own menstruation was the result of her sadomasochistic relationships. She sensed a sexual vacuum, death. In her imagination, the final abortion was associated with her fantasies about her own imaginary abortions: "They aborted my womb. I have the impulse to destroy it totally time and time again. Maybe by means of those humiliating fucks. Men destroy everything inside me." Every month Ella fantasized that she had forgotten to take the pill, so that she was always in a panic near the end of the cycle. She experienced this fantasy compulsively, and when her menstrual blood at last arrived, she felt released; then the whole thing repeated itself again.

Ella described her own menarche as a black day: "I was half dead; it was a physical effort to deliver the menstruation." This she associated with a black night, her mother crying in the bedroom, the punishment she got for listening to what was going on there, and fantasies about my black room. Ella believed that after delivering her, mother pushed her away as if she was just a placenta. She pushed her away again when her sister was born. "Why did mother not abort my sister? Abortion is murder. I abort every month. My sister's accident reminds me of her delivery. She was reborn after the accident." I interpreted to Ella that, as a child, she had repeatedly fantasized the destruction of her sister, who kept on reappearing intact. She wished to believe that her sister was aborted in mother's menstruation. Then she wanted to find out whether her mother's menstrual blood contained parts of her sister, at the same time trying to make sure that this was not true, and that Ella did not induce this act of violence. This was an analogue to hyperemesis gravidarum, where the double wish of the pregnant woman is to find pieces of the fetus in her vomit and, at the same time, to make sure that the fetus remains inside her. Through the repetitive imaginary act of becoming pregnant, aborting, and becoming pregnant again, Ella each time expressed her murderous wish anew in order to undo it. By imagining her own abortion, she also turned against herself the wish to murder her sister inside her mother. Sometimes the need to look at her mother's menstrual blood expressed Ella's wish for fusion: "If she is my mother, there should be no physical boundaries. There should be a blood treaty between us. I wanted to get proof 'red' on white that she is my mother." By association, fusion fantasies brought Ella to express the undifferentiated state of her organs: "Last night I had pain while urinating. It is like feeling pain in the womb. It reminds me of mother's operation on the womb, of the bladder. Having intercourse is like playing with urine, with menstrual blood, with feces. Delivering a baby is disgusting, like defecating." Sometimes Ella described the inner space as full of feces, an overflowing with dirt.

Later, when she referred to her mother's womb, the symbol of the vagina dentata cropped up. She described a mouth full of teeth, comparing me with a dentist, and getting frightened by the idea that I would straighten her teeth. She dreamed about a structure that reminded her of a snail shell. She was going to be swallowed by it. In fact, she denied her vagina and referred only to the uterus. (Perhaps I should therefore speak here of "uterus dentatus" rather than "vagina dentata.")

Ella's sexual behavior was an important indicator of her problems with her body and its intactness. She feared penetration, often remaining dry during intercourse. Recurrent inflammations of the urinary tract often followed. In her masochistic way, she let the inflammation develop to the point where she could imagine that pus was flowing all over. Only then was she willing to consult a gynecologist. Parallel to the tendency to hide and protect her inside, she was then taking the opposite course by revealing the inside totally. Everything was on the surface. This was not just a way of self-punishment; Ella wanted to find out to what point I would be able to accept her murderous imagination. She revealed to me all her mud in order to find out if she really was as dirty as she used to think. After doing this for some time on the physical as well as on the mental level, she realized that she did not lose me after all, which calmed her down a little.

After showing herself and me in analysis her bad inside, reliving predominantly masochistic fantasies, and turning against herself, Ella approached the phallic-sadistic stage. She had many more overt and direct aggressive fantasies. This phase was characterized by her imaginary penis, which protected her from the outside as well as from the inside. This was a dangerous penis. "I do with men whatever comes into my mind." She compared her nose excretions with semen. She described orgasm as climbing Mt. Everest up to 7,000 meters and then falling. She could not make up her mind whether she reached the climax, as she could not feel a short and sharp point of excitation like in male's orgasm. I interpreted to her that she was trying to see herself in a man's role, and therefore could not enjoy herself as a woman.

Ella feared that she would not be able to control herself during orgasm. She thought that her sexual feelings expressed her aggression against men, whom she treated ruthlessly. She excited them, dragged them to bed, and then drew back, feeling powerful and full of revenge. In parallel, this open aggression was also expressed against me. She declared that I was sexually dead for her. She deprived me of good news concerning her improvement, like being more in harmony with her body, no longer suffering from asthmatic attacks, being able to separate from her family by taking her own apartment, etc.

Simultaneously with the increasing capacity to bear her own aggression in reality as well as in her imagination, she was prepared to deal with her aggression against her sister. She dreamed that she was wheeling a cripple in a wheelchair. She lost control, and the wheelchair ran into a streetlight, with the result that the cripple was killed on the spot. She felt guilty. In her associations, she drove her sister to commit suicide, recalling the accident her sister had had some time before Ella began her analysis. If something serious had happened to her sister, she feared the blame would undoubtedly have fallen on Ella. In another significant dream during this period, the dog jumped from a window. Ella, fearing her mother's reaction, was happy to realize that the dog jumped on its own initiative. Among her associations were: "When she was 8, the cat jumped from the window. There was a time when she took revenge on the dog. The dog crashed to the ground and all its parts spread all over." I connected this dream with Ella's fantasy that mother's menstrual blood contained parts of her sister. The wish for the dog's suicide corresponds with the wish to see her sister aborted by her mother. (It was by means of her dangerous penis that she could induce such an act.)

Ella was able to understand the displacement to the dog and the need for the repetitive fantasy about her sister's annihilation, finding out every time anew that she was resurrected. In a series of dreams, she hit her sister and even killed her. In the climax of her rage, she asked me whether I would be on her side in the event that she killed her sister. She wanted to find out whether I was able to bear her fantasies. The fact that she was able to express all these terrible thoughts and yet remain alive without being rejected gradually calmed her, and her aggression decreased. My curtains no longer bothered her.

Ella gradually lost interest in her sadomasochistic fantasies and impulses. She began to feel more feminine and started to get acquainted with gentler men, like her father. She was no longer willing to have humiliating sexual relationships. It was only at this stage that she could afford to pay attention to the breast. She had denied her own as well as her mother's breasts. She would not let men touch them. She did not feel they were a sexual organ and denied their existence. Now it also became clear that the penis partially symbolized the good breast, which always turned out to be disappointing. It was father's penis that should have compensated her for losing mother's breast to her younger sister. The more the breast recovered its real meaning, the more the penis could represent a penis instead of a breast. (She was no longer interested in fellatio.) Ella gradually began to develop and enjoy her feminine identity.

DISCUSSION

It is striking how little knowledge we have about the inside of our bodies as reflected in fantasies and unconscious material. We hardly have any substantive material derived from analysis which could give us a significant picture of how a human being perceives his or her inside—in spite of the fact that the inside contains the most vital organs and seems to be a significant source of our bodily sensations (Spitz, 1955). In part, this is understandable because of the different ways in which the inside and outside of the body are innervated; moreover, the inside is much less differentiated and sensitive. The hidden inside should stimulate the most flourishing fantasies, but they are repressed, at least if we take the clinical psychoanalytic material as a criterion. This raises the question whether the inside is too dangerous a subject to be uncovered. My patient had the need, the strength, and the courage to make this trip into the inside. Her analysis taught me something about a subject which is for the most part *terra incognita;* in addition, it implies reasons for the fear of the inside.

Kestenberg (1968) has written about the profound difficulty of the human being to relate to the inside of the body. While this is generally true, males, due to their anatomical structure, seem to be more capable of dampening and repressing their anxieties about the interior than females. For the female, the discovery that there is a difference between the sexes is another proof that the inside of the body is dangerous, dark, and full of aggressive elements. Irrationally, femininity is associated with bleeding holes; and masculinity, with intactness.

In Ella's analysis, the body language and symbolism were translated in terms of inside/outside. The obsessive need for the preservation of the intactness of the surface, the danger of being pushed from the inside to the outside, and the ambivalence toward the inside were leitmotivs throughout her analysis. The skin functions as the border between the inside and the outside and fulfills an important symbolic role. Similarly, the skin serves as a defense against the outside world and as a means of primary communication (Pines, 1980), but there are two more factors which play a role in the perception of the skin. One is the containing function of the skin. According to Bick (1968), "in its most primitive form, the parts of the personality are felt to have no binding force amongst themselves and must therefore be held together in a way that is experienced by them passively, by the skin functioning as boundary" (p. 484). The symbolism of the skin in Ella's analysis supports Bick's theory. The skin prevents the annihilation of the inside by protecting parts from falling into the outside, breaking apart, and disintegrating. When the skin is injured, the inside is prone to be expelled. Then the skin does not hold the self anymore. The intact skin is essential for the preservation of the inside self, for prevention of disintegration.

In the transference situation, Ella found herself a place under my skin. If the primary skin relations with the mother had been satisfactory, Ella would not have insisted on her hermetically closed system which did not permit exchange between inside and outside. She used rigid defense mechanisms excessively when there was not enough trust, self-cohesion, and adaptive ego functions.

There is an additional factor: the skin does not merely serve as a container and holder. It is supposed to protect the self from dangerous and dirty inner content which might come to light. Ella's decompensation started with the fungal disease of the skin which, in her imagination, spoiled the intactness of the surface and endangered her self-sufficiency. Even the smallest lesion could bring to light the terrible inside. In the same way, the denial of the vagina served the need to think of the body as a hermetically closed system. This was not just a defense against the dangerous penis but a defense against the menstrual blood with all its terrifying meanings.

The transference situation in the different phases of the analysis gave us a good picture of the fight for autarchy and intactness. In the first phase of the analysis, Ella was flooded with fantasies about my room which turned into a dangerous womb in which the primal scene and the sadomasochistic fantasies were overwhelming. This was an externalization of what she feared might happen inside her mother and inside herself (at this stage of analysis she could not express these fantasies directly). In the second phase, she was capable of closing herself again in a narcissistic cocoon. This was the antithesis of the exposed position she took in the beginning. After a while, the scenario changed again; she became capable of looking inside herself, and there she observed the sadomasochistic scene *in vivo*. She tried to solve the problem of being harmed by building herself a penis which not only protected her and restored her sense of intactness, but also enabled her to intrude into other objects and weaken them, an act which restored the feeling of intactness in herself (the illusion that by this aggressive way of showing her power and intactness she could deny the fear of the inside).

What is so frightening about the inside of the body? The main themes that came to light throughout the analysis were: (1) the dangerous content of the inside, mainly the menstrual blood; (2) the dangerous uterine space; and (3) the symbolism of the pregnancy-abortion-pregnancy cycle.

The dangerous menstruation also symbolizes abortion and super-menstruation (fetus), which is well known from anthropological observations. Ella's urge to see mother's menstruation has the double meaning of her being convinced that the mother aborted the sister, and at the same time she tries to make sure that her sister's pieces are not in the menstrual blood which would prove her mother's (and her own) innocence. This leads to the idea of the pregnancy-abortion-pregnancy cycle, which may be a common fantasy in women. This fantasy is a life-death symbol. Abortion is connected with the idea that there is a basic fear of falling in space, falling endlessly, and falling apart. This can be seen in Ella and in anthropological material.

Menstruation and blood in general are still a mystery in psychoanalysis. Talking about the instinctive fear of blood, I wonder what we mean by that and at which developmental stage it occurs. Is the fear of blood in general equal to the fear of menstrual blood? The menstruation reveals itself as a condensation of various factors: the fear of not being a woman (delay of menstruation); the masochistic identification with the mother; the wish for a symbiotic unification with the mother; the wish for a blood treaty between the guilty (according to Freud

[1913], the blood treaty is connected with the first crime); the double wish to see pieces of the sister in the menstrual blood and to find evidence to the contrary; and, above all, the idea of the condensed life-death symbol interconnected in the menstrual blood. Via the different meanings of menstruation, one can understand many of the central drives and conflicts of the patient. Ella connected menstruation with defloration, sexual intercourse, pregnancy, delivery, death, bleeding, hysterectomy, artificial and natural abortion, and all of these with mother's inner space which is filled with babies and blood—these elements which Devereux (1950) also found in the Mohave tribe. Ella's unusual and desperate insistence on seeing the mother's menstruation is of special interest. It has several meanings: (1) Ella did not believe that her mother wanted to unite with her through blood, which brought her into a state of painful loneliness (Deutsch, 1944); (2) the wish to share with her mother the guilt or the innocence; (3) the frightening idea that menstruation means life and death at the same time. Mother is losing parts of herself; is this the beginning of the end or does it mean a new child? It could also be both at the same time. When Ella referred to the menopause of her mother, she felt that she herself, with her menstruation, lived on account of her mother, who was going to die.

Associating to her own first menstruation, she said "I was born and dying at the same time." Menstruation meant abortion, delivery, and dying. The abortive element of menstruation was the link between content and space. The content might fall out into space (when the intactness was threatened). Falling had a very frightening connotation. It meant losing the good old womb; it meant falling apart, crushing, and falling into dark holes; falling meant to be pushed away by the mother and from the mother; it meant losing parts of the body; it meant not having any sort of control.

Falling in space therefore had the quality of dying, of annihilation. Not remaining with the mother was synonymous with death. Coming out of the mother, coming to life, meant at the same time dying. Ella's fear of being aborted, of falling, was not just guilt feelings about her aggressive fantasies. It was partly a very primitive, primary, psychobiological fear, the basic fear of being dropped. The very early anxieties described by M. Klein (1932) are based on an early superego and object relations. But for the sensations of falling, disintegration, and falling apart, one does not need a superego and hardly any object relations. My patient was talking in terms of clinging or sticking when she wished to stay under my skin in order to escape her fear of being dropped. It was Bick (1968) who spoke about adhesive identification as a form of holding oneself together by the attachment to the object in which there is no projection or introjection, only sticking.

This sticking is an analogue to the grasp reflex which prevents the baby ape from falling from his mother's breast under the tree. The womb, as it is described by the patient and by Erikson (1968), is Janus-faced. It represents the holding versus the expulsive womb, the protective darkness of the inner space versus the hyperstimulating effect of the dangerous outer world to which the bad womb is pushing, the soft place in which one can hibernate versus the "uterus dentatus." Pregnancy, too, has two faces, especially when it becomes part of the pregnancy-abortion-pregnancy cycle, as in Ella's case.

This is an endless cycle in which the pregnancy fantasy immediately awakens the drive to abort, and the wish to abort brings with it the renewed wish to become pregnant. In the clinic, we can see women who get pregnant, abort, and very soon become pregnant again, and this can repeat itself. It is a wish to create, destroy, and be re-created in an endless cycle. It has two sides. The wish to murder, to undo, with an omnipotent fantasy of re-creating. But the fetus is a part of the mother and the mother identifies with it (Ella is the aborter as well as the aborted subject). Devereux (1976) explored abortion in many different cultures. In various areas, suicide was a technical means for abortion, especially when other means proved impossible. One of the ways to abort successfully was by jumping from a high place which caused the death of child and mother. There is an unconscious link between abortion and suicide. The common fear that the child will be born with a defect is the fear of the annihilation of the self at the same time.

Fears connected with pregnancy, abortion, and delivery are at the same time fears concerning an object and the self, and they are in fact inseparable.

The pregnancy-abortion-pregnancy cycle represents the inseparable connection and link between life and death, which are so closely tied together. The womb, the menstrual blood, and the pregnancy represent all three of them, the condensing symbols of life and death. We should remember in this connection that anthropology pointed out a triad of taboos—the menstrual taboo, the pregnancy taboo, and the taboo of parturition.

The inside of the body, pregnancy, and parturition symbolize the condensation of contradictions. Menstruation is sacred and profane. It cures and kills; it represents the reproductive qualities of the woman versus the evidence for the destruction of the fetus. Pregnancy and parturition symbolize the living child versus the dead child, birth of the perfect child versus birth of a monster. These double symbols are meeting points of life and death. They suggest a partial answer to the basic question why it is so difficult to refer to the inside of the body.

CONCLUSION

In this paper, I show how a psychoanalytic patient views the inside of her body. Further studies could enable us to gain more specific knowledge about the different areas of the body inside. The dangerous content and the dangerous space are united by the pregnancy-abortion- pregnancy cycle which represents the perpetual mobile fantasy of the life-death unit. Annihilation and resurrection are endlessly interconnected in active as well as in passive terms (referring to the object as well as to the self). The content of the inner body is the plot, the inner space is the arena in which it takes place. The skin represents the boundaries which can either protect the self or allow the catastrophe to occur. The skin protects from the inside no less than it protects from the outside. The fear of the menstrual blood reflects the drama going on inside the body. When the blood is seen, this equals a flowing out from the inside, and the drama cannot be concealed. The blood symbolizes the unity of life and death.

How can my hypothesis be explained in connection with the head? The mouth is the opening of the head, and the mouth and the vagina are interchangeable in the unconscious. We see displacement from above to below and vice versa. In the second place, the idea of being born from the head is not strange to the human mind. After all, Athena was born from the head of Zeus.

BIBLIOGRAPHY

BICK, E. (1968). The experience of the skin in early object-relations. *Int. J. Psychoanal.*, 49:484–486.

DEUTSCH, H. (1944). *The Psychology of Women.* New York: Grune & Stratton.

DEVEREUX, G. (1950). The psychology of feminine genital bleeding. *Int. J. Psychoanal.*, 31:237–257.

——— (1976). *A Study of Abortion in Primitive Societies.* New York: Int. Univ. Press.

ERIKSON, E. H. (1968). Womanhood and the inner space. In *Identity.* New York: Norton.

FREUD, S. (1913). Totem and taboo. *S.E.*, 13:1–161.

KESTENBERG, J. S. (1968). Inside and outside, male and female. *J. Amer. Psychoanal. Assn.*, 16:457–520.

KLEIN, M. (1932). *The Psychoanalysis of Children.* London: Hogarth Press.
PINES, D. (1980). Skin communications, early skin disorders and their effect on transference and counter-transference. *Int. J. Psychoanal.*, 61:315–323.
SPITZ, R. A. (1955). The primal cavity. *Psychoanal. Study Child*, 10:215–240.

CLINICAL APPLICATIONS

"I Ain't Nobody"

A Study of Black Male Identity Formation

HELEN R. BEISER, M.D.

SEVERAL YEARS AGO, WHEN I WAS NO LONGER SEEING CHILDREN PROFESsionally, I participated in programs my church sponsored for a nearby black housing project. My experiences in tutoring a 9-year-old boy who never knew a father, and whose mother was murdered when he was 7, stimulated my interest in the processes by which such a child would develop his identity. Although there is considerable literature about fatherless children, there is nothing based on case studies of illegitimate orphans, especially poor black ones. Neubauer (1960) reviewed the psychoanalytic literature, quoting the speculations as to the possible effects of fatherlessness. For example, Aichhorn was concerned about the lack of an adequate ego ideal for a young, fatherless boy; Ferenczi felt the absence of oedipal conflict would lead to homosexuality; and Melanie Klein stated that an inverted oedipus complex would be reinforced. Nunberg gave two alternatives, either the transfer of a fantasied father to an actual man, or else resentment without guilt and a wish for revenge. In their war nursery, A. Freud and Burlingham observed the development and persistence of a fantasied father. Neubauer added the case he saw of a girl without a father, and described analytic cases of adults who had lost a father. All stress the overinvestment and seductiveness of the remaining parent. Schalin (1983) described in detail the struggles throughout latency of the boys' attempts at identifying with a male figure.

Training and supervising analyst (child and adult) at the Institute for Psychoanalysis, Chicago, Ill. Past president of the American Academy of Child and Adolescent Psychiatry.

A modified version was presented at the Vulnerable Child Workshop of the American Psychoanalytic Association, May 7, 1987.

In a very different approach Adams et al. (1984), dealing with the ever increasing social problem of single-parent families, questioned the psychoanalytic emphasis on the necessity of fathers. Cross-sectional anthropological and psychological studies failed to show a consistent effect on gender identity, masculine behavior, or psychopathology. They stressed the number of variables that might have an influence, such as age at loss, type of loss, race, social and economic levels, ordinal position, type and number of siblings, mother's attitudes, and the availability of surrogates. Constitutional differences may also have an effect. Even variations in patterns within a seemingly uniform cultural group, such as black, low-income, single-parent families (Lindblad-Goldberg and Dukes, 1985) can make a difference depending on the type and quality of support networks.

Although I have analyzed some children who have lost a parent by death and have been involved with a clinic whose purpose is to help children with such problems, the emphasis was on how to deal with loss. It was a totally new experience for me to try to understand how a child who had never known a father, and then also lost a mother who could give little or nothing, went about building an identity. The paper also raises a number of interesting and important questions regarding the effects of severe deprivation and trauma, as well as about the process of recovery and its limits. Further studies might be indicated as to how special education or individual tutoring might be combined with psychoanalytic theory and clinical skills in helping these children.

THE SETTING

The church is in a high-income area with a mainly white, well-educated congregation. It developed a relationship with a housing project which is within walking distance, and the elementary schools serving it. As far as I know, the population of the project is all black. The representative to the state legislature from this very disparate district is a black physical education teacher who has formed a tumbling team with an excellent reputation. The church, with the cooperation of the schools, offered a one-on-one tutoring program for about 150 children twice a week, for an hour and a half. The volunteer tutors were mostly white, not all members of the church, and of both sexes and all ages. An older woman, Debbie, hired by the church, and assisted by her husband and a number of black teen-agers who were paid a small amount, was in charge. Maxine, a grandmother from one of the project buildings, was the moving force in bringing the children and keeping them coming. She was paid a small salary to cook a simple supper for the tutors at the start of the evening. Debbie made announcements, oriented new tutors, and arranged some workshops with professionals to instruct them in some techniques of tutoring as well as an understanding of cultural differences. By experience, Debbie had made rules that no gifts were to be given unless all tutors were giving them, of the same value at the same time, like at Christmas. Children were not to be taken out of the building on an excursion or for a treat during tutoring time, and at least half of the time was to be used for some sort of schoolwork. She knew every child, and could be loving or tough, as the occasion demanded.

Tutors were asked for a commitment to the same child for the entire school year. If an absence was unavoidable, the child and Debbie were to be notified as far in advance as possible, so that a substitute could be arranged. Work sheets, books, games, and art materials were provided. The tutor and child had a small table to work on, but there were a number of tables in each of a number of rooms scattered throughout the church. Chocolate milk was passed out by the teen-age helpers in the middle of the evening, and occasional parties or excursions were planned well ahead. Parents or guardians were invited to meet the tutors at the beginning of the school year, and the children's public school teachers had that opportunity at a group supper at the end of the school year.

ZEKE'S BACKGROUND

In this setting, I was introduced to Zeke, aged 9, and to his guardian, Rose. She was the younger sister of Maxine, who later gave me a more extensive history. Zeke was the second of five children, and the older of the two boys. His mother had been raised in the south by a blind mother. She came to Chicago to live with the sisters, who were her cousins, but Maxine said she was "restless," and always in some sort of trouble. The children each had a different father, none of whom was a part of the household. Zeke's mother was investigated for abuse or neglect a number of times, but would threaten or beat the children, especially the oldest girl, into defending her against the investigators. Zeke responded by silently withdrawing. She sometimes locked the children in the apartment, telling them to open up to no one, not even Maxine, and would not come back for a week, by which time they were almost starving.

When Zeke was 7, his mother was found murdered in an alley on the other side of the city. Rose took the two boys, adding them to three children of her own, one a teen-aged boy. Maxine took the three girls, adding them to an indeterminate number of her children and grand-children. As far as I know, there were no permanent adult males in either household. A grandmother lived in a town 30 miles away, and there were brothers of Rose and Maxine, but their roles were hazy. The whole family gathered at grandmother's for big holidays. The children attended a Baptist church in the project, and Zeke described a trip to Florida in the church bus once during our first year.

Zeke had been seeing a young male lawyer once a week for two years. He told me that after his mother was murdered, Zeke was harder to manage for some time. He wondered about the possibility of retarda-tion, and could only get him to try to read by bribing him with candy. As a particularly tough learning problem, and because Debbie felt sorry for him, he as well as some other children were to have tutoring twice a week. He continued with the lawyer, and we continued to exchange our experiences with him. Quite against the rules, the lawyer bought him a jacket after he came without one on a cold night. He was a handsome boy, with big brown eyes and long lashes, dimples, a shy smile, and not very active physically. His language was almost impossi-ble for me to understand, and our verbal communication was minimal, even after two years. One evening I met his youngest sister, whose language was much clearer. However, Zeke's charm was undeniable. Some visiting black teachers fell in love with him on sight, as well as a past teacher whom I met at the supper after the first year. He also seemed to be a favorite of the teen-aged helpers who always gave him extra chocolate milk. One evening, after drinking four cartons, he had a stomachache. Rose, who did not seem too bright, was quite fond of him, and pleased that now he had a doctor and a lawyer for tutors.

THE FIRST YEAR

At our first meeting, child therapy style, I suggested he draw his fami-ly. After a number of attempts, with constant erasing and growing distress, he threw the pencil down and said, "Ah cain't draw." I then asked him to copy a diamond, which he couldn't do either, making me wonder if he did not have a true learning disability. Although I could have arranged for psychological testing, he didn't want it, and the cousins didn't cooperate. As time went on, however, we drew greeting cards on holidays, and he traced and copied simple forms, showing gradual improvement. As far as reading was concerned, he could not read a complete sentence without stumbling on at least one word. However, with flash cards, he would sing out the words with me and would recognize them the following week. He had considerable skill with numbers, and doing arithmetic work sheets gave him some sense of success. Because of this, I introduced him to dominoes, which he picked up very quickly, and he introduced me to Sorry. In either game, if I made a good move or insisted on following the written rules rather than his private ones, he frequently withdrew into silence. Sometimes he would slip into a wordless fantasy in which his motions indicated that he was fighting someone. It would end by his shooting the imaginary opponent and then, with a smile, himself. Although I could usually coax him back into the game, toward the end of the year, when I did not succumb to his desire to start over again to erase his failure, he told me he was leaving and walked out of the room. I told him he wasn't coming for my benefit, and I certainly couldn't stop him (although I knew Debbie would). Before I had finished packing up our materials, he came back, saying he had changed his mind, and I told him I was glad.

During the year I got some of his ideas relating to male identification. I had brought a tape recorder, thinking it might help him with his language and pronunciation in reading, but he chose to sing into it. I finally realized that the songs were those of Michael Jackson, a popular black singer, who seemed somewhat effeminate. That probably was related to his coming a couple of times with his hair done in corn rows, complete with beads. Another indication that he was trying to identify with some male figure was when he failed to come to tutoring one night (the only unplanned miss in two years) because he wanted to see a Bruce Lee movie. With the help of the Analytic Institute's Chinese librarian I obtained a number of articles about Bruce Lee, hoping he would get interested in reading them, but to no avail.

Gradually through the year his relationship to me improved, although erratically. Early in the year I could not recognize him in the mass of children waiting, and he gave me no help. Slowly, his friends would recognize my dilemma and helped me to locate him. He enjoyed this game. At the end of the school year, we took all of the children to a live performance of Hansel and Gretel. Although he had never seen a live show before, he enjoyed it, and identified with the lost children. When I said good-bye, I told him I wasn't sure if I could continue as his tutor in the fall. He fixed me with a stare and said, "You *do*."

THE SECOND YEAR

The second year was markedly different. At first we continued with our old activities of flash cards, a work sheet, and dominoes. When we began to plan for Halloween, which fell on a tutoring night, I got some real insight into his problems of identification. I asked him who he would like to come as, "if you had all the money in the world." With urging, he reluctantly said, "A football player"; and when pressed to be more specific, "Walter Payton." Walter has played many years for the Chicago Bears team, holds many rushing records, and has the nickname "Sweetness." Having carefully studied the Bears' uniforms, I came prepared on Halloween to turn a paper bag into a mask of a Bears helmet. At first Zeke acted uninvolved, just eating the candy all of the children had been given, while I drew and colored. When I urged him to participate in the work and reminded him of his wish to be Walter Payton, he resisted, but finally said, his head hanging down, "I ain't *nobody*." I found myself saying in a firm voice, "Oh yes you are. You are Zeke Johnson, and tonight you can be Walter Payton." At that, we began working together, he filling in the outline of the helmet with black crayon, and I constructing shoulder pads with Walter Payton's number on them. The teen-aged helpers, who acted as judges, awarded him first prize. As usual, he showed no emotion, but ate his prize chocolate bar with relish, and several times throughout the year asked me if I remembered Halloween.

At about the same time, I decided that one reason he didn't read was that he got so bogged down in the mechanics that he couldn't follow a story. I decided to read to him, and did so for about a half hour each evening for the rest of the year. I started out with "The Little Engine That Could." He listened to that and a few other stories of a similar nature, but made no comment. Around Christmas I read him "Twas the Night Before Christmas." This time he commented, "Reindeers can't fly." I agreed, but said it was fun to imagine that they could. After Christmas I looked for something else. I couldn't find anything at his level relating to black heroes, so, with some hesitation, started a book I just happened to have, "The Lion, the Witch, and the Wardrobe" by C. S. Lewis. Could this little black boy living in a housing project relate to a story about well-to-do English children evacuated to the country during World War II and their adventures in a fantasy land with a lion representing a Christ figure? I began, a chapter at a time. He got so engrossed that I increased to two chapters, and once to three. The lion allowed himself to be killed to save a bad little boy just before Easter. I reassured him, as we broke for two weeks, that the lion would come back to life, but asked him curiously if this reminded him of anything. With no hesitation he said, "Jesus." I was impressed not only by his ability to translate symbols, but by his training in the project's Baptist church.

During the Christmas vacation I invited him to go downtown with me to see the city Christmas tree and have lunch at McDonald's. He wouldn't come alone, and finally settled for his companion on a much younger cousin, a grandson of Maxine. The boys got lost trying to find my address, but Zeke called me collect from a store, and I went there to meet them. At lunch he finished up his cousin's half-eaten Big Mac. It was a very cold day, so we spent most of the time in the toy departments of the big stores. While his little cousin was attracted to big trucks, Zeke shyly touched furry stuffed animals. On our way out, I saw him looking in fascination at a mannequin modeling a maternity dress, and whisked him away as he was about to pull up her dress. On the whole, he was less demanding than his cousin.

Aside from reading, we continued with work sheets and dominoes. I noted that his handwriting on the score sheets was much improved over the previous year, with some attempt at embellishing the letters. He was able to tell me the names and ages of his siblings. Although I mentioned his mother's death occasionally, he made no apparent verbal or affective response that I could determine. In February I was out for a few weeks for an operation. I prepared for my absence by wanting to give him explanations, but he did not seem interested. However, he changed his play, and I realized that he wanted me to win in dominoes. If I had a poor move, he encouraged me with the same words I had used with him. With the help of Debbie, he sent me a "Get Well" card to the hospital. At the final party of the year, we stood in line a long time for ice cream. He invited more physical contact than he ever had, using me to hold him while he performed acrobatic tricks.

In the spring, I told the Halloween story to a church committee which included a former White Sox baseball player. He said he knew Walter Payton's manager and would ask for an autographed photo. I received it after tutoring was over, a great action picture, signed "To Zeke. You're a winner, Walter Payton." I called him with the news that I had something special for him and invited him for a morning at the beach and lunch. He made very little response to the photo, but the beach was an interesting experience. He stood with his feet in the water and would go no further, complaining that the water was too cold. I went in and tried to encourage him, along with two white boys, but he stayed glued to the shore. Finally he said, "Can I wear your cap?" Putting my white bathing cap over his very short hair, which certainly did not need protection from the water, he got the courage to go in, playing vigorously with the two boys. For lunch I offered him a roast beef sandwich, which he refused, eating only peanut butter and jelly. We had one more swimming party before I left for vacation. He again used my cap, but spent more time playing in the sand. I encouraged him to dig down to water and use the wet sand to build a castle. Although he had obviously never done this before, he did a good enough job to attract the admiration of passing children. This time I had hot dogs for lunch, stopping him after three with a reminder of the stomachache he got after four cartons of milk. He knew about my allergy to chocolate, so when he conversationally asked me if I ate "grains," I thought he was asking about other allergies. He realized I had misunderstood him and persisted until I got it clear that what he wanted to know was if I liked "greens," a popular food in the black community.

FOLLOW-UP

That fall I found I had too many conflicting meetings on tutoring night, and reluctantly told him I could not continue. He was assigned a male tutor, and I was both surprised and pleased when Debbie told me later that year that he had won a book review contest. I asked to see his work, a form with questions to be answered. Although his answers were short sentences, he had captured the meaning or purpose of the story very well, just as he had seen the symbolism of the lion the year before. In the spring I talked to him briefly when I went down to the hall where the tutors picked up the children. He helped me to find one of Maxine's daughters, who was to help me with a family party. She told me that Rose and all of the children in her household had moved out of the housing project, so probably would not be able to continue tutoring. Zeke was pleased that the new home was near a swimming pool. On the negative side, this meant he could not become a teen-aged helper, which had been his ambition. That fall I sent him a card for his thirteenth birthday, including a stamped envelope and paper, asking about his progress. I repeated that at Christmas, but have not heard from him. In the meantime, Maxine has left the project, and Debbie has retired. Her replacement does not know Zeke, so l have no way to follow him. Adolescence could certainly test the results of the tutoring program.

DISCUSSION

Although this experience was not set up as therapy, it is obvious that something therapeutic happened. Over a two-year period, this deprived black orphan developed a meaningful relationship to me and allowed me to observe both some of his strengths and his weaknesses. Fatherless, and with a cruel and depriving mother whom he lost by murder when he was 7, what possibilities are there for his future? His situation is quite different from most in the literature. He never knew a father at all, so didn't lose him, and his mother certainly didn't overinvest in him, although he was her first son. Rose also did not have the time or energy to make him feel special. When I observed his fantasy play of shooting someone, and then himself, I could not help but wonder if he would end up being murdered or being a murderer. What elements might go into a boy like this to give him a sense of not only being a male, but a "somebody"?

First let us look at the positives, or strengths, in the situation. Luckily, he was not only physically attractive, but seemed to arouse many people in the environment to take an interest in him. Although a poor reader, Zeke had important abilities with numbers as well as in understanding symbols. His ability to telephone me collect showed a practical side that could accomplish something he wanted. His cousin Rose had taken him into her family, and he had not only his real brother there, but foster brothers and sisters who were also cousins. Next, he had a whole extended family, the older sister Maxine with all her children and grandchildren, Rose's mother and a number of brothers. When he said "Hello" to some other child, and I asked if it was a brother or sister, it was usually a cousin. I finally did meet his siblings, and the older sister was much less likable, whereas the younger sister seemed the least disturbed and was much more verbal and easier to understand than he. I was also impressed by the relationships in the tutoring group as a whole. When we took the children to Hansel and Gretel, any child who had food or candy shared with whoever asked, with no holding back. This was probably the origin of the need to regulate gift giving by tutors, as if one child succeeded in getting a gift, all felt entitled to receive the same. In the broader community, his church and mine were important supports for him.

On the negative side were his chaotic early life and the probability of some kind of a language disability. This latter could not be explored as he and his cousins resisted testing. The adults in his life had had very limited education but aspired to more, at least for their children. The housing project not only had the meaning of poverty but also violence, and the mothers were the main protectors of the young children. The one thing that could cancel tutoring was gang warfare. He not only suffered a lack of individual care and nurturing, making him suspicious of it when offered, but had actually been hungry and continued to show an enormous appetite for any food available.

It seemed that the first step was to try to make some relationship on which he could grow. At first he probably came just to get what he could of a material nature, and his first tutor went along with this. I probably scared him with my interest in his family at our first meeting. I also allowed him to demonstrate his ability with numbers and introduced a game which used this ability. His withdrawal when he did not do as well as he wished, or even when I did well, was probably transference from battles he had with his mother, as described by Maxine. Because the reason for coming was reading, I persisted in doing some work with him in this area, his worst, and developed some hope when I found that he could learn by imitation. Near the end of the first year he threatened rejection, but did not follow through, and indicated he would like me to continue tutoring him. A marked change occurred when I accidentally had an opportunity simultaneously to support his own identity and help him to identify with an appropriate ego ideal. I am not sure whether this was an important preliminary to his using the nurturing experience of reading to him and revealing his ability to understand symbolic material. He let me know of his enjoyment by saying when the book was finished, "They should make a movie out of that." He showed evidence of identifying with my teaching and caretaking functions in playing dominoes when he knew I was facing an operation. Perhaps the most interesting evidence of identifying was his use of my bathing cap to get the courage to enter the water. When I presented this case at a workshop, one of the members pointed out the similarities in shape of my cap with a chin strap and a football helmet, although one was white and the other black.

After a boy feels nurtured by a woman and shows some signs of identification with her functions, how does he become identified with someone his own sex? Is biology enough, especially in the absence of a biological father in the boy's life? The little boys in the wartime nurseries had fantasy fathers, but there was an actual father somewhere in the background. Other boys seemed able to transfer their fantasied father to an actual man. In this housing project males seemed either weak or violent. The one thing that could cancel tutoring night was an outbreak of gang warfare. Although a male "friend" of Maxine helped for most of one year, there were no stable, strong males in Zeke's family. The teen-aged helpers were mostly female. The one male, who had started college, did not relate well to the boys, although all the girls were enamored of him. I am not sure if Zeke encountered any significant males at his Baptist church. In the tutoring setting, he encountered white males, racially and educationally very different from him. Debbie's husband was a stable figure, but Debbie was the one in charge.

It was interesting to observe Zeke's process of finding a suitable ego ideal. He had resisted identification with his white tutor of two years, and even with his teen-aged foster brother, who liked boxing. When he came with his hair in corn rows, I thought he was moving toward a feminine identification, but, in retrospect, it could have been part of his imitation of the popular singer, Michael Jackson. Actually he showed some talent in music during his enthusiastic participation in a Christmas Carol sing. I was fascinated by his brief interest in Bruce Lee, who was violent, but in a good cause. In a state clinic, I observed that many black families related better to Asian professionals than to white ones.

Another area to consider is the black youth's opportunity to "be somebody" by excelling in sports. Zeke rejected not only his foster brother's boxing but my interest in baseball. He showed an interest in basketball by trying to toss his milk cartons into the waste container from a distance, but he showed no talent in this direction. His most persistent athletic interest was football, and his chosen ego ideal in this field was not very big but fast and quick, known for his ability to avoid attackers in the form of tacklers. Although certainly not effeminate, with the nickname "sweetness," he had a reputation of being a very pleasant person. Since then the whole Bears team has shown considerable talent in singing and dancing. I think his choice was a good one, allowed by his ability to fantasy himself as Walter on Halloween, my support, and finally the gift of the personally autographed photo. Most importantly, this must have been instrumental in allowing him to learn from, and possibly identify with, a new white male tutor the following year.

What I am not sure of is the relationship between his ability to accept nurturance and the attaining of a male ego ideal. They seemed to proceed in almost parallel fashion in the second year. Maybe the first step has to be simply a determined and sustained effort to make a relationship despite resistance and distrust. Perhaps it took the first two years with the first male tutor, as well as my first year, to convince this boy that people could really care about him. I do feel that the turning point was Halloween, on which he could admit his sense of being "nobody." This is a holiday which stimulates trial identifications, and imagination, as well as a desire for sweets. With this shift, I concentrated on broadening his imagination by reading to him obviously unrealistic stories, and he found them enjoyable. It is interesting that he responded more to this kind of "food" than to candy. How solid this trial identification will prove to be is a matter of speculation.

It would be tempting to generalize from this experience. Could a significant improvement in personal relationships and learning be expected from a prolonged one-on-one experience of a seriously deprived child with any well-meaning adult? Other children in this particular program have responded, and the church offers a scholarship to a boarding school to one such child each year. Not all children do, however, and it would be interesting to study the factors which lead to success or failure. I do not think that my psychoanalytic background was as important in achieving the result obtained as much as in understanding and following the themes which developed over time. Perhaps the most important thing I learned was that an older woman from a different culture and race can be helpful in guiding a boy in his search for an appropriate male identity.

Summary

A two-year-long experience tutoring a 9-year-old deprived, illegitimate, black boy whose mother was murdered has been described. He resisted the efforts of a white male tutor, and also the additional efforts of a white female psychoanalyst for a year. Some trial male identifications with entertainment figures were observed during that year, but some significant changes in his relationships and learning occurred after he was encouraged, in the context of a Halloween costume, to identify with a prominent football player, who sent him an autographed photo. During the second year I read to him stories with a highly imaginative and symbolic content which he seemed to grasp. At the end of the time, he was able to use a combination of identification with his tutor and ego ideal in order to embark on a new and apparently frightening experience. In a follow-up, he demonstrated markedly improved reading skills.

BIBLIOGRAPHY

ADAMS, P. L., MILNER, J. R., & SCHREPF, N. A. (1984). *Fatherless Children.* New York: Wiley.
LINDBLAD-GOLDBERG, M. & DUKES, J. L. (1985). Social support in black, low-income, single-parent families. *Amer. J. Orthopsychiat.,* 55:42–58.
NEUBAUER, P. B. (1960). The one-parent child and his oedipal development. *Psychoanal. Study Child,* 15:286–309.
SCHALIN, L. J. (1983). Phallic integration and male identity development. *Scand. Psychoanal. Rev.,* 6:21–42.

Communal Upbringing in the Kibbutz

The Allure and Risks of Psychoanalytic Utopianism

EMANUEL BERMAN, Ph.D.

> It is a paradox of Freudian psychoanalysis that, whilst consistently struggling against Illusion, it somehow activates it.
> CHASSEGUET-SMIRGEL AND GRUNBERGER (1986, p. 14)

THE FANTASY OF AN IDEAL SOCIETY AND AN IDEAL HUMAN BEING RUNS deep in the history of humankind. Any theory exposing some sources of human misery tempts us to consider its potential usefulness as a springboard for the elimination of that misery. Marx saw himself as an enemy of utopianism, but, as Ernst Bloch and others could demonstrate (Hudson, 1982; Lukes, 1984), utopian elements do appear in Marxist theory.

Psychoanalysis is no exception to this rule. Freud himself may not

Senior lecturer, department of psychology, University of Haifa; faculty, Israel Psychoanalytic Institute; faculty, postgraduate department of psychotherapy, Tel Aviv University.

Dedicated to the memory of Shmuel Nagler, Ph.D., a beloved teacher and friend.

Earlier versions of this paper were presented at a conference of the Sigmund Freud Center of the Hebrew University (May 1984); at the First National Conference of Kibbutz Researchers (University of Haifa, June 1986); and at a colloquium of the Postdoctoral Program in Psychoanalysis and Psychotherapy, New York University (December 1986). I wish to acknowledge the contributions of Dana Biran, Zafrira Dgani, Benny Gleitman, Eleanor Herschlag, Ethel Kadishevitz, Adina Keesom, Doron Lulav, Sarita Ringel, Ruth Segel, and Orit Sheri.

have been completely immune.[1] Consider, for example, his prediction regarding the impact of psychoanalysis on the reduction of overall repression. "The success which the treatment can have with the individual must occur equally with the community," Freud (1910, p. 148) said. Later on, he expressed the hope that "all the energies which are to-day consumed in the production of neurotic symptoms serving the purposes of a world of phantasy isolated from reality, will, even if they cannot at once be put to uses in life, help to strengthen the clamour for the changes in our civilization through which alone we can look for the well-being of future generations" (p. 150f.).

This hope was much more extensively elaborated in the work of the major psychoanalytic utopians: Wilhelm Reich, Herbert Marcuse, Erich Fromm. Their grand schemes deserve careful theoretical scrutiny, but nothing can be said about their actual results; like most universalist utopias, they were never realized.

When social scientists wish to study the real-life impact of utopian visions, they turn to their "patent office models" (Bestor, 1951). Pitzer (1984) suggests: "If we agree that no nation has ever achieved the utopian ideal, we might also recognize that, however briefly, in communal societies, and in communal societies *alone,* human relations and institutions have approached the realisation of utopia as 'now here' rather than 'no where'" (p. 122f.).

The Israeli kibbutz is one such communal society, and it was indeed characterized by Buber and others as a utopia that has been materialized. Most of its aspects have much more to do with socialism than with psychoanalysis. One aspect, however, was conceived under the influence of psychoanalytic ideas as well: its method of communal upbringing of children. Therefore, an examination of this system—its initial rationale and its actual outcomes—should be of interest to psychoanalysts, and could supply us some data for the study of that intriguing question: Can psychoanalytic insights contribute to the design of an improved society? Can the undeniable elements of social criticism present in Freud's work be translated into constructive proposals?

PSYCHOANALYTIC RATIONALES IN COMMUNAL KIBBUTZ UPBRINGING

The "classical" version of kibbutz collective upbringing was described in detail by several authors (e.g., Spiro, 1958; Rabin, 1965; Bettelheim, 1969). Its essential features were: all children live and sleep in a special

1. Here I find myself in disagreement with Chasseguet-Smirgel and Grunberger (1986) who portray Freud as lacking utopian illusions and are therefore overstating the contrast between Freud and the utopist Reich.

children's house from the age of a few weeks; they are arranged in small groups, and cared for by a special caretaker ("metapelet"); they see their parents once a day for a brief afternoon visit.

When communal kibbutz child rearing was established along these lines, it had numerous motives, such as: socialization of the young generation into collective life and collectivistic values; freeing women for work, for both ideological and economic motives; saving on building expenses, so that members could live in rooms (one room per couple or for a group of single members) rather than in family apartments; freeing the members' evening hours for group activities and community meetings; etc.

Nevertheless, psychoanalysis did play a role, whether as a rationale or as a rationalization. This is particularly evident in the literature of Hashomer Hatzair, a movement directly influenced by Freud's thought (at times in an attempted integration with Marx), but it can be detected in the literature of other kibbutz movements as well, starting with the 1920s. A good background picture of the idealistic combination of psychoanalysis, socialism, and progressive education among young European Jews after World War I can be found in Hoffer (1981). These developments in Europe, in which Siegfried Bernfeld played a central role, had a direct impact on the kibbutz movement in Israel.

Let me quote briefly from a programmatic statement:

> . . . after a stubborn war we overcame in our movement—in the kibbutzim of Hashomer Hatzair—the danger of children sleeping jointly with their parents . . . the dangers involved in it were discovered by modern psychological science with such great certainty, that they need not be repeated . . . separate sleeping arrangements for parents and children are one of the guarantees of correct sexual education [Zohar et al., 1937, p. 31].

The words "stubborn war" give this statement a dramatic coloring, and the repeated emphasis on dangers suggests a rescue fantasy is in operation. The hope was "to abolish the pathogenic bridge between generations" (Kaffman, 1971). What are the children to be rescued from? The literature of the period reveals three major issues:

1. Children should be kept far from their parents' bedroom, to avoid the pathogenic and traumatic influence of the primal scene (Nagler, 1963a).

2. Due to their lesser involvement with their parents, these children develop less intense oedipal feelings, and are thus rescued from the pathogenic impact of the oedipus complex, known to be a central source of neurosis (Gerson, 1968).

3. Due to the separation of parental functions, with socialization and disciplining turned over to the metapelet, the parents can offer during their daily meetings with their children "pure love," not marred by demands (Hurwitz, 1963),[2] and thus generate more harmonious parent-child relationships.

"Disappointments the child experiences with the parents are much more painful . . . when the difficult demands involved in the education of the instinctual drives come from the metapelet and not from the parents, this is an educational advantage" (Gerson, 1968, p. 51f.). The existence of a number of identification figures allows the child to divide his feelings among them, and so to reduce the ambivalent fluctuations regarding his mother (Levin, 1960).

It should be noted, however, that parental love was also seen with some suspicion. Golan, a psychoanalyst who played a leading role in the formation of kibbutz education and in the formulation of its psychological rationale, said,

> Psychoanalytic theory taught us that the gratification of the need for affection, when it is uncalculated and libidinous, will end up with destructive exaggeration; we know that it often stems from the ungratified needs for love of the parents themselves, which find a dangerous and purposeless substitute in libidinal ties to the children. Here are the roots of traumatic developmental distortions and of a heavy burden regarding the oedipus complex. Just as we saw a need to remove children from the intimate ties between their parents, which were discovered to have a traumatic impact (by establishing the children's houses), so we also found it necessary to set limits to the parents' expressions of affection. . . . We do not approve of endless hugging, caressing and kissing [1948, p. 47].

Golan proceeds to discuss how excessive physical contact with parents leads to masturbation, and to explain why it is better for children to be put to sleep by their metapelet and not by the parents.

Some extreme kibbutz ideologists suggested that the maternal instinct should be opposed as stemming from capitalistic possessiveness (Sitri, 1959). This position was not common, but parents' wishes for a close and unique tie with their children were generally viewed with

2. Hurwitz is a well-known Jungian psychologist, who held for many years a central position in one of the kibbutz movements (Ichud). The unique combination of Jungian individualism and kibbutz collectivism requires further exploration. It may have been aided by the joint tendency toward idealization. Paradoxically, while early kibbutz psychologists see themselves mostly as Freudian or Jungian, their emphasis on the commitment of each individual to his or her social group often brings Adler to mind, as Cafri (1985) astutely observes.

reservation and defined as neurotic and narcissistic (Golan, 1948). Parents were also warned not to respond to their children's exhibitionism.

The puritanical undercurrents of these formulations put them in clear contrast with central aspects in the utopian vision of Reich or Marcuse, in spite of their common wish to combine Freudian and Marxist concepts. Moreover, I believe that these puritanical elements are foreign to Freud's own belief in the heavy emotional price for the individual whenever sexual freedom is curtailed. Freud's complex, dialectical, and tragic view of the unavoidable tension between individual happiness and the requirements of civilization is translated by his utopian students into one-directional (though opposite) prescriptions: the bliss of polymorphous sexual fulfillment in Marcuse's utopia, the benefits of inhibition and "required sublimation" (Levin, 1961) in the kibbutz. In this vein, kibbutz educators, particularly again in Hashomer Hatzair, were convinced that the prevention of any direct sexual activity in adolescence is a crucial prerequisite to successful sublimation, to the development of social, scholastic, and artistic interests.

Paradoxically, these educators also supported joint showers for boys and girls (at least through preadolescence); this was a remnant of the joint showers for all members which had existed in the early stages of the kibbutz movement. These arrangements were justified as creating a more rational, natural, and demystified attitude to the other gender. Similar formulations can be found in the literature of organized nudist colonies in the U.S.; nudism is described as suppressing sexual stimulation. We may indeed speculate that the combination of nudity (as well as joint bedrooms through the age of 18) with a puritanical ethic could produce powerful repressive forces (Nagler, 1963b, p. 212). This may be relevant to the finding that marriages do not occur between men and women of close age who grew up in the same kibbutz.

Many kibbutz founders wished—at least consciously—to create a society which would negate all traditional values of their families of origin[3] (Nagler, 1963b, p. 203). They rejected the authoritarian control of the patriarchal nuclear family (Golan, 1946), but may not have realized that they unconsciously re-created a Spartan, puritanical au-

3. Several historians pointed to the fact that the founders of the kibbutz movement rebelled against their own parents, often abandoned them in Eastern Europe when immigrating alone to Palestine. They usually never saw them again, as the parents became victims of Nazi extermination. The guilt involved was forcefully repressed, and only in recent years some of it became expressed, as in the poetry of Avot Yeshurun, a major Israeli poet.

thoritarianism of their own. This group authoritarianism also became
a model for harsh mutual control within the children's peer group.
Indeed, in my view, the superego of kibbutz-born persons represents
to a considerable extent an internalization of the peer group, and its
harshness may at times be very difficult to modify.

Attention must also be drawn to the enormous differences in emotional atmosphere that exist among kibbutzim, a topic not studied
systematically so far. Generalizing about the impact of "the kibbutz" is
parallel to generalizing about the impact of "the family" and equally
risky.

HISTORY OF THE DEBATE

The initial hopes for the impact of kibbutz upbringing were high.
Kibbutz educators of the 1920s and 1930s believed they were molding
a new, better person, and expected to find less pathology among their
children than in pathogenic urban families. They had to face resistance, however, from some members, in particular young mothers
who felt deprived of their maternal role and who were concerned
about the capacity of the metapelet to take care of their child. Some
recently published diaries from the early days express these experiences powerfully. At times opposition was public even then, as in the
following view from a kibbutz publication (Yatzker, 1924): "just as
grown-ups, in addition to their public life . . . , have a valuable corner
in their private room, so the little one too needs this corner, which will
teach him to think alone, to be an individual, not to always need society . . . otherwise our children will be superficial."

These resistances were overcome by the strong political-educational
leadership within the kibbutz, and the method remained unchanged
for several decades. However, when we follow the relevant literature,
we notice that the claims for the unique mental health of children
gradually appear to disappear, apparently with the realization that
kibbutz children actually do exhibit various forms of disturbed behavior—even schizophrenia and homosexuality which at one point had
been reported to be nonexistent. "The fact that within the kibbutz
movement the percentage of disturbed children compared to other
societies is not considerably lower has caused much disappointment
among leading kibbutz educators" (Nagler, 1963b, p. 204).

Moreover, in the 1950s kibbutz educators and psychologists faced a
rather threatening challenge, when the psychological literature in the
West, now less preoccupied with oedipal issues, started to emphasize
the central impact of mother-child relations and the pathogenic influ-

ence of maternal deprivation. The formulations of Spitz and Bowlby in particular put kibbutz educators in a defensive position, though its first manifestation is in Golan's 1948 review of *Infants without Families* by Dorothy Burlingham and Anna Freud. Bowlby visited Israel and his observations of communal upbringing led him to predict an increase in depression in kibbutz populations (Nagler, 1984, personal communication).

Papers published in kibbutz journals in the 1950s and 1960s, rather than claiming superiority, deny inferiority. They show how the partial separation of mother and child cannot and should not be defined as maternal deprivation (Lavi, 1967); how collective caretaking may compensate for the pathogenic impact of certain destructive mothers (Katzir, 1958); and how pathology that does appear in kibbutz children should be attributed to particular families rather than to collective upbringing (Alon, 1966). In other words, once the hope to "rescue the child from the family" was to a large extent frustrated, the family became portrayed as the destructive element which may cause observers (particularly foreign) to blame the kibbutz educational system unjustly.

This process should be familiar to us as psychoanalysts and therapists. Greenacre (1971, p. 760f.) portrays the analyst's rescue fantasy and the analyst's self-image as substitute parent. "In such rescue operations the analyst's aggression may be allocated to those relatives or therapists who have previously been in contact with the patient and are, in fact or in fantasy, contributors to his disturbances. The analyst then becomes the savior through whom the analysand is to be launched." The various forms of such fantasies, especially among child therapists, were reviewed by Esman (1987). The complex dynamics of the mother-metapelet relationship were illuminated by Nagler (1963b).

The first comparative surveys of psychopathology appeared to indicate that the prevalence of most symptoms is rather similar in the kibbutz and in the Israeli city, thus giving support neither to utopian hopes nor to alarmist fears. Neubauer's (1965) and Rabin's (1965) books provided a balanced view. They indicated some difficulties in early development which tended to disappear at later stages.

When Bettelheim published his book *Children of the Dream* (1969), based on clinical observations during a short stay in a kibbutz, the controversy intensified. Bettelheim's book aroused intense anger in many kibbutz circles. Shner (1986, p. 37) spoke of "a compulsive apologetic attempt to disprove Bettelheim's claims." Bettelheim's work was characterized as biased, superficial, impressionistic, and unscientific.

In addition, he opened up a "second front" of the old debate. While the psychopathology "battle" ended with a tolerable compromise, the new "battleground" related not to symptoms but to personality development. Following the work of Erikson, Bowlby, and Spiro's (1958) earlier observations, Bettelheim spoke of a "flatness" in the personality of the kibbutz-born child, due to a certain shallowness of early experiences of both trust and mistrust. "In the kibbutz, with its multiple mothering, the infant has neither the utter security that may come of feeling himself at the core of his mother's existence, nor will he know the bondage it can bring" (p. 306).

RECENT CONTRIBUTIONS

In view of the fact that Bettelheim's work was indeed impressionistic, it may be of interest to examine what support his assertions found in more systematic, controlled studies. I will try to list some central findings of more recent research (1974 to present) without covering *all* relevant studies or doing full justice to the complexity of the studies quoted.

Sharabany (1974) found that preadolescents in the kibbutz developed a less intimate and less exclusive relationship with their closest friend than a matched sample of city children. In a later study Sharabany (1982) found, contrary to her expectations, that comradeship, defined as a less intimate form of social relating, was also less developed among kibbutz adolescents, in spite of the centrality of the peer group in their lives.

Regev (1976) found that emotions expressed by kibbutz children toward significant others, including their parents, were of lesser intensity than those expressed by city children. This included in particular negative and ambivalent feelings. Bitan (1978) found less openness of kibbutz girls, 17 years old, toward significant others, although no parallel difference was found between kibbutz and city boys of the same age.

Dana-Engelstein (1978) showed that kibbutz adults expressed fewer emotions in recounting their earliest memories, in comparison to moshav members (a less communal agricultural structure). Studying the same sample (a follow-up of Rabin's earlier sample), Kaminer (1979) found a less emotional tie of kibbutz members to their parents (see also Rabin and Beit-Hallahmi, 1982).

Arnon (1980), in a study specifically comparing two styles in contemporary kibbutz life, found that family-raised kibbutz children rated their best friend higher on frankness and spontaneity, knowing and sensitivity, and exclusiveness and taking (all being subscales of Sharabany's intimacy scale) than communally raised children. Adelist (1980) found less creativity among the kibbutz-born, accompanied (especially among girls) by greater conformity in comparison to city-born controls.

Biran (1983) found that kibbutz-born adolescents (aged 14 to 15) reported less self-revelation in social contacts, and had fewer and less complex emotional expressions in their TAT stories, in comparison to city-born counterparts. It is interesting that when questioned about their conscious views regarding self-revelation, the two groups did not differ at all.

Herschlag (1984) studied kibbutz and city married couples. She found no overall difference in degrees of intimacy within the two groups of couples, concluding that marriage in the kibbutz may be a stage when intimacy is finally achieved, compensating for earlier stages; she did find, however, greater emotional complexity in her city sample.

While, as mentioned, this list condenses and oversimplifies many complex findings, it gives us some sense of the gradual accumulation of empirical findings which give support to the sensitive clinical impressions of Spiro (1958) and Neubauer (1965). My own reading of the data is that communal kibbutz upbringing (the traditional form, including communal sleeping), while not producing pathology in the narrow sense, does have a visible impact on personality development, causing a subtle but consistent interference with emotional experience, creativity, and the quality of object relations as expressed especially in intimate relationships.

Such a conclusion is also supported by voices from within the kibbutz movement in recent years. The intensive debate about its present state includes many references to the emotional and psychological dimension. I quote a few of these critical views.

Shner (1986), a kibbutz member and educator, emphasizes the infantilizing impact of kibbutz life, which damages personal autonomy and the development of full adulthood. Public opinion evolves into an external conscience, with "a destructive influence on the development of an internal conscience and internalized self-criticism" (p. 29). Anxiety about losing the group's approval and affection, he suggests, creates "a dependent personality, lacking in basic security." The child is alienated from his natural drives, individual uniqueness is stigmatized, and intimate involvement becomes impossible. The result is "emotional shallowness to the degree of becoming a mental cripple" (p. 32).

Rosental (1985), a journalist and kibbutz member, writes, "The phenomenon of 'emotional shallowness' . . . derives directly from the continuous involvement in a uniform society and in one life circle. . . . The need to function and to relate incessantly to the social group, to defend yourself and your status, and the lack of intimate circumstances allowing the expression of that which cannot be expressed in an exposed society, all diminish the capacity for emotional expression" (p. 39). Rosental also describes the phenomenon of "the mute kibbutz member," whose speech is laconic and limited, and expresses concern about the lack of both initiative and rebellion among kibbutz-raised individuals. He brings up the contributory influence of the army—the first external setting encountered by kibbutz youngsters—to all these phenomena.

The observations of Rosental and many other commentators stand in direct contrast to the belief of Golan (1946) that kibbutz education will prevent "the authoritarian-masochistic character formed by education in capitalist society" and will instead foster independence and rebelliousness.

The most direct linking of specific child-rearing practices to personality development is suggested by Cafri (1985), a writer who presents herself as one of the first generation of kibbutz children. She speaks bitterly of "the infants' house sterilized of bacteria, dirt and parents." She describes "Nights, with no grown-ups and not a single light; days full of orders and instructions and prohibitions; endless cleaning projects; Mom and Dad who barely existed; softness and warmth which were a nameless dream; . . . the insoluble problem of individuation in the 'sibling' group controlling 22 out of 24 hours; the denial of the sensuous, the libidinal . . . the I" (p. 11).

Intense night fears were reported by many kibbutz-born analysands of Pelled (1964), but they were reported with considerable shame and guilt. "For most of them these are 'silent traumas' from which they suffer for many years without giving expression to their feelings" (p. 157). Other studies of children raised by schizophrenic parents (Nagler, 1985; Marcus et al., 1987) suggest that those raised in the city were less disturbed than those raised in a kibbutz.

My impression is that some awareness of this emotional price has contributed—in conjunction with numerous economic, social, and ideological factors—to the gradual shift within the kibbutz movement to family living arrangements. By now, most of the kibbutzim of the largest kibbutz movement decided to implement this shift, and it is advocated by a strong minority even in the more radical kibbutz movement of Hashomer Hatzair, whose leadership opposes it. In the new model, the children's house becomes mostly a school and a center for extracurricular activities—no longer a home.

THE PSYCHOANALYTIC RATIONALES IN RETROSPECT

In retrospect, the belief of kibbutz founders that they were applying Freud's views appears to have been misguided from the start. To the best of my knowledge, they were not aware of Freud's own skepticism about similar experiments. Sterba (1982) reports a hitherto unknown discussion at the Vienna Psychoanalytic Society in 1929 or 1930. Wilhelm Reich praised in that meeting the Russian sociological experiment of taking infants away from their families and raising them in social centers, thus preventing the development of a strong attachment to the parents, since he felt that it would prevent the development of an oedipus complex.

Freud's response, as reported by Sterba, was quite skeptical. He mentioned his own critique of sexual morality, but questioned the chances of attempts to reform the situation. (Some of his 1910 enthusiasm must have waned.) Then, Sterba quotes Freud as saying:

> There is a second point in Reich's presentation against which I have to raise objections. He claims that if, in Russia, marriage and the family are abolished consistently, there will be no development of an Oedipus complex and, consequently, there will be no neuroses. This can be compared to treating a person's intestinal disorders by having him stop eating and at the same time putting a stopper into his anus. The family is, after all, based on a biological foundation. Besides, we have to say that the Oedipus complex is not the specific cause of neurosis. There is no single specific cause in the etiology of neurosis [p. 111].

Indeed, the formulations of early kibbutz educators lend psychoanalytic insights an alien, mechanistic, causal simplicity. A concept such as "the education of instinctual drives," central in their writings (e.g., Golan, 1948), sounds to me more behavioristic than psychoanalytic. What Skinner chose to adopt from Freud in his own utopian *Walden Two* (1948) sounds similar. Skinner also envisions communal child rearing, and when defending this attenuation of family life (Kateb, 1963, p. 209), he mobilizes both Plato and Freud: "By balancing the sexes we eliminate all the Freudian problems which arise from the asymmetrical relation to the female parent; . . . In the family, identification is usually confined to one parent or the other, but neither one may have characteristics suitable to the child's developing personality. It's a sort of coerced identification, which we are glad to avoid" (p. 120).

In order to reevaluate communal upbringing from a psychoanalytic perspective today, we cannot, of course, rely exclusively on Freud; we must utilize in full the growing complexity of the psychoanalytic understanding of early childhood, including the work of Spitz, Winnicott, Mahler, Kohut, and especially Anna Freud. I will not attempt such a full reevaluation, but only indicate some points which cast doubt on the old psychoanalytic rationales for communal child rearing and may explain some of its subtle detrimental impact on personality development.

For example, the view of the oedipus complex as solely a source of pathology appears today strikingly narrow and one-sided. We have learned to value the positive impact of a successfully resolved oedipal stage for future development. An inhibited or moderated oedipal stage may be detrimental to identification processes and to sexual identity formation. We also know that failure in achieving oedipal resolution is often related to disturbances in preoedipal stages which make the child less equipped to deal with oedipal issues. Therefore, the reduction of oedipal intensity (as reported in the kibbutz by Rabin and others) seems a doubtful blessing, while the possibility that the mother-infant dyad is not allowed to develop fully and freely seems more disconcerting than it did a few decades ago, even in terms of its impact on the later triangle of mother, father, and child.

Parallel and related questions must be raised regarding the pathogenicity of primal scene experiences. Strong concerns regarding their danger were based on an oversimplified model of psychic trauma as related to a single incident and its direct impact. From Ferenczi (1933) on we have learned to look at such events with a greater emphasis on the way they were presented, talked about, and experienced on a fantasy level. Khan's (1963) concept of the cumulative trauma gives a more central weight to overall processes in comparison to single events. We may assume, for example, that the lack of a successful sexual relationship between the parents may be more traumatic to the child, and have a more disturbing impact on his or her future sexual development, than an occasional coincidental exposure to parental sex occurring on the background of a successful sexual tie which in general maintains intergenerational boundaries rather than erodes them. Sleeping far away from the parents' bedroom seems a relatively minor change in comparison to the more central issues.

From our contemporary psychoanalytic perspective, another proclaimed gain of communal upbringing, the separation of discipline from love, appears as a very mixed blessing. Couldn't it contribute to an increase in splitting and to a greater difficulty in the integration of object and self representations? Couldn't the limited hours spent with the parents become an artificially idealized segment of one's life, in which aggression should be avoided, even denied? Is there enough continuity of contact with one significant object to make it possible for the child to go through a full cycle of frustration, aggression, distance, and reunion?

Such cycles play, of course, a central role in many newer psychoanalytic models of early development. Whether conceptualized within Mahler's scheme as central to the rapprochement subphase, or seen in Kleinian terms as an opportunity to experience depressive anxiety and reparation, their importance appears great. There are additional issues regarding the separation-individuation process in communal upbringing. Is there a unique process of separation and individuation from the peer group (Aronzon, 1984, personal communication)? The intensified crises related to separation-individuation in the kibbutz are also described by Pelled (1964).

Winnicott (1972) raises the issue of difficulties in separation faced by an infant who has three nurses in the course of a day in an institution. Flarsheim, in his annotation, spells out the implication:

> The integration of hate and love in relation to objects is facilitated by survival of the object love and of the loved object during periods of frustration, hate and aggression. The opportunity to make reparation for one's own hatred, and to gain reassurance against the destructive fantasies associated with hatred, depends on continuity of maternal care. If there is a discontinuity of maternal care and no opportunity to make reparation for the aggressive component of the primitive love impulse, one consequence can be an inhibition of the primitive love impulse, and an inhibition of all instinctual excitement. The continuity of maternal care which frees the development of spontaneous object related instinctual impulse, is one aspect of the "holding environment" [p. 470f.].

It may be of interest to mention here the study of Sagi et al. (1984) who observed infant-adult interactions in various situations in the kibbutz and city. They found an increased number of insecure-resistant attachments in the kibbutz sample in comparison to American norms, and an increased number of anxious-insecure attachments relative to that observed among Israeli city children. Considerable differences were found according to the metapelet—some metaplot appear to enable more secure attachments.

It appears self-evident that the personality of the metapelet is a relevant factor in the development of a kibbutz child. Yet psychotherapists working with kibbutz-raised children are often puzzled by the marginal role the metapelet plays in treatment; her actual centrality in one's childhood appears to be erased in inner reality (Nagler, 1963b; Pelled, 1964). It would seem that even the best metaplot cannot offer any equivalent to the unique investment created by primary maternal preoccupation. Without such attention, significant moments are trivialized. "What could make Mom joyful may annoy the metapelet when it delays bedtime" (Sheri, 1984, personal communication).

The degree of interaction with the metaplot, who may be changed often, as well as with the peer group with its intense pressures for conformity, raises the issue of possible false self characteristics in the communally raised child. Therapists of kibbutz-raised patients often speak of their strong need to fulfill expectations, combined with a difficulty in pinpointing and verbalizing their own genuine needs.

Of course, some alternative, more benign interpretations have been offered to such observations and findings. Regev (1976), for one, speaks of "emotional moderation" as an adaptive quality, related to the decrease, in the kibbutz, of sources of emotional conflict.

Personally I find this explanation apologetic and unconvincing. Our knowledge of kibbutz life does not support the hypothesis of fewer sources of conflict. The lack of emotional depth is, I suspect, defensive in nature; and while it may be adaptive in a superficial sense of smoother social functioning, it is not genuinely adaptive due to the heavy price one has to pay for it in emotional blocking and in loss of intimacy.

If this "shallowness" is indeed defensive, what kind of defense does it convey? I tend to believe that this is not necessarily a neurotic defense against drive derivatives, as described by Freud. It may belong more in the category of "prestages of defense" postulated by Stolorow and Lachmann (1980) as related to cases of developmental arrest on the background of early deficits in the environment's capacity to meet the child's emotional needs. If this line of thought is correct, we are not dealing with a specific defense vis-à-vis a specific conflict, but rather with a global defensive style necessary in order to cope with an environment lacking in cohesion and continuity, while overcrowded with sources of stimulation related to transient superficial social contact. This reaction, while it is in my view quite global and pervasive, is *not severe* in terms of interference with daily functioning.

SOME IMPLICATIONS

If these conclusions are correct, they may lead us to a much more sober evaluation of attempts to improve our emotional life by "mental hygiene" and "preventive mental health." Radical psychological experiments appear to have something in common with the enthusiastic scientific projects of improving life through building dams, rechanneling rivers, or spreading pesticides—all of which proved to be naïve due to their disregard of their subtler destructive impact on natural ecology.

We are reminded of Anna Freud's (1965) conclusion that

> . . . psychoanalytic education did not succeed in becoming the preventive measure that it set out to be. It is true that the children who grew up under its influence were in some respects different from earlier generations; but they were not freer from anxiety or from conflicts, and . . . other mental illnesses. Actually, this need not have come as a surprise if optimism and enthusiasm for preventive work had not triumphed with some authors over the strict application of psychoanalytic tenets. There is, according to the latter, no wholesale "prevention of neurosis." . . . By definition, the various psychic agencies are at cross-purpose with each other, and this gives rise to the inner discords and clashes which reach consciousness as mental conflicts" [p. 8].

Chasseguet-Smirgel and Grunberger (1986, p. 213) suggest that the tendency of ideologies to foster an illusory belief in perfectibility is linked with their projective aspect:

> Once it is purged of evil, be it represented in the form of the Jews, private property, capitalism, patriarchal society, character and muscular armor, or any other projected object [I would add here the primal scene, or, in a more contemporary context, sex roles or child abuse], the purified ego can exist without conflict, man can be united with God. In Aden Arabie, Paul Nizan says, when man shall be whole and free he will no longer dream at night. In other words he believes that all desires will be fulfilled. Psychoanalysis, however, maintains that human incompleteness, and thus human desire, will never disappear. Humanity is destined to dream from here to eternity.

BIBLIOGRAPHY

ADELIST, M. (1980). Creativity among kibbutz children. M.A. thesis, Univ. Haifa.

ALON, M. (1966). On Spiro's book *Children of the Kibbutz. Hachinuch Hameshutaf*, 17(3):2–7 (Hebrew).

ARNON, A. (1980). Intimacy and interpersonal relations. M.A. thesis, Tel Aviv Univ.

BETTELHEIM, B. (1969). *Children of the Dream.* New York: Avon.

BESTOR, A., JR. (1951). Patent-office models of the good society. *Amer. Hist. Rev.*, 58:505–526.

BIRAN, D. (1983). Emotional experience and its verbal expression among kibbutz and city adolescents. M.A. thesis, Univ. Haifa.

BITAN, N. (1978). Openness: a comparison of kibbutz and city youngsters. M.A. thesis, Tel Aviv Univ.

CAFRI, Y. (1985). Stamping or stamped? *Al Hamishmar,* November 15.

CHASSEGUET-SMIRGEL, J. & GRUNBERGER, B. (1986). *Freud or Reich?* New Haven: Yale Univ. Press.

DANA-ENGELSTEIN, N. (1978). Repression-sensitization and interpersonal relationships among adults in the kibbutz and the moshav. M.A. thesis, Univ. Haifa.

ESMAN, A. H. (1987). Rescue fantasies. *Psychoanal. Q.,* 56:263–270.

FERENCZI, S. (1933). Confusion of tongues between adults and the child. *Int. J. Psychoanal.,* 30:225–230, 1949.

FREUD, A. (1965). Normality and pathology in childhood. *W.,* 6.

FREUD, S. (1910). The future prospects of psycho-analytic therapy. *S.E.,* 11:139–151.

GERSON, M. (1968). *Education and Family in Kibbutz Reality.* Merhavia: Sifriat Poalim (Hebrew).

GOLAN, S. (1946). The means of communal upbringing. *Ofakim,* 3(4):47–58 (Hebrew).

——— (1948). Psychological evaluation of communal upbringing. *Ofakim,* 5(2):65–75; 5(3):45–57 (Hebrew).

GREENACRE, P. (1971). *Emotional Growth.* New York: Int. Univ. Press.

HERSCHLAG, E. (1984). Intimacy and mutual awareness of emotions among married couples in the city and the kibbutz. M.A. thesis, Univ. Haifa.

HOFFER, W. (1981). *Early Development and Education of the Child.* London: Hogarth Press.

HURWITZ, E. (1963). In favor of communal sleeping. *Igeret Lachinuch,* 26–27:15–17 (Hebrew).

HUDSON, W. (1982). *The Marxist Philosophy of Ernst Bloch.* London: Macmillan.

KAFFMAN, M. (1971). Psychological problems of the kibbutz child. *Hachinuch Bakibbutz,* 1:23–25.

KAMINER, H. (1979). The linkage between socialization and relationships of adults toward their parents. M.A. thesis, Univ. Haifa.

KATEB, G. (1963). *Utopia and Its Enemies.* New York: Free Press.

KATZIR, H. (1958). Thoughts on communal education. *Hachinuch Hameshutaf,* 10(2):16–17 (Hebrew).

KHAN, M. M. R. (1963). The concept of cumulative trauma. *Psychoanal. Study Child,* 18:286–306.

LAVI, Z. (1967). The theory of maternal deprivation in a new light. *Hachinuch Hameshutaf,* 18(5):24–35 (Hebrew).

LEVIN, G. (1960). Identification with numerous figures in infancy. *Hachinuch Hameshutaf,* 12(4):2–6 (Hebrew).

——— (1961). The education of instinctual drives in infancy. *Hachinuch Hameshutaf,* 13(1):13–16 (Hebrew).

LUKES, S. (1984). Marxism and utopianism. In *Utopias,* ed. P. Alexander & R. Gill. La Salle, Ill.: Open Court, pp. 153–167.

MARCUS, J., HANS, S. L., NAGLER, S., AUERBACH, J. G., MIRSKY, A. F., & AUBREY, A. (1987). Review of the NIMH Israeli kibbutz-city study. *Schizophrenia Bull.*, 13:425–438.

NAGLER, S. (1963a). Is communal sleeping at the children's house a pathogenic factor? *Igeret Lachinuch*, 26–27:6–14 (Hebrew).

—— (1963b). Clinical observations on kibbutz children. *Israel Ann. Psychiat. & Rel. Discipl.*, 1:201–216.

—— (1985). Overall design and methodology of the Israeli high risk study. *Schizophrenia Bull.*, 11:31–37.

NEUBAUER, P. B. (1965). *Children in Collectives*. Springfield: Thomas.

PELLED, N. (1964). On the formation of object-relations and identifications of the kibbutz child. *Israel Ann. Psychiat. & Rel. Discipl.*, 2:144–161.

PITZER, D. E. (1984). Collectivism, community and commitment. In *Utopias*, ed. P. Alexander & R. Gill. La Salle, Ill.: Open Court, pp. 119–135.

RABIN, A. I. (1965). *Growing up in the Kibbutz*. New York: Springer.

—— & BEIT-HALLAHMI, B., eds. (1982). *Twenty Years Later*. New York: Springer.

REGEV, E. (1976). Emotional moderation and de-focusing as outcomes of kibbutz communal education. M.A. thesis, Univ. Haifa.

ROSENTAL, R. (1985). The kibbutz—B minus. *Politika* (Hebrew).

SAGI, A., LAMB, M., LEWKOWICZ, K., SHOHAM, R., DVIR, R., & ESTES, D. (1984). Security of infant-mother, -father, and -metapelet attachments among kibbutz-reared Israeli children. In *The Strange Situation*, ed. I. Bretherton. Monographs of the Society for Research in Child Development.

SHARABANY, R. (1974). Intimate friendship among kibbutz and city children and its measurement. Ph.D. dissertation, Cornell Univ.

—— (1982). Comradeship. *Personal. & Soc. Psychol. Bull.*, 8:302–309.

SHNER, M. (1986). The kibbutz towards the year 2000. *Sdemot*, 66–67:25–37.

SITRI, Y. (1959). Basic assumptions of communal education. *Igeret Lachinuch* (Hebrew).

SKINNER, B. F. (1948). *Walden Two*. New York: Macmillan.

SPIRO, M. (1958). *Children of the Kibbutz*. Cambridge: Harvard Univ. Press.

STERBA, R. F. (1982). *Reminiscences of a Viennese Psychoanalyst*. Detroit: Wayne State Univ. Press.

STOLOROW, R. D. & LACHMANN, F. M. (1980). *Psychoanalysis of Developmental Arrests*. New York: Int. Univ. Press.

WINNICOTT, D. W. (1972). Fragment of an analysis. In *Tactics and Techniques in Psychoanalytic Therapy*, ed. P. L. Giovacchini. New York: Science House.

YATZKER, S. (1924). On communal sleeping. *Mibefnim*, 1(8):135–138 (Hebrew).

ZOHAR, Z., CHAZAN, Y., YUDKES, M., ROSENZWEIG, Z., & GOLDSTEIN, M. (1937). Proposal for basic lines in sexual education. *Hachinuch Hameshutaf*, 1 (Hebrew).

The "Golden Fantasy" and Countertransference

Residential Treatment of the Abused Child

YECHESKEL COHEN, Ph.D.

THIS ARTICLE ATTEMPTS TO DESCRIBE AND CLARIFY A CERTAIN RELA-
tionship that may develop between abused children referred for residential treatment and the treatment staff. An understanding of this
relationship with its distinct stages and phases can obviate additional
traumas in an abused child's development.

The object relations that develop between therapists and patients are
known to be exceedingly complex, are based on many processes, some
of which contradict one another, and undergo many transformations.
In this study I intend to illustrate one process only—"the golden fantasy"—and to follow its expression, the changes it undergoes, and how
it manifests itself during the various stages of treatment of the abused
children, on the one hand, and in the care workers, on the other.

The "golden fantasy" is awakened in the abused child and his care
workers simultaneously at the outset of the therapeutic process. As it
proceeds, however, a sharp break in the fantasy takes place, often
resulting in a premature disruption of the therapeutic process.

I use the term "golden fantasy" essentially as it was described and
explicated by Sydney Smith (1977):

> . . . it is the wish to have all of one's needs met in a relationship hallowed by
> perfection . . . it is always passive, always tied to the conviction that some-
> where in that great, unbounded expanse called the world is a person

Director of the B'nai-B'rith Women's Children's Home, Jerusalem, Israel; president of
the Israel Psychoanalytic Society; supervising and training analyst.

capable of fully meeting one's needs. The wish is to be cared for so completely that no demand will be made on the patient except his capacity for passively taking in [p. 311].

This fantasy is common to all men, but it does not harm personality integration. However, those whose personalities have been in one way or another damaged are liable to be negatively influenced by the functioning of the fantasy since for such individuals the fantasy may become so central as to determine motivations, interpersonal relations, fateful decisions, and at times even the essence of one's sexual relations.

Placement of the abused child in a residential treatment center powerfully evokes his "golden fantasy." The child senses that he has reached a paradise in which everything is good; all his wishes will be fulfilled; he is no longer the victim of violence; and, somewhere in this paradise, there is someone who is utterly at his disposal and who will gratify all his needs while he, the child, remains totally passive. Facing the child is the care worker who takes in the abused child. The care worker devotes himself completely to the child's needs to the point where his own golden fantasy is evoked. Through countertransference and projective identification, he fulfills it through the child he is treating. By means of different processes, especially the mechanism of splitting, the parents are perceived as evil creatures to be avoided, as opposed to the benevolent and omnipotent therapists.

After a certain time the entire process enters its second stage which I term "disappointment and despair." Again by means of the mechanism of splitting, the child perceives his care workers as the evil persons who do not fulfill his golden fantasy (and this fantasy functions on an "all or nothing" basis). He again turns to his parents and attributes to them the ability to fulfill his fantasy. The therapist who devoted his entire self to the abused child is disappointed and in despair. Through projective identification the child succeeds in bringing the therapist to fulfill the role of the abusing parent, even though the therapist refrains from any physical abuse.

In what follows I attempt to describe these processes as they occur in a residential treatment center for emotionally disturbed latency children.

The removal of an abused child from his home and family and his placement in a residential treatment center can evoke powerfully complex, emotional reactions in the abused child and his family as well as in the therapists. The abused child may develop feelings of guilt stemming from the conviction that he has been beaten and placed in the residential center because he is "bad." He may use the mechanism of denial to ignore the phenomena of abuse to which he has been subjected over a long period of time; he may project all "evil" onto the residential center and its staff; or he may regard the center's staff as he did see his abusive parents.

The various emotional reactions of the parents and the therapists to the placement of an abused child in a residential treatment center are well known. I have chosen to focus here on only one phenomenon singled out from the entire array of emotional reactions. The process described should not be perceived as isolated or assumed to exist in each and every such meeting between abused child and treatment center and its staff.

An "abused" child is one who was the victim of violent behavior on the part of a parent over the course of a long period of time. The child may have required hospitalization as a result of the physical injuries caused by the parent. Placement in a residential treatment center occurs as the result of intervention by the authorities responsible for the child's welfare. The treatment center also provides an opportunity to treat the child's emotional problems which have been diagnosed prior to placement. It has the function of protecting the child physically by separating him from a violent social environment.

THE AWAKENING OF THE "GOLDEN FANTASY"

First and foremost, the abused child views the center as a haven, a refuge. During the first stage of therapy, he does not understand that the intention is to treat his emotional problems; all he perceives at the outset concerns physical defense, since the framework is so different from his past. He is not moved to a different family or foster family; rather there is a substantially different living space. His initial expectations are therefore directed at that narrow aspect of the trauma to which he was subject: the beatings, the violence, the rejection, the denial of his basic needs.

The child turns to the institution and its staff members in a general and unspecific, nondistinct way, either openly and verbally or in a disguised manner. This is perceived as a cry for help and evokes feelings of omnipotence in the staff, feelings which are intensified because of the child's condition, his suffering, and his distress. Feelings of transference and countertransference develop in every therapeutic situation, and certainly in an educational situation, but in the case of an abused child who relates to it openly, these feelings develop immediately and to an extreme.

I shall examine the changes that occur during therapy. If the changes are not understood and the phases of therapy ignored, treatment may be terminated before it is complete. I give two examples of children's reactions in the first encounter, i.e., in the evaluation and assessment interview in the center.

An 8-year-old boy entered the interview room after a short tour of the center and turned immediately to the interviewer with these words: "Can I stay here? It's awfully nice here, everything is green and the pool is wonderful. I saw two children who asked me if I was a new boy and they were on their way to the pool." Later, when the interviewer confronted the child's immediate wish to remain in the center, the child rolled up his sleeve and pointed to burn marks and scars on his arm while he went into a long explanation of how his father had hurt him, adding, "He never hurts my sister, but he beats me to death. If I ask him to buy me ice cream, he says no; and if I ask him again, he hits me and tells me that he's sick of me. So, sure, I want to be here in the center."

A 7-year-old boy sat down in a chair in the interview room and folded his arms as if waiting for something to happen. The interviewer asked a neutral question, something like, "Well, what's up?" The child answered, "It'll be okay. Once I'm here in the school, I'll get hold of myself and I'll learn to read, I promise you; as soon as I'm here, I'll get hold of myself." The examiner's response to this sudden statement was that Daddy certainly often demanded that the child take hold of himself. The boy replied, "Oh, he's always saying that and then, when I start to cry, he takes the belt and hits me; here, see for yourself, look what he did to my back."

In these two examples the child's golden fantasy is expressed by means of the mechanism of splitting and denial. The two children ignore reality, even if confronted directly with it. Should we explain to them that in a treatment center children do not sleep with their parents, that parents' visiting hours are limited, that bigger children are liable to hit them, that the food is rationed? In each of these cases the children's reactions will be based on massive denial and will take approximately the following form: "So what, I want to stay here, it's good here, everything's great here, I've already seen it and I know everything."

Even after the child has been admitted into the center, he continues to express his golden fantasy to the staff. He may go from one staff member to another, pointing to scars or other injuries on his body, at the same time praising the treatment center and the way various staff members worry about him, care for him, and love him. He may name a certain staff member and comment that "he loves me more than anyone else, and I don't want to go home for vacation at all. It's great fun here."

These direct expressions of regard for the center and its staff indicate special object relations. The object is perceived as superior, as the omnipotent defender and gratifier, caring for and protecting the child; and, indeed, quite rapidly the object—the staff—responds to these object presentations. As a teacher expressed it in a discussion of an abused child: "I am ready to come to work every day just for this child." In a further supervisory session the teacher clarified that the child elicited in her the feeling that he was an empty vessel and she was full of things she could give him; from the very outset he had sent her looks of longing for warmth, caressing, hugging, and the like. This was followed by intense condemnation of the child's father: "How could he be so cruel to such a sweet boy?"

The teacher's statements expressed several areas of her own emotional constitution and should not be perceived only in terms of her ability to empathize. As Lieberman and Pawl (1984) state, "It is as if we could now magically undo reality and redo it in accordance with our dreams. In the long process of trying to protect a child, our small measure of power to bring about changes also makes us vulnerable to the illusion that we can erase the harsh realities of the child's circumstances."

Thus the teacher seems to have been activated by those of her own emotional tendencies that characterize countertransference. I view this phenomenon according to Ogden's (1983) definition, who clarified the term used by Racker (1957). Racker claims that countertransference is the unconscious identification of the therapist with one of two aspects of the patient's ego: complementary, i.e., identification with the aspect of the patient's ego identified with the object; and concordant, i.e., identification with the self component of the patient's internal object relations.

This distinction is especially important since identification with the abused child is likely to be interchanging, as in any process of identification: sometimes with the self part of the abused child, and at times with the internalized object. The object that has been internalized and has become part of the ego is not necessarily the realistic object, but rather the representation of the object as it is perceived by the internalizer or as he would like to see it and feel it. The therapist on his part identifies with the abused child, with the self part of the abused child (concordant countertransference), simultaneously fulfilling his own golden fantasy, but with the object of this fulfillment being the abused child with whom he has identified.

In the initial meetings between therapist and abused child, complementary countertransference takes place, i.e., the therapist's identification with the internalized object which will realize the child's golden fantasy. In addition, the therapist projects onto the child the self component in himself which seeks the fulfillment of his own golden fantasy. The therapist wishes to give the child that which he himself desires. Because of the tremendous responsiveness of the child, each "completes" the other: the therapist complements the child, and the child complements the therapist. I believe, however, that the child is assisted here by the mechanism of projective identification as well, by means of which he imposes on the therapist an identification with the object projected onto him. The therapist's countertransference is closely related to the child's mechanism of projective identification.

It must be noted that the therapist also feels superior to the child's parents: "I am better than they and I will succeed where they have failed in reforming the child."

It may of course be that the processes of projective identification in the child and of countertransference in the therapist or child worker may be facilitated by the special personality of those who choose child care and child therapy as a profession. Ilan (1963) has noted personality traits characteristic of such persons, traits which facilitate these processes:

> . . . education [is] a field of activity particularly attractive to specific drive constellations. It shows an affinity for people who have a particular love or hate for the child, people who have not completely grown up yet, who have not mastered certain conflictual situations, and who are therefore driven to repeat them in one form or another within the process of education [p. 272].

Two examples may serve to describe what happens at the outset of therapy of an abused child and how the golden fantasies of child and therapist work in concert. They also show how projective identification of the child and the countertransference of the therapist operate.

A. was placed in a residential treatment center through legal intervention after his father's violent attacks ended in the child's hospitalization. A.'s parents were both previously divorced with two children each; each took one of the two children and left the other in the care of the former spouse. A.'s parents were married following a brief acquaintance. The marriage soon began to founder, arguments became heated and were accompanied by A.'s father striking A.'s mother. As the marriage deteriorated, the mother sank deeper into herself and her own problems and became increasingly incapable of looking after A. She eventually abandoned the home, leaving A. with his father. The problems between child and father worsened and deteriorated into violent beatings and hospitalization. Eventually, the court had to intervene and the child was placed in a residential treatment center, both because of his severe emotional state and for protection and supervision.

In treatment, A. evoked the therapist's golden fantasy. The therapist summed up the initial period of therapy as follows:

> A. began his therapy by evoking in me the feeling that I was the most important person in the world for him. On the way to his first hour with me he told me that the hour of therapy was an unmatched pleasure where he could do everything he wanted.
>
> At the second meeting he brought his books and phonograph record with him and made me feel that from now on this was his home, this was his refuge. In fact, I felt that he was giving himself entirely to me. He made me feel that I was the only person he had on earth, I was the only one who gave to him unconditionally, the only one he trusted.
>
> In fact, I felt a great deal of sympathy for him, a great desire to give him everything I could, and I also felt sorry for him. I sensed in this initial period of treatment that I was dealing with the question of how I could give him more.

The therapist, as object, was not perceived as constant, as whole, and as having her own self. The therapist was perceived at this stage as a gratifier, as a giver, and, in Kohut's terms (1971), as a mirror and ideal.

The therapist informed us that "A.'s performances are solo performances since he fills the entire space and time of the session and I must take the role of observer who enjoys these performances and admires his roles, such as Superman, Judah Maccabi, and others." The therapist had no reservations in regard to the role assigned to her; she was not uncomfortable with it. On the contrary, she felt herself to be entirely at the disposal of the child, whom she perceived as a passive vessel (even if he performed active roles such as Superman, he was viewed as passive in that he must receive praise, support, admiration, affection, and love).

At this stage of treatment there was a realization of the golden fantasy for both child and therapist. The child felt that the therapist was realizing his fantasy for him, and the therapist realized her fantasy by means of countertransference while she served two roles: the gratifier of needs, on the one hand, and the receptor of gratification by means of countertransference. The case of D. further illustrates this point:

D. was 8 years old when he was placed in a residential treatment center. He was the second child and first son in a two-parent family of six children. The mother was described as suffering from a severe personality disorder. She could not cope with her daily duties, was depressed and subject to frequent outbursts. She rejected D. openly, stating that it was hard for her to touch him since she was "revolted by boys." She exaggerated demands in regard to tidiness and cleanliness, was preoccupied with herself, and generally lost in memories of her own difficult past, memories that she was willing to share with anyone willing to listen. She clearly favored her three daughters over her three sons; with the girls she was exacting and demanding in regard to order and cleanliness, but did not exert physical force, which she did use severely with the boys, especially D. She even starved him and openly expressed how repelled she was by him. For this reason she did not touch him. As soon as he was born, she adopted a special technique of bottle feeding him that obviated the need to touch the baby directly. The father claimed that the mother blamed D. for everything that happened in the house and severely restricted him: "D. is like a hostage in my wife's hands."

In the initial interview D. asked various questions about life in the center: How many children are in each room? Do they get to eat ice cream? What games do they play? He talked easily about his mother's outbursts, her beatings, and his being blamed for everything. Upon his acceptance into the institution his care workers noted that he was "cute and adorable." When he showed up in the dining room he was usually carried by a worker who added that the child waited for her near her apartment on the premises, jumping on her as soon as she came out the door, and that she immediately hugged him and carried him into the dining room. The rest of the staff added that D. was accepted, integrated quickly, and evoked affection and love from everyone.

During the first stage of treatment D.'s therapist noted that D. was anxious at every meeting lest he do something wrong, cause some damage. "I'd better just sit here like a robot, otherwise I'm bound to do some damage here, I'll break some toy." The therapist noted that the boy's fear and anxiety made an impression on her, that she found it hard to look the child in the eyes—eyes which, she claimed, seemed to be begging: "Just don't hurt me." She felt a need to be with the child; she had difficulty ending the session at the set time. She saw the child care worker carrying D. in her arms, hugging him, and she felt jealous of her. The therapist understood that because of her role she could not act like the child care worker; but at that stage she was ready to give up her role as psychotherapist and be the boy's foster mother.

DISAPPOINTMENT AND DESPAIR

Smith (1977) claims that the second aspect of the golden fantasy is the preservation of the fantasy, as if one's very existence depended on maintaining it. This was indeed obvious in the ensuing stages of therapy and in the eventual relationship that developed between the child and his care workers or other staff members, in whom the golden fantasy was aroused through countertransference. In other words, the realization of the fantasy would all too soon end, first and foremost because of the child himself, who was not capable of accepting its fulfillment. The more the fantasy was realized, the more two forces within him operated toward ending this "adventure": (1) the child's inability to relinquish his first wish—that his golden fantasy be realized in the person of his parents, and especially the abusing parent; and (2) the fact that realization of the golden fantasy was illusory, since he would always be aware of its gaps. By means of splitting he would therefore reject any additional attempt on the part of the therapist and other staff members to realize the fantasy.

The first factor—the inability to relinquish the parent—serves as a central force in the changes that take place in this stage of the treatment. Recognition of the treatment center in general, and its staff members in particular, as realizers of the golden fantasy, is tantamount to relinquishing the possibility that the abusive parent is also the benevolent parent, the gratifying, protecting, omnipotent parent. The mechanism of splitting operates intensively here, and any recognition of the therapists and care workers as ideal gratifiers was tantamount to annihilation and utter rejection of the parent.

Not relinquishing the parents as potential realizers of the fantasy also has its roots in the child's own intrapersonal constellation, since renouncing the parent represents renouncing the internalized object, the introject, as if a part of himself were being relinquished. As Cath and Cath (1978) have stated,

> Having invested in a painful relationship, such children paradoxically "prefer" an abusive parent to a kindly stranger or to nonsibling peers. Furthermore, a battered child may later identify with this aggressive aspect of his parent. . . . Giving up such an introject, however negative, would be like giving up an integral, "protective part" of the self because the negative introject has become part of the cohesive self (ego and superego) [p. 629].

Galdston (1981) has dealt with the complexity of the abused child-abusive parent relationship, both from the point of view of the parent vis-à-vis the child and the child vis-à-vis the abusive and rejecting parent. These relations are not consistent and the relationship is beset by great contradictions at different times. It has been noted that after a while, sometimes weeks and sometimes months, the child directs all his yearnings toward the parents. He begins to describe his parents, his family, and his home in rosy hues, as if he had left behind him the best of all possible worlds. He increasingly expresses his resentment against the treatment center and staff members who "forcibly" removed him from his parents' care, "harming" his parents in the process. He complains more and more of his life in the treatment center and begins to ask his parents to do all they can to have him returned to them, to all the "good things" of which he has been robbed because of some "bad judge, bad social worker, bad school principal." This stage is parallel to the one Rinsley (1974) termed the "resistance stage" in institutional therapy.

At this point the child uses the mechanism of projection vis-à-vis the therapist, but he no longer projects onto him the realization of the golden fantasy; rather, the therapist now serves as a target for the projection of aggression and violence. Suddenly the child perceives the therapist as the abuser, the bad person, the rejector, someone out to "get him," and any act on the part of the therapist (or other staff member) is interpreted as intended to harm the child. He enlists his parents, asking them to save him from the violence and aggression he feels in the center and its staff. In other words, those very factors which brought about his removal from home in the first place have become his saviors. Now, when the child projects his aggression onto the therapist, his violent and aggressive internalized object, something also happens in the object relations between child and therapist. Through projective identification, the child activates and controls the therapist so that the therapist performs the part projected onto him.

At the same time, the therapist's countertransference is also activated. He has ceased to see himself in the abused child and can no longer realize his golden fantasy by means of concordant countertransference. Now complementary countertransference takes place; i.e., the therapist begins to identify with the violent object of the child. From this point on we are likely to hear increasing expressions of rejection from the therapists in regard to those same children for whose sake, in the first stage of treatment, they were "ready to come to work every day" and give of themselves completely. A.'s therapist, for example, after several months of therapy, said,

> A. appeared increasingly angry, furious, and disappointed. During one
> of the meetings he decided to build a box, which he wanted to use at

home. In the course of the session he worked on the box, sawed, measured, glued, hammered, nailed. My feeling—in contrast to the feeling I had during the first period of therapy—was that I was totally superfluous here, as if I were just another item in the room that he used.

At the end of the session A. opened his cubby hole in the therapy room and took out the books he had brought to the second therapy session to keep here forever and took them from me—out of the cubby hole, out of the room. I felt insulted, hurt, and betrayed. I seemed to be saying, "How could you do this to me?"

At that same time a conference was being held with the participation of A.'s child care workers, therapists, and others. One of the care workers opened the discussion as follows:

> It's hard to believe that this is the same child that arrived four months ago. I'm sure you remember what I said about him, how he was so cute and adorable. How I sat next to his bed every night before he went to sleep. I honestly don't know what happened to him and how he's changed. Now he's become a real pest. He sticks to me like glue and doesn't leave me alone. He always complains about what's going on. He bothers me all day long with nonsense and squabbles with the other kids. I have to admit that yesterday he had a quarrel with another kid and I actually felt myself standing aside, not getting immediately involved, as if I said to myself: he deserves to be hit a bit. But I really don't understand what happened to him. I would like to understand how he could have changed so much. He was my favorite kid of all, the one I really dedicated myself to. And what gets me even angrier is that several times a day A. threatens to get his father to come here and "straighten things out"—that same father who, we well know, caused A. so much suffering all those years.

It appears that this care worker had already gone on to the stage of complementary countertransference, i.e., he had already identified with the internalized object, the abusive and rejecting parent; in fact, he even used the same method, physical violence, albeit by means of postponing intervention in a quarrel during the course of which A. was hit. The therapist, on the other hand, has not yet reached this stage, i.e., projective identification has not yet made its full impact on her; she is still in the "hurt" stage, although this stage itself indicates that complementary countertransference is taking place, since the abusing parent as the child's introject is not merely the abusing object but also the abused object.

The second factor is the fact that the golden fantasy cannot ever be realized. The child can never be so passive as to be gratified without the benefit of any active intervention on his part; he can never have all his needs and desires immediately gratified without even having to ask. The fantasy cannot even be partially realized, a circumstance that provokes several reactions in the child. First of all, he is no longer prepared to accept anything from the therapist, since the therapist is perceived as disappointing. The mechanism of splitting operates here as well: "Either all or nothing." The child rejects the therapist totally, exhibiting a tremendous amount of aggression toward the therapist. Since the abused child identifies aggression with violence and cannot distinguish any other form of aggression, he expresses his own aggression violently, but this arouses feelings of being "bad." The following are a few examples of such behavior:

> I am bad, I am a dangerous criminal. At my first school I even threw the teacher into the pool. If anybody swore at me, I would beat him to death. One boy had to be brought to the hospital because of what I did to him.
>
> During therapy H. played with a baby doll and said, "He needs an operation. He has to have his heart and all his blood switched. All the pills that we gave him didn't help, and now we have to bring him to the hospital for a long time until everything is replaced."
>
> They buy my brother everything, everything he wants, but they don't buy me anything because I've ruined everything. I've ruined all sorts of toys. I even remember that I broke some jar and everything spilled out on the floor, and my sister was set on fire and cried awfully and then my mother beat me terribly.

Whenever the child receives attention or evidence of concern from the staff members, he is unable to perceive it as something he deserves by virtue of his humanity. As Galdston (1981) states,

> Nothing ever can be earned as deserved. Nothing is ever enough, not because of insufficient quantity but because of the quality of having been stolen. These children are deprived of the experience of contentment, the equitable satisfaction of their own desires through their own efforts on their own behalf. . . . When they do get what they want, it appears to be either the result of luck, and therefore subject to equally fortuitous loss, or as the result of having violated another and therefore at the cost of a guilty conscience [p. 399f.].

Conclusions

The discharge of many cases of abused children from treatment in residential centers before the conclusion of their therapy takes place during the second stage of treatment, which I have called the stage of disappointment and despair. At this stage strong pressure is exerted by those staff members whose countertransference has resulted in their identification with the abusing parent. The stronger the countertransference, and the less control and supervision in the treatment center—processes which permit the functions of countertransference to be diagnosed—the greater is the danger that the child will be discharged prematurely. It is therefore a major task of the residential treatment center to pass this second stage of disappointment and despair successfully. The quality of a residential treatment center can be measured by the degree to which it is able to provide suitable resources to facilitate and enhance its ability to meet the problems that arise in the second stage of treatment. These resources are of two sorts:

1.   The entire staff must be prepared and trained to cope with negativistic expressions of the abused child. These expressions can be verbal or behavioral, or they may take the form of the child ignoring the staff members.

2.   Through controls and supervision, the treatment center must be made aware of countertransference in those of its staff members who come into direct therapeutic contact with the abused child. The processes of identification with the abusive parent are unconscious and therefore require the presence of machinery by means of which they can be "caught" before they can be exerted directly on the child and possibly result in his premature removal from the center and cessation of treatment.

In the absence of resources such as these, the residential treatment center loses its therapeutic character and becomes no more than a framework for boarding children, a shelter. I believe that when Bettelheim (1950) claimed that "love is not enough," he meant, among other things, this process of treatment within a residential center. The removal of an abused child from a residential treatment center and his transfer to another framework because of "deterioration in his condition after a period of good response" only exacerbates the child's problems and decreases the chances of his rehabilitation.

BIBLIOGRAPHY

BETTELHEIM, B. (1950). *Love Is Not Enough*. Glencoe, Ill.: Free Press.

CATH, S. H., & CATH, C. (1978). On the other side of Oz. *Psychoanal. Study Child*, 33:621–640.

GALDSTON, R. (1981). The domestic dimensions of violence. *Psychoanal. Study Child*, 36:391–414.

ILAN, E. (1963). The problem of motivation in the educator's vocational choice. *Psychoanal. Study Child*, 18:266–285.

KOHUT, H. (1971). *The Analysis of the Self*. New York: Int. Univ. Press.
LIEBERMAN, A. F. & PAWL, J. H. (1984). Searching for the best interest of the child. *Psychoanal. Study Child*, 39:527–548.
OGDEN, T. H. (1983). The concept of internal object relations. *Int. J. Psychoanal.*, 64:227–241.
RACKER, H. (1957). The meanings and uses of countertransference. *Psychoanal. Q.*, 26:303–357.
RINSLEY, D. B. (1974). Residential treatment of adolescents. In *American Handbook of Psychiatry*, vol. 2, ed. G. Caplan. New York: Basic Books.
SMITH, S. (1977). The golden fantasy. *Int. J. Psychoanal.*, 58:311–324.

Fantasies of Gender

E. KIRSTEN DAHL, Ph.D.

ENCOUNTERING FRANKIE IN CARSON MCCULLERS' *THE MEMBER OF THE WEDDING,* we recognize a familiar dynamic in this prepubertal girl masquerading as a boy—a regressively oriented fantasy constructed in the attempt to solve conflicts generated by the progressive forces of development. As McCullers helps us to understand, Frankie is afraid of the psychological separation implied by the move into puberty (Dalsimer, 1986) as well as the increasing pressure of the drives as her body begins to mature. The crisis from which she is attempting to retreat has been precipitated by her largely fantasied sexual activity with a boy. Frankie wishes for an ideal world where people can "instantly change back and forth from boys to girls which ever way they felt like and wanted." Frankie does not want to be "caught," as she puts it—she wants to feel "loose," unseparate, mutable. Perhaps it is not surprising either that her next transformation is as F. Jasmine, the *femme fatale* who unwittingly seduces a soldier. Frankie sees herself as a freak, but to the reader her inner crisis precipitated by the demands of approaching puberty is familiar territory, as is her representation of the dimensions of this crisis through the mutability of gender.

In contrast, we are shocked and profoundly disturbed when we slowly realize that the archly feminine Divine of Genet's *Our Lady of the Flowers* recalls her childhood as the boy Culafroy. We struggle to understand Divine as a symbolic transformation of Culafroy's childhood—that in his metamorphosis as Divine he has become the miraculous virgin he adored. He/she has become himself/herself by becoming the Other. Although the character Divine gives literary form to Genet's idea of the infinite possibilities for metamorphosis in any given identity at any given moment (Coe, 1968), Divine's organization around fantasies of degradation, asceticism, and masochism seems fixed, immutable; an abyss seems to separate her from the boy Culafroy.

Assistant clinical professor, Yale University Child Study Center, New Haven.

These two novels vividly depict aspects of the construction of gender. Part of their appeal lies in their ability to capture our imaginative sense that it may not be an impossible leap to become "the other." Most of the time we equate sex and gender; since the former is a biological given, we assume the latter to be immutable as well. These creative works remind us that gender is a construction of the mind and as such potentially transmutable. A much earlier developmental period is touched upon, a period before the certainty of the constancy of gender. The capacity of such works of art to resonate with childhood fantasies of gender mutability tells us something about our curiosity about "transsexuals" and other disorders of gender.

Gender is one area where the interrelationship between body and mind can be examined. The psyche is the main organ of adaptation to the outside world and to the needs and demands of the body. Gender is a complex psychological construction formed from the individual's adaptations to the demands of external reality and social conventions, as well as from subjective efforts to find compromise gratifications to satisfy instinctual drives. Gender draws together aspects of ego development and libidinally driven derivatives of infantile sexuality in the context of object relations, narcissism, and aggressive desires. The pathway to a final gender organization is influenced by development along all of these lines in interaction with one another. Difficulties or distortions in one area will contribute in significant ways to the final apparently seamless, largely unconscious, gender organization. Fantasies are a major expression of the psychological efforts involved in the construction of gender.

Unfortunately, little is known about normal gender development. The attainment of a sense of "gender constancy" develops over time beginning with the ability to categorize persons by gender and concluding at a developmentally later point with the realization that gender is resistant to change. However, as Frankie's story suggests, the cognitive acceptance of the immutability of gender may coexist with wishes for, fantasies of, mutability.

We know that genital experiences begin very early. The emergence of genital awareness during the second half of the second year is followed by the discovery of the genital anatomical difference (Galenson and Roiphe, 1971, 1980; Kleeman, 1971). Heightened genital arousal spurs the child toward schematization of the genital outline of the body along with increasing consolidation of self and object representations (Galenson and Roiphe, 1980). The construction of gender appears to be linked both to the development of object relations and to the vicissitudes of aggression (Pruett and Dahl, 1982). Gender develops out of the matrix of bisexuality (Freud, 1905, 1925); the latter powers fantasies of gender mutability. The earliest reported observations of cross-gender behavior date its occurrence during the latter half of the second year (Steiner, 1985), coinciding with a period of rapid development of the capacity for symbolization (Stern, 1986). Recent infant research suggests that the beginnings of gender identity belong to a developmental time period in which the small child is already capable of complex mentation and symbolic thinking. The heightening of aggression observed during the second year probably contributes to the construction of gender as well. I think these data support the notion that the vicissitudes of gender identity can be viewed as potentially conflictual, complex fantasy configurations. It seems plausible therefore that cross-gender behavior in young children may represent a complex intrapsychic reaction to the discovery of the anatomical differences and an effort to contain anxiety generated both by heightened aggression and the complemental processes of separation-individuation (Person and Ovesey, 1983). However, it is important to keep in mind the possibility that earlier meanings may become transformed retroactively in light of newly acquired libidinal and aggressive aims—a psychological situation so well illustrated by Frankie.

In this paper, I offer three brief clinical vignettes in an effort to use the expression of fantasy configurations to illustrate the underlying complexity of gender identity. Fantasies as they were reported in the psychotherapy sessions of an adolescent girl, a latency-age boy, and a preschool boy are presented. This material is limited to the narration of specific fantasies and does not pretend to convey a sense of the course of the respective treatments. Rather, the vignettes are intended as windows into complex fantasies about gender that may help us understand something of the vicissitudes of gender and the ways in which an individual may develop such constructions in the service of resolving conflict in the inner world.

CASE ILLUSTRATIONS

1. Marty, age 16½, was referred for psychotherapy following a brief psychiatric hospitalization which had occurred after a suicidal gesture following an argument between Marty and her mother. She was described as depressed, with low self-esteem, but not acutely suicidal. In addition, she expressed concern both about her sexual identity, stating that she was "a boy trapped in a girl's body," and about her father who she felt had abandoned her after divorcing her mother when Marty was 7.

Marty's early developmental history was reported as unremarkable. She did well in grade school and had friends. Her parents' marriage was extremely stormy, and Marty witnessed her father beat her mother on several occasions. The mother terminated the marriage when she discovered that the father was involved with another woman. The mother also believed the father had been sexually active with her homosexual brother. It was not clear whether Marty knew of these accusations, although it was useful to assume that she had some sense of them. Contact between father and his children ended at this point.

At age 12, Marty initiated contact with her father. Two years later when Marty was 14½, the mother consulted a mental health clinic because of Marty's expressed concern that she was homosexual. Marty had become sexually involved with a girl who lived near her father. At that time Marty was seen as masculine, walking, talking, and sitting "as if she were a boy." Her descriptions of female figures in her life were "sexualized": she described her younger sister as "a whore" and her mother as overly feminine and obsessed with her looks. She was aware that her mother disapproved of her attachment to another girl but stated that her mother was just going to have to accept it. Psychological testing at this time showed her to be of average intelligence but did not reveal a conclusive diagnosis of homosexuality. Although psychotherapy was recommended, it was not utilized.

When Marty entered psychotherapy at age 16½, she was a junior in a high school to which she commuted because of its excellent athletic record. She was on the basketball team, had a large circle of friends, both boys and girls, worked part time after school, and did poorly academically. Since the age of 9 she had had a number of accidents and sustained multiple injuries, the most notable being four fractures of limbs, three concussions, and one dirt-bike accident in which her leg required multiple sutures.

Evaluation found her to be articulate and coherent with no loose thinking; her affect was frequently constricted, although at other times she appeared sad. She spoke of fearing her own anger and her difficulty in controlling outbursts of temper, which resulted in her hitting other people and punching inanimate objects like doors. She stated that she felt rotten about herself because she could not be a man. She thought that her problems would be solved if she could undergo sex reassignment surgery.

Marty was a short, overweight girl with moderately short curly hair; she dressed in jeans, pastel sweatshirts, and white hightop sneakers. During sessions she sat as a boy might with her legs spread apart, but she also frequently arched back in her chair revealing a bosom. She looked alternately like a young adolescent girl and a prepubertal boy. Marty described herself as part of a group of active "partying" girls. She reported having male friends, too, but these never figured prominently in her narratives. During the 18 months of psychotherapy, Marty had two girlfriends with whom she was sexually active, although neither girlfriend was allowed to touch Marty's body. She reported that these girlfriends accepted her as "a guy" and was insistent that they were "straight," not lesbian. During one hour Marty became quite excited as she imagined the possibility that her girlfriend might be in a situation in which she could be raped by a man. Marty felt enraged that any guy would dare to do such a thing and tried to imagine what she would do to protect her girlfriend. Although she talked of wanting to "punch the guy out," what was most striking was her excited helplessness as she imagined the various ways in which the man might try to rape her girlfriend.

Marty remained insistent that her problem was that she was "a guy in a girl's body." Her fantasies about plastic reconstructive surgery bordered on the miraculous: she would go away Martha and disappear. Instead Marty, a man, would take her place and no one would wonder about what had happened to Martha. She imagined that surgery would give her an unscarred, genitally correct, and potent male body. When confronted with the reality of the surgery, Marty became angry, storming from the session. However, she never made any effort to explore the possibility of surgery, preferring to imagine that therapy would result in some kind of certification for surgery, although she knew this was not the case.

The metaphor Marty used in her psychotherapy was that she was "stuck"—she was neither a girl nor a boy and she could neither move forward developmentally nor go back to being a child. Marty felt that being stuck was the safest place to be. During one session, Marty talked about how her girlfriend Jane's mother had asked if Marty were gay. Marty felt very angry about that. What should she do? She couldn't really talk to Jane's mother; what would she say? She wanted to say she was not gay. That's for sure. But how could Jane's mother understand Marty was really a guy? Jane knew that. Jane said she wouldn't go with Marty otherwise. She could tell Marty was just like a guy. When I commented that Marty wanted to be with Jane sexually like a guy but that sex was hard for her because she was then confronted by the fact of her female body, Marty said, "That's why I don't let her touch me. If she touched me, it'd feel like a guy touching me. I'm not gay. If I were gay, I think I'd want to go with guys." Marty then fell silent. After a bit she said she felt stuck. I commented that the stuck feeling had to do with her body and sex—that Marty seemed to feel that the only way to grow up and allow herself sexual feelings was if she were turned into a man, which wasn't possible. Marty looked depressed and fell silent again. After a bit she stretched, revealing her large breasts. Then she picked up a wooden chair and put it between her legs, steering it as if she were driving a car, making automotive sounds. After a bit she said she wished she could have another dirt bike, but she couldn't because of the accident. In a tone of excited horror she then recounted an earlier accident: Marty was riding with her very first girlfriend on the way to see her father, when she hit a patch of water and spun out. Marty did not realize anything was wrong, even though a car had run into her and flipped her against a tree, until her girlfriend asked her what was wrong with her leg, which had been torn open. Marty fainted and regained consciousness as her father was getting her into an ambulance. She kept saying, "My mother is going to kill me," and the attendant said, "I don't think anyone will hurt you with that guy around," meaning her father because "nobody's going to mess with him." Marty smiled broadly at me as if she had just reported a romantic encounter. After a pause she said in a low engaging voice, "I often think of dying like that."

2.   Jack was first referred at 4¾ years because of concern about his lack of interest in peers and his unusually feminine behavior including cross-dressing (Pruett and Dahl, 1982). Jack's developmental history revealed that at age 2½ his mother suffered a miscarriage of a much wanted second child whom she had imagined to be a girl. The mother became depressed, angrily blamed her husband, and turned to her young son for solace.

Jack and his parents were seen for 18 months in treatment aimed at modifying Jack's feminine behavior, encouraging his identification with his male therapist, and altering the familial interpersonal dynamics that were thought to have led to his feminine behaviors. Jack appeared to improve, developed more of a relationship with his father, and gave up much of his effeminate behavior. Treatment ended when his therapist left the clinic.

Jack returned for treatment at age 7½ because of concern about his poor school performance and unhappy mood. The parents reported that although Jack's effeminate behavior had been "programmed out of him," they continued to feel that his masculine identity was weak.

Jack began treatment preoccupied with witches who were either all good or all bad, and not easily distinguished. Responding to my comment that it must be scary never to know "which witch is which," Jack began to elaborate fairy tales characterized by dominant female figures who were competent, intrusive, and destructive toward the weaker males. For example, in Jack's version of "Little Red Riding Hood," the roles were reversed, so that the little girl was a tough gangster named "Little Red" who continually tormented the ineffectual wolf. The wolf was described as sad and helpless in the face of his insatiable hunger. When I commented that perhaps the wolf felt afraid of his "gobbly feelings," Jack agreed, saying that it was like "being crazy." He then said he remembered feeling hungry all the time as a baby. This association was followed by Jack's interest in "Peter," a helpless rabbit, punished for not obeying his mother. Peter failed to listen to his mother because he felt compelled to find his missing father who, he imagined, would protect him from his intrusive domineering mother. As I clarified how a child might feel with such an intrusive mother, Jack began to attribute increasingly angry feelings to Peter. The story reached a climax when Peter, enraged and starving, destroyed his home, demanding a new one.

Jack's fantasies during the second year of treatment suggested that he felt men were ineffective compared to the primitive omnipotence of women. The year was dominated by the story of "The Pink Panther" who shared a deteriorated house with invisible monsters. This story led Jack to associations about his mother whom he depicted as thoughtless, cruel, and controlling. When some of Jack's realistically based angry reactions to his mother's behavior were supported, Jack decided that the Panther would fix up his house and "get rid of the monsters."

Eventually, the Panther disguised himself as a woman in order to escape the nagging and intrusive "inspector," explaining, "It's safer for the Panther to be dressed as a girl." When I commented that perhaps Jack felt angry at the intrusive inspector, Jack remembered that when he was younger, he had loved to dress up in his mother's clothes: "I felt so good and safe." Thereafter, the Panther became more feminine in appearance, though he always carried a "jet-powered broom." Jack added, "Underneath he's a boy and feels very scared. He doesn't want to have to give up his broom because then he'd really be done for." Jack thought about how angry his parents made him; they were always letting him down. He then returned to the story, saying the moral was "Don't mess with a boy who can be a girl!" Jack went on to tell an "uproarious" story about a boy who was only a head. The boy head searched for a body, but as soon as he found one, he was run over by a truck. Jack said with great laughter, "And the moral of *this* story is— quit while you're a *head*—get it?! Quit while you're a girl!" Jack grew serious and said he remembered how he used to think a lot about witches because you can't tell which witch was which—good or bad. He said he used to wonder what kind of witch his therapist would turn out to be.

During subsequent sessions, Jack returned to the ways in which he felt enraged with his mother. When I suggested that it might be hard to know what to do about a mother who always knew what was best, he repeated, "Don't mess with a boy who can be a girl!" Whenever his rage mounted, Jack feared that his attempts to become independent from his mother would result in the death of one of them. At that point he would become acutely anxious, announce that there was "no escape," and conclude, "I'll just have to grin and bear it."

3.   Colin was referred at age 3½ for an evaluation because of his parents' concern about his exclusive preference for very feminine dolls.

Colin was the result of an unplanned pregnancy when his older brother, Mark, was 3 months old. Mark had been a very difficult, colicky baby who had trouble achieving state regulation, and the mother found herself exhausted with the unexpected pregnancy; she recalled thinking it was terrible timing and wondered how she would manage two babies. The pregnancy was full term and uncomplicated. Birth was easy. From the beginning the mother found Colin to be a darling, lovable, cuddly, and easy baby. The parents thought Colin a quick, responsive baby whose development seemed precocious. They were thrilled with his early walking and talking.

At ages 2 and 3 respectively, both boys entered the same nursery school program. Colin quickly surpassed Mark both cognitively and in skill development. Mark, always a stormy child, became increasingly aggressive in nursery school. The parents speculated that Mark's outbursts might have been a reaction to his fear of being outdistanced by his precocious younger brother. However, by the time the parents sought consultation for Colin, Mark's outbursts had subsided and he was reported to be doing well in school.

The parents reported that Colin was a cheerful outgoing child, well liked by other children, visually alert, sensitive to colors, already identifying letters and numbers, and expressing an interest in reading. Mark was very aggressive toward him and seemed to be very jealous of him. Mark continually took Colin's toys away.

During the summer in which Colin turned 3, both parents became aware of Colin's increasingly exclusive interest in very feminine dolls. Although the father thought Colin might originally have chosen such toys in an attempt to find playthings that Mark would not appropriate, he agreed with his wife that by age 3 Colin did not seem to be interested in any other kind of toy. In addition, the parents noted Colin's growing attachment to Sandy, the daughter of mother's best friend. Sandy was midway in age between Mark and Colin and initially had played more with Mark; gradually the relationship between Colin and Sandy had become exclusive of other children, including Mark.

Colin was reported to have no interest in feminine clothing or make-up, although he was very complimentary of his mother's appearance. His parents described him as appropriately assertive and masculine looking. Nevertheless they felt very uncomfortable with his preoccupation with dolls and decided to get a consultation.

At the time of the consultation, Colin was a short, attractive little boy, sturdy in his manner, who came to his appointment dressed in a stylish athletic outfit. Very well related, he was both appropriately reserved and extremely appealing. Although quite verbal, his articulation seemed somewhat babyish and in his initial presentation there was a sort of "performance quality" as if he might be an adorable television character.

During one evaluation session, Colin began thinking about his brother Mark. At first he talked about how he and Mark had been separated that weekend for the first time when Colin spent the night at the grandparents. He reported that Mark had cried very hard when Colin was away and wondered whether he could have heard Mark. Very shortly, having noticed what he thought was a broken chair, his thoughts turned to Mark's hitting him and how he cried, "A lot, a lot, a lot." Colin recounted, while clutching his genitals and with a good bit of intensity, how Mark one time hit him in the throat, and how Colin had hit Mark "in the same place." Although Colin seemed to be crowing with pleasure at this recollection, he looked anxious.

His thoughts turned from his brother to Sandy, as he imagined calling her on the toy telephone. He then became interested in a picture book, *Bambi Gets Lost*. As he examined an illustration of Bambi and his friends, he became quite insistent that Bambi's mother must be in the picture too. Unable to locate her, Colin claimed that a part of Bambi's ear was his mother. Colin did not seem to have lost touch with reality, but rather it looked as though his need to place Bambi's mother with Bambi was so great that he would have to set aside his own good judgment.

Although Colin protested his mother's leaving the room with a loud whine, "I don't want ya to go!" there was no follow-through, leaving the impression that his complaint was rather pro forma. Immediately upon his mother's departure, however, Colin turned his attention to carefully feeding himself the snack his mother had packed for him. This done, Colin picked up a pig and duck puppet and had them announce, "We like to BIIITE!" They then began to compete with one another over who was higher, "No I'm higher and I don't care." This seemingly insoluble dilemma was resolved with both animals declaring, "No we're the same height."

Nibbling more from his snack, Colin began to examine the mirror. Making a big mouth, he announced, "I have lipstick. From Sandy." He glanced provocatively at me, "Do you?" When I said no, Colin turned his attention back to the mirror, and after a long dark gaze, he said softly, "I have a bigger mouth than you." This introduced a long fantasy in which Colin imagined he was "a real bad guy" who would eat me for dinner. "And you'll do nothing! I'm not going to let you go anywhere! I'm going to eat you for dinner! I'm not going to let you have any of your other parts," Colin said as he imagined breaking off parts of my body and making me dead. As he imagined possessing me completely, he announced that this would make me bad; "We'll get the other bad guys," he whispered. He became quite conspiratorial as he invited me to join him in getting the "real real bad guys"; he pointed out that "really" I would have to do it, "Because I'm just a kid." Colin went on to enumerate how the two of us would break every part of the bad guys' bodies—arms, necks, "everything." Still whispering, he told me, "If they come to our house, they'll take our dolls and toys away." As Colin circled around me whispering conspiratorially about the dangerous bad guys and how the two of us would get the bad guys, he began to clutch his genitals and then his bottom. Shortly he announced that he had to go to the bathroom.

Colin and I left the room so that he could use the toilet. Once there he told me with great animation how he and Sandy got to be friends. She had been his brother's "girlfriend," Colin said, and they were always leaving him behind to climb walls and things. "You can't come you're too little, they were always saying." He didn't like that and so he practiced and practiced his climbing until he could climb "anything." Then one day he just went along and climbed what they climbed. And "Sandy saw" he could climb things and so, Colin crowed, "She said I could be her friend and we just left Mark behind!" With this Colin beamed and sighed. It was as if he had told me what needed to be said. He finished his business in the bathroom and went back to the playroom where he finished the session arming the knights with weaponry, helmets, and flying horses.

During a subsequent meeting with Colin's parents, they reported that Colin had lost interest in his dolls and had become a good bit more aggressive, challenging his brother to various tests of strength, being furious when he lost. Recently he had announced, "There'll be two first places—me and Mark—and one last—Daddy!" The father wondered whether Colin's interest in the dolls might have been "fetishlike." He revealed that Colin's interest in the dolls seemed to be primarily an interest in their hair; he wanted only those with the longest hair. The father confided that the parents adored Colin's great mass of curls—so like the father's once had been (he was now losing his hair) and had often told Colin that his hair was "just like Daddy's" had been and that his father had loved his own so much during college that he had worn it in a then-fashionable pony tail! The mother then recalled that Colin had never complained about getting his hair cut until very recently. She reported that Colin had noticed one fish hiding in the aquarium at the barber's and had asked about it. The barber had said the fish was hiding so the other fish "wouldn't take a nip out of him." Colin had paled, grabbed his hair, and said, "And I don't want my penis cut off either!"

DISCUSSION

Although Marty presented herself as having achieved a fixed but pathological gender identity, that of a man trapped in a woman's body, in fact the central dynamic in her fantasy had to do with feelings of being "stuck," of refusing to "choose," and of being neither male nor female. The fantasy of a man trapped in a woman's body appeared to be a highly organized and condensed construction, ego syntonic and successful (although maladaptive) in keeping out of awareness Marty's intensely conflictual sexual fantasies. Paradoxically the apparent fixity and rigidity of the fantasy of being a man in a woman's body mask her insistence on gender mutability, allowing Marty to experience herself as simultaneously a boy and a girl. The incompatibility of these two stances is kept from awareness by Marty's use of externalization—outside reality "forces" her to be a girl because of her body. In order to maintain this split, Marty is forced to disavow her own sexual pleasure; if she became aware of her capacity for sexual pleasure, she would be reminded that the body she represents as belonging to external reality (social convention) is hers and part of her inner world as well. Further, in her statement that if she allowed her partner to touch her, "I would feel like I was being touched by a man," there is a hint of highly conflicted heterosexual fantasies, experienced as extremely dangerous perhaps because of their preoedipal, sadomasochistic valence. It is possible that another source for her self-destructive behavior—besides giving representation to fantasies of a damaged and hated body—lies in an effort to reclaim her disavowed body; hurting her body gives dimensionality to it and serves to remind her that she is contained in and by her body. By report Marty's gender dysphoria began with the onset of puberty, suggesting that her most intense conflicts may have been stimulated by the dangers of the transformation of preoedipally colored erotic fantasies in the context of the sexually maturing body (Laufer and Laufer, 1984). Marty illustrates the ways in which it is possible retroactively to transform previous meanings in the light of newly acquired libidinal and aggressive aims. Unfortunately because of the rigidity and complexity of the fantasy, "man trapped in a woman's body," Marty, although unhappy, is not very amenable to treatment.

Jack's gender pathology is the end path in a quite different sequence. His cross-gender behavior appeared in the third year of life, during a period in which we would expect his strivings for autonomy and control to be heightened. I think it is difficult to know whether Jack entered this phase with a constitutionally based vulnerability to anxiety. Certainly by age 7 he exhibited both a vulnerability to anxiety and disorganization in his thinking under the press of anxiety. At any rate, his mother's angry depression during this early period resulted in her being less available to him as an age-appropriate container for his anxiety and aggression and more available to him at a regressive level at which Jack experienced himself as no longer autonomous and differentiated. Conflict over autonomous strivings seems to have been poorly resolved for Jack, probably from a combination of environmental and constitutional factors. This unfinished developmental task then seemed to become entangled with somewhat later age-typical castration anxiety. Phallic strivings became distorted by the poorly resolved anal conflicts over autonomy and his experience of his own aggressive drive derivatives colored by fantasies of annihilation and fusion. It was as if there was no way to be separate and autonomous from his mother without giving up his penis. Jack's fantasies suggest that he attempted to preserve his endangered penis through identification with a phallic, bisexual woman.

Colin's fetishlike attachment to the very feminine dolls appears to be a compromise formation at the oedipal level. The dolls give symbolic representation to both his identification with his father via his hair and displacement upward. It is as if the dolls function as a talisman to keep the identification and displacement viable and thereby ward off the experience of castration anxiety. One can speculate that the identification with his mother and Sandy represents his attempts to possess them as oedipal objects: "I'll show you how much I love you by being you." In addition, the identification simultaneously masks his aggression and contains it; the feminine identification allows him to be his mother's adored, competent, good boy, not the damaged bad boy. It is also possible that this compromise formation contains the fantasy of "the price of victory." After all, Colin has bested his brother twice—with his mother and with Sandy—and the dolls represent toys for which his brother has contempt. It is as if Colin were saying, "I will take second best here and then perhaps you won't notice my victory there." By accepting the appearance of castration, Colin is able both to protect his penis and preserve his oedipal victory. It is interesting that after the session in which he revealed his oedipal victory with Sandy and the force of his aggressive strivings to possess his mother, Colin became openly competitive and aggressive at home with both his brother and his father, simultaneously relinquishing the dolls.

These vignettes give us a window on the highly individual and complex dynamics of gender construction, a construction that evolves over time and involves various subjective states especially as revealed in fantasy configurations concerning the body, objects, and the drives. "Gender identity" is not a fixed normative end point in a linear developmental sequence but a complex construction involving the interrelationships between body and mind and between inner and outer reality. It includes the possibility of retroactive transformation of previous meanings in the light of new libidinal and aggressive aims. The mind must find a balance between the needs and demands of outer reality and the needs and demands of the body (Ritvo, 1984); it does so through the creation of the configuration of fantasies we subsume under the term "gender identity." Although apparently seamless by adulthood, gender develops from the matrix of bisexuality and so contains within it the capacity to resonate with fantasies of mutability (Freud, 1905, 1925).

It is for these reasons that I question Stoller's formulation that the pathologies of gender are the result of the child's failure to differentiate from a primary feminine matrix contained in the symbiotic union between mother and child (Stoller, 1974, 1985). This view seems both too simple and simply wrong. It is too simple to view gender as the result only of the process of identification and its vicissitudes. And it is incorrect to suggest that the child's identification with mother is monolithic. Stoller himself seems to recognize this in his more dynamic formulations concerning the mothers of gender-dysphoric boys (Stoller, 1985); here he depicts the mother's identity as composed of multiple identifications developed from the matrix of bisexuality and woven together in a highly idiosyncratic whole. Clearly the child identifying with the mother has multiple aspects of the mother from which to pick and choose.

Our task is to understand how a particular child constructs his or her gender—how the highly individual, subjective sense of maleness and femaleness comes into being. Our emphasis must be on the process and the inherent variability of outcome, not on gender as a dichotomous variable. We need to ask: what kinds of problems have been entertained and what possibilities were available for their resolution? What lines of development and conflict resolution have been favored and at the expense of what others? It is in this context that the question of the sex of the therapist should be examined (a question so often raised as a technical issue in the treatment of the gender pathologies). If we reject the view of gender development as the result of social learning or identification, then we should not expect therapeutic action to lie in the sex of the therapist. On the other hand, we can expect the sex of the therapist to have great importance in the therapy as it is used by the child to represent some of the meanings of gender. Obviously this is not an argument in favor of choosing one sex over the other, but is a plea for us to attend to gender as a process that favors something at the expense of something else (Grossman and Kaplan, 1986).

The developmental endpoint of that aspect of identity called gender gives it the appearance of fixity that obscures the fact that gender organization is not a dichotomous variable, male/female. Gender identity is a complex psychological construction centering on the body, interactions with the bodies of others, and the drives. These psychological constructions, often expressed in fantasies, spring from the bedrock of human bisexuality that allows us to try on in our imagination, and so experience within ourselves and in interaction with others, efforts to find gratifications and to solve conflicts originating between the needs and demands of the body and outer reality. As a developmental pathway it draws together aspects of ego development and derivatives of infantile sexuality in the context of libidinally driven object relations, narcissism, and aggressive desires. The so-called "final" patterned organization is influenced and integrated by development along all of these lines. Difficulties or distortions in any area make significant contributions to the final, apparently seamless, and largely unconscious mosaic of gender organization.

BIBLIOGRAPHY

Coe, R. N. (1968). *The Vision of Jean Genet.* New York: Grove Press.
Dahl, E. K. (1986). Reflections on the development of gender identity and its vicissitudes. *Contemporary Psychiatry*, 5(4):233–236.

DALSIMER, K. (1986). *Female Adolescence.* New Haven: Yale Univ. Press.

FREUD, S. (1905). Three essays on the theory of sexuality. *S.E.,* 7:123–247.

—— (1925). Some psychical consequences of the anatomical distinctions between the sexes. *S.E.,* 19:241–258.

GALENSON, E. & ROIPHE, H. (1971). The impact of early sexual discovery on mood, defensive organization and symbolization. *Psychoanal. Study Child,* 26:196–216.

—— —— (1980). The preoedipal development of the boy. *J. Amer. Psychoanal. Assn.,* 28:805–828.

GENET, J. (1963). *Our Lady of the Flowers.* New York: Grove Press.

GROSSMAN, W. I. & KAPLAN, D. M. (1986). Three commentaries on gender in Freud's thought. Unpublished.

KLEEMAN, J. A. (1971). The establishment of core gender identity in normal girls. *Arch. Sex. Behav.,* 1(2):103–129.

LAUFER, M. & LAUFER, M. E. (1984). *Adolescence and Developmental Breakdown.* New Haven: Yale Univ. Press.

McCULLERS, C. (1950). *The Member of the Wedding.* Toronto: Bantam Books.

PERSON, E. S. & OVESEY, L. (1983). Psychoanalytic theories of gender identity. *J. Amer. Acad. Psychoanal.,* 11:203–226.

PRUETT, K. D. & DAHL, E. K. (1982). Psychotherapy of gender identity conflict in young boys. *J. Amer. Acad. Child Psychiat.,* 21:65–70.

RITVO, S. (1976). Adolescent to woman. *J. Amer. Psychoanal. Assn. Suppl.,* 24(5):127–138.

—— (1984). The image and uses of the body in psychic conflict. *Psychoanal. Study Child,* 39:449–469.

STEINER, B. W., ed. (1985). *Gender Dysphoria.* New York: Plenum Press.

STERN, D. N. (1985). *The Interpersonal World of the Infant.* New York: Basic Books.

STOLLER, R. J. (1974). Symbiosis anxiety and the development of masculinity. *Arch. Gen. Psychiat.,* 30:164–172.

—— (1985). *Presentations of Gender.* New Haven: Yale Univ. Press.

Family Intervention and Parental Involvement in the Facilitation of Mourning in a 4-Year-Old Boy

ELISABETH MUIR, B.SC.,
ANN SPEIRS, BA.Hons., and GINNY TOD

THE THEORETICAL CONTROVERSY SURROUNDING CHILDHOOD MOURNING includes some differing views regarding the necessary levels of cognitive and ego development which have to be achieved before mourning can occur. This is reflected in the contingent controversy over the age at which mourning can take place. It has been variously argued that mourning in children is possible from as early as 6 months (Klein, 1946; Winnicott, 1954; Bowlby, 1960, 1980), from 3½ to 4 years (A. Freud, 1960; R. A. Furman, 1964), from 7 to 8 years (Anthony, 1973), or not until adolescence (Wolfenstein, 1966). In 1974 E. Furman argued that 2- to 3-year-olds appropriately guided and taught can mourn, and drew our attention to the mediating effect of the environment on the process of childhood mourning. It is now widely accepted that in bereaved families a surviving parent's unresolved mourning with its defensive behavioral consequences *does* interfere with a child's capacity to mourn.

There is strong evidence to support the belief that the circumstantial aspects of a bereavement can profoundly affect the family and thus the capacity of the surviving parent to help the grieving child to accept and integrate the reality of a parent's death and to adjust to life without him

Elisabeth Muir was senior child psychotherapist, Otago Hospital Board, Dunedin, and clinical lecturer, department of psychiatry, University of Otago, Dunedin, and is currently in private practice in Dunedin, New Zealand. Ann Speirs is child psychotherapist, specialist services, department of social welfare, Dunedin, New Zealand. Ginny Tod is child psychotherapist, specialist services, department of social welfare, Christchurch, New Zealand.

or her (Adam, 1982). That this is necessary in order to avoid a pathological outcome (Wolkind and Rutter, 1985; Adam, 1982) is of clinical significance.

This paper will describe the assessment and treatment of a child in a situation where that child's arrested grieving was not only a reflection of his mother's difficulty in mourning but was also, in part, being perpetuated by the mother's need to project into him her disowned and disavowed grieving self. Her defenses established within, and perpetuated by her own family, not only directly impeded her capacity to mourn adequately, but also made her parents and friends unavailable to her, effectively depriving her and her children of the supportive network so necessary to a bereaved family. Her recourse to projective mechanisms prevented her from objectifying, and therefore helping, her son with his struggle to accept and integrate the death of his father.

The setting in which we worked was a developmental center which specialized in the assessment and ongoing therapy of preschoolers and their families. A formulation and treatment plan would follow a minimum of three assessment sessions, including a home visit. Frequently we found it was necessary to extend the assessment process when an adequate formulation could not be reached.

THE CASE STUDY

Four-year-old David was referred by the family doctor following a consultation with his mother. She had been having difficulty managing her elder son's angry tantrums and demanding, clingy behavior, which had been a problem for a year following his father being killed by a falling tree—something David had witnessed. David's behavior was described as becoming worse since the death of his father. He was also exhibiting extreme jealousy toward his younger brother; although he attended preschool, he was reluctant to mix with other children.

DEVELOPMENTAL HISTORY

David's mother, Mrs. X, was the younger of two girls brought up in an intact family. She had little to say about her city childhood, but remembered always feeling inferior to her sister, 6 years her senior. After leaving school, Mrs. X worked in a shop for some time, continuing to live at home. At 17 years she met John, a farmer some 6 years older; they were married when Mrs. X was only 18 and moved to live on his farm 150 km. away. David was born soon afterward and Mark, her younger son, 2 years later.

David was conceived around the time of his parents' marriage. The pregnancy was complicated by high blood pressure and Mrs. X spent some weeks before the birth in the city maternity hospital away from her husband and new home. Labor was long and difficult, and eventually a forceps delivery was necessary. However, Mrs. X remembered that David was given to her straight after the birth. Breast-feeding was established and continued until David was 10 months old, when he weaned himself. Mrs. X reported that he was a colicky baby. His development and milestones were average.

When David was 3 years old, Mr. X suffered the farm accident which caused his death. Following this, Mrs. X attempted for a time to manage the farm on her own. She felt conflicting pressures. On the one hand, her father offered little comfort to her in her grief, but advised her to sell the farm. An estrangement between father and daughter dated from this period. On the other hand, she felt an obligation to her dead husband and his family, for whom the farm and the land had special meaning. The farm had only been marginally profitable and proved too much for the young widow. Three months after the accident she sold the property, reluctantly and with feelings of guilt, and returned to her home town. She bought a house and settled with her two small sons not far from her parents' home.

ASSESSMENT

David's mother was a subdued young woman who became easily tearful and appeared particularly irritable toward David, whom she described as a demanding, naughty child. She spoke of a depression pervading all her activities and revealed that although she had family and friends close by, she was unable to talk with them about her husband's death for fear of overburdening them. She also conveyed a strong need to cope by herself; because of this she failed to ask her family for emotional support and yet was resentful that they seemed unaware of her needs. She also let us know that she was planning to go on a holiday without the children in three weeks' time.

Throughout the assessment we observed that the boys played independently and appropriately, but were watchful of their mother and responsive to her mood. It became clear that Mrs. X was discriminating between her sons. Mark was able to get physically close to her; she would voice her pleasure and enjoyment of him, saying, "He's a charmer." David, however, was watchful, often keeping himself at a distance. Mrs. X was unable to respond to his attempts to interest and impress her, and she in turn tried to get him to play with her when his attention was elsewhere.

David's play revealed his preoccupation with his father's death when he failed to find a place for the father doll in the doll's house. He repeatedly bumped into things and stumbled, strenuously denying any hurt to himself. He was seen to clutch his penis frequently and displayed an unusual degree of concern and solicitousness for Mark. He armed himself and Mark with toy guns and was preoccupied with a wolf puppet and with a Sendak wall frieze depicting some wild monsters.

PROVISIONAL FORMULATION AND TREATMENT PLAN

We understood that Mrs. X's stated need to establish her independence was probably due in part to her having married and had children while she was still quite young. In addition, her late husband had had responsibility and independence thrust on him at an early age, thus providing a powerful model for her to emulate, and a way for her to internalize an aspect of him. Her father, by urging her to sell the farm, had painfully exposed his daughter's conflict regarding autonomy: at this period we assumed that a regressive pull toward a renewal of dependency would battle against fears of dependency. Mrs. X's wish to cope without falling back on her family might be understood in these lights, but her strong fear of overburdening people, and her family in particular, needed further understanding. Whatever the reasons, it was clear that by not sharing her grief she was failing to work through the mourning process and was thus depriving herself of the understanding and acceptance she needed. Something prevented her from responding empathically to her children's, and especially David's, distress. We decided to offer Mrs. X some individual sessions to help work through the mourning process. We also decided that since David had been able to use the playroom well during the assessment, this work could continue on an individual basis to address his own difficulties. Because we felt Mrs. X could benefit from participating in her son's work on his unresolved grief, we decided to offer her the opportunity to share her son's sessions by observing them through a one-way screen along with another therapist.

It was felt that Mrs. X's reluctance to share her grief with her family reflected some conflictual issues from within her family. We decided we needed to explore this further and to assess her family's capacity to provide the necessary support and containment. Within the wider family there was a precedent of children going into care following a parental death; we felt there was a risk that this could be repeated and that our intervention should focus on cementing the integrity of this fragile family. Accordingly we made a decision to extend the assessment to include a joint family session with Mrs. X, her children, and her parents, Mr. and Mrs. J.

In our formulation meeting with Mrs. X we presented her with these conclusions and treatment options. She accepted the offers of individual help for herself and the opportunity to view David's individual therapy. Our suggestion that we hold a joint family session with her parents met with resistance. She expressed doubt that her father would want to come and let us know that she was not even sure she wanted him to be involved. She finally agreed to a joint family session on condition that the emphasis would be on the forthcoming separation of Mrs. X and her children while she was on holiday and the implications of this for David.

FAMILY SESSION

Initially this three-generational family session concentrated on the relatively safe issue of child care over Mrs. X's forthcoming three-week holiday. A discussion of the possible effects the separation might have on David was brought to a close when Mr. J. said he was more worried about his daughter than his grandson. Both his wife and daughter began to cry, and Mrs. J. described feeling helpless with regard to her daughter's tragedy; she felt she always said the wrong thing. Mr. J. said he thought his daughter would have "a breakdown" if she kept on the way she was. He added angrily that thousands of widows had had to cope with bereavement in the war and that one shouldn't dwell on death. During this time David was shooting everyone in the room with a toy gun and was finally reprimanded by his grandfather. The therapist intervened, commenting that she wondered if David's behavior might not be connected to what they were discussing. She asked David what he felt about his father. David said he was sad; and then clearly stated he was angry too. This obviously shocked his grandparents, and it was only when the therapist reassured them that such feelings were in fact normal that Mr. J.'s rigid posture flagged and tears came into his eyes. He then talked about his never forgotten experiences of atrocities and death during the war. He said he had seen his friends die, but had not had "even half an hour" to think about them before having to get on with the fighting. Toward the end there was more warmth between all the family members, and Mr. J. was able to say he had not wanted to come but had appreciated the session and felt relieved to have unburdened himself. The session ended with this acknowledgment of the need for time to mourn properly and thus permission for Mrs. X and David to do so within the therapeutic setting.

Mrs. X in the next session reported feeling better about her father, saying that things between them were easier.

INDIVIDUAL AND FAMILY FORMULATIONS

From the history it seemed likely that David had experienced a satisfactory infancy. However, the colic suggested a possible early element of anxiety and tension in the mother-infant interaction. Mrs. X had to make several major adaptations within a few months: from city life to a rural life of isolation, physical challenge, and sometimes hardship; from child status in her family of origin to that of partner in a marriage; and, finally, to the demanding task of motherhood. This was a happy period, according to Mrs. X, but it must also have been a stressful one.

The fatal accident took place when David was aged 3 and his brother Mark was close to a year in age. By then, David could be expected to have achieved libidinal object constancy (Mahler et al., 1975), and to have acquired some fusion of libidinal and aggressive impulses following the intense ambivalence of anal sadism (A. Freud, 1963). Recent intrapsychic achievements are fragile, however, and major stress would lead to regression. The conflicts and tantrums reported by Mrs. X appeared to indicate renewed ambivalence. David's anxious watchfulness suggested a loss of object confidence regarding his mother.

The death of David's father provided the realization of one half of the oedipal fantasy. David would both cognitively and psychologically experience that death as in some way his doing. Cognitively, in Piaget's terms, David's thinking was egocentric. The psychological aspect of egocentrism is omnipotence under which the child experiences his personal power as boundless. Normally, this omnipotence is challenged by the parents' rules and by the vicissitudes of the child's experience. Reality testing develops and gradually the child is able to relinquish both his omnipotence and his oedipal hopes. For David, however, this process was disrupted by the death of his father. Because he was the frequent recipient of his mother's angry projections, his fantasies of destructive omnipotence were confirmed. These would be accompanied by powerful unconscious fears of paternal retaliation. David's frequent "accidents" in the playroom, accompanied by an anxious denial of hurt, seemed indicative of such fears and fantasies.

The other half of the oedipal fantasy had not been realized, however. Mark, a charming and assertive toddler, clearly afforded his mother pleasure. Equally clearly Mrs. X derived little pleasure from David. David's exaggerated concern for his younger brother defended against

angry oedipal rivalry. Resolution of the oedipal conflict would be difficult for David in the absence of a male object with whom he could
achieve a comfortable latency identification. Moves to resolve the conflict would be impossible while there was an apparent splitting between
a "good" boy and a "bad" boy in Mrs. X's perception of her sons. Mrs. X
had always perceived herself as being the inferior child in her family of
origin. Now, because of projective processes, this inferior status
seemed to be passing to David.

David was also struggling with issues of autonomy (Erikson, 1950).
But the violent death of his father was a fearsome example of what can
happen to strong, assertive male figures. Moreover, Mrs. X often set
overfirm limits and reacted negatively to David's desire for independence. It seemed that David's developmental task was being hampered
by his mother who had only limited experience of personal autonomy
and for whom the issue was conflictual. The mode and timing of her
presentation seemed to reflect this ambivalence regarding dependency: Mrs. X had sought help shortly before leaving on holiday, thus
providing herself with a way to terminate the contract, should help
become too conflictual for her to accept.

The multigenerational family session provided insight into Mrs. X's
difficulties with mourning. In her world people avoided emotional
expression lest it overwhelm them. She herself described to us her fear
that if she abandoned herself to grief, she "would never get up again."
After the death and up to the time of referral, she felt emotionally
isolated because of her mother's "helplessness" when faced by powerful feelings and her father's rigid lack of sympathy, masking feelings of
helplessness.

Mrs. X had been unable to own or express anger with her husband
for his abandonment of her by death: instead David's anger seemed to
express this for her through the process of projective identification
(Klein, 1946). Because her anger could not be owned, David's had to be
punished. David's caretaking of his mother and brother appeared to
express the care for herself which Mrs. X longed for but denied.

Our additional understanding of the family's emotional restriction
reassured us that our plan for individual sessions for David, observed
by his mother, was appropriate. The therapist working with David,
encouraging him to own and express the full range of his feelings,
would be able to show that powerful, even violent, feelings could be
expressed safely. This example of therapeutic containment might in
turn render it easier for Mrs. X to acknowledge and express her own
conflictual feelings. She had in fact begun to do this in the few individual sessions she agreed to have, where she revealed her guilt over

not wanting to see her husband after he had died and described how exhausted she had become trying to run the farm by herself. After sharing this with the therapist, Mrs. X decided not to have any more sessions for herself. This was accepted because it was felt that she had begun the mourning process and that by sharing with and understanding her son's mourning in a safe environment, her tentative steps in this direction would be reinforced.

DAVID'S INDIVIDUAL SESSIONS

David had six sessions with a child psychotherapist during which he described, often in detail, the journey he had traveled since the day that the tree fell and killed his father. His material showed a striking preoccupation with powerful and dangerous creatures, with his father, with death and destruction. His fantasy world was so vivid, and his ability to explain it so good, that the therapist often felt she was the observer, and even sometimes a participant, in six 50-minute dreams that began as soon as he entered the room and ended when he left.

David responded to his therapist's initial tentative explorations of his thoughts regarding his father by talking about "dress-ups," saying his father had a lot of them, "a dragon, a fox, a lion, and a wolf one." He said he wasn't scared of them because he had some himself and, pointing to the wall frieze with its wild-looking monsters, said his Dad was the sea dragon and that he was safe "because no sharks could get him."

The trees in the wall frieze provoked the memory of his father's death, and David talked of the "big nasty tree" which started to fall on his Dad until David shot it with his gun, causing it to fall in another direction, so saving his father. Here David commented that he had to be very strong and look after his father. In describing another accident, he talked of a tree that had prickles on it and a horrible monster face and which fell on his father. There was a lot of "muddy yucky blue and red sort of stuff" around after the tree had hit his father.

In recalling the accident, David described his parents both going away in the ambulance while he went off to play with his friends. This was "alright," but he had to look after his little friend too. "It's really hard work caring for people."

The theme of David's role as protector of his father was a recurring one, poignantly related in a story in which a "nice man" was saved (by David's gun), and safely placed in a locked room "where the monsters couldn't get him." David's relief was marred by sadness at his inability to get in to reach the nice man because the door was "only a tiny one." His solution, that the boy should get smaller, was qualified: "Not baby size, just middle size." David tenderly placed a cover over the baby doll in the pram as he talked of the boy getting into the room and being really happy. At this time he asked for the therapist's help in doing up his shoe lace, something that developed into a repeated interaction between him and his therapist. In subsequent play he revealed the extent of his awesome task. He needed to dig "the biggest hole [in the sandpit] in the world"—to stop his Dad feeling sad. He had to be "really good" for fear his Dad would be sad and go away; that is why he was never naughty. He had to look after the therapist too because she might cry, although he reassured her that if she did she wouldn't die. He had to look after his mother and his friend Mark for the same reason. And he mustn't show he'd hurt himself because *he* might die. Following a reassurance that in the playroom it was his therapist's job to look after him, not for him to look after her, David practiced putting himself at risk by climbing repeatedly onto a barrel and eliciting his therapist's help to prevent him hurting his leg.

In the middle of his therapy David shared with his therapist his fantasy that there were big birds with no wings at kindergarten and they could kill people, including him. He added that it was his job to protect his friends from these birds; and he seemed really worried. Later he said that the birds had died, but he still didn't want to go back to kindergarten, because they were lying on the floor and it was still "yucky." He thought he might be able to go back later. The following week David informed the therapist that she had been wrong about the dangerous birds, and that they weren't at kindergarten at all.

The termination of David's sessions had been carefully planned, and at this time his therapist clarified with him that there would be two more sessions in which to say good-bye. In these final sessions he was able both verbally and through his play to reveal his anger at his therapist. Having said he was angry, he added that he wanted to be bigger than she was so that he could make the rules; he went on to talk about digging a hole and putting her in it, commenting that since she wasn't as strong as his father, he, David, must now be stronger than she. Amidst repeated testing of playroom rules he talked of an angry wild wolf and proceeded to "cook" the wolf puppet in a pot on the toy stove. When the therapist remarked that people sometimes had feelings that seemed like wolves inside them—angry feelings—David asked if she had an angry wolf inside her. She acknowledged that she did sometimes feel angry, and he went on to talk about his own angry wolf feelings, placing the wolf puppet on his hand and threatening to eat the therapist up. He added that he had used his angry wolf to eat and kill the dangerous birds at kindergarten.

In the final session David reassured his therapist that he could "now swim" and he was safe (in reference to a story about a man falling into the sea). He had spent most of the session playing in the doll's house. In this play he had laid the boy doll (which he identified as himself) on a bed, then placed the father doll on the floor beside him. In the drama that unfolded the father doll sometimes went through to his wife's bedroom, but there was always a struggle to get through the small door to her room. The David doll went downstairs, followed by the father, who had an accident on the way and fell out of the house. Although he tried to climb back in, he couldn't. David tried to get the father to hold a gun, but it was too big. The David doll was put in the kitchen with a gun beside him. Another gun was placed next to the mother doll in her bedroom. The father doll was left outside.

As this session was coming to a close, David gave some magic medicine to an imaginary "bad and nasty" shark, changing it into a fish that "would not hurt anything." He then commented that they hadn't played with the wild things all that week.

Initially David had avoided talking about the end of sessions, threatening to shoot the therapist if she mentioned the subject. Toward the end of the session the therapist talked about the sad feelings people often had about finishing, and said that she would be sad not to see David in therapy anymore. David said he would be sad too—he had wanted to keep coming, but next week he would be going to kindergarten.

DISCUSSION OF INDIVIDUAL SESSIONS

David's material made it plain that he believed his behavior could affect the life and death of people around him. The anxiety caused by omnipotent fantasy had led David to create fantasies of benign destruction, with protection of the father as their aim.

In an early session David explained that unless he was good, people would get sad and go away. This statement came shortly after the holiday separation from his mother and was a clear indication of the stress David must have experienced at this time. No disturbance was acknowledged, however, by either Mrs. X or her parents—an example of the family's mode of denial and perhaps also of David's struggle to repress anxiety.

David's omnipotent fantasies meant that he felt responsible for the safety of those around him, as his caretaking activities indicated. His tender play with the baby doll, and the request to the therapist to do up his shoe, showed the yearning for care for himself that lay behind his activities. In therapy David started to take care of the therapist—but also hinted at how hard it was to take on an adult, invincible role. When the therapist insisted that *she* was the caretaker, David showed immense relief: he was able to practice being held safely while he climbed the barrel. While thus held he played out the issue in a more appropriate manner with a toy car, which was constantly in danger of falling from the barrel, but was kept safe by David. In a later session he passed over responsibility for the dangerous birds which had made kindergarten unsafe to the therapist—and in so doing seemed to shed much of his burden of guilt.

The biggest challenge to David's omnipotence came with the process of termination. Here David was again confronted with impending object loss. We believed that through the experience of a planned termination, the most beneficial part of therapy would be for David to understand that the end of the therapeutic relationship was not brought about by him. David acted out his conflict in his fantasied attacks on and threats to the therapist. Her task was to survive these attacks, to show that she was neither saddened nor angered by them, and to insist that it was her decision to finish the sessions because the work of therapy had been done. At this time she also frequently emphasized that just as David was not responsible for the end of therapy, so he had not been responsible for the tree falling on his father.

At the beginning of therapy David had needed to deny the angry side of himself. Anger was kept at a distance and figured in his fantasies of angry, destructive monsters. Gradually David allowed his own dangerous anger to come closer; he handled the guns, devoured the therapist with a wolf puppet, and once the therapist had owned her "angry wolf," was able to acknowledge and discuss his angry feelings. In the final session he turned a fierce shark into a harmless fish, showing an awareness that his impulses could also change, that they were not dangerous, immutable monsters.

Like his mother, David struggled with issues of dependency. These were explored over several sessions, often focusing on David's shoes. David would ask or order the therapist to put on his shoes, then reject her angrily or kick them off again. These battles had their counterpart at home in fights over clothes and food. David's desire for autonomy was in conflict with his ambivalence regarding growing up. To be small was to be safe. To grow up meant to assume power but also uncomfortable responsibilities. It meant facing the ambivalence of his objects. David's shrinking in size to get close to his father suggested an anxiety with his destructive oedipal wishes. Fear of retaliation from the father of the oedipal fantasy was masked behind descriptions of the "nice man." As his sessions progressed, David quickly developed an intense oedipal transference with his therapist, indicating the importance of oedipal concerns. He swaggered in front of her; addressed her in a lordly manner; was alternately coy, charming, and demanding; and angrily spoiled the playroom for other children.

David's rich fantasy illustrated his level of cognitive and psychological development, characterized by a fluid merging of fact and fantasy, symbol and object, which in adult life finds its expression in dreams. The monster trees, the dress-ups worn by the father, the sea dragons in the Sendak frieze, the bears, the wingless birds, the wolves and sharks and gentle fish—all enjoyed a complex reality. They had a vivid existence in play and fantasy, where David controlled them. They were both symbolic and representations of David's object world. They also were clear embodiments of David's internal objects.

OBSERVATIONS OF DAVID'S SESSIONS BY MRS. X AND CO-THERAPIST

Mrs. X was immediately absorbed in the new experience of watching her child from behind the one-way screen. Her initial reaction was amazement at the confidence and competence with which David related to another adult without her help. This amazement extended to the detailed account of the accident provided by David and to the fantasy that he had woven round the event. Mrs. X expressed surprise that she hardly figured in David's account. (This sense of not being seen and the concern regarding being needed were repeated themes in her presentation, clearly related to her own neediness and anxiety about competence. These concerns had been projected onto David—and Mrs. X was suddenly seeing that they did not fit.) Despite some ambivalence regarding this evidence of David's growing autonomy, there was a new note of respect for her son in Mrs. X's voice. She was also moved to realize how much David had been, and still was, affected by the death and touched by the loving concern he expressed for his father.

During these sessions Mrs. X frequently made embarrassed, apologetic, or disparaging remarks about aspects of David's behavior which she viewed negatively. But there was already less resentment of David's behavior than there had been during the assessment sessions. She became more able to explore peaceful resolution to conflict: allowing David some choice over his clothes, preparing foods he liked, not insisting he finish everything. Comments such as "I suppose it's a phase kids go through" became more frequent.

Mrs. X expressed consistent concern with any evidence of aggression and with the violence of David's fantasy. The co-therapist explained the defensive connection between this fantasy and the accident, the fear of another accident, and the fears of hurt that lay behind David's posture of invulnerability and omnipotence. The connection between David's caretaking activities and his feelings of responsibility for the accident was made. These explanations provided relief for Mrs. X, who responded by citing remarks made by David at home which were related to the same issues. She also asked questions about child development, was relieved to hear that much of David's behavior was age-appropriate, and commented with surprise and admiration on the range of his imagination.

Gradually Mrs. X became more confident in talking about David and her handling of him. By the fourth session a note of pride was clear in her accounts of his assertiveness, both at home and at kindergarten, where she reported that he had a definite status as one of the "noisy big boys." She felt confident that David would be able to cope with the move to school in a few months. During this session David assumed a demanding, oppositional posture with his therapist, who had to set firm limits, particularly in response to his messing of the playroom. Mrs. X was able to observe this calmly. She reported similar home behavior and the strategies she used, without resorting to disparagement or blaming of her son.

The next session the co-therapist brought Sendak's book, *Where the Wild Things Are*, for Mrs. X to read. David still frequently talked about the wild monsters and touched the frieze illustrating the rumpus scene in the book. The popularity and value of the book were explained in terms of its expression of wild, angry feelings, its rich fantasy, and the safe boundaries it provided for fantasy and behavior. We felt that Mrs. X still had difficulty accepting the angry side of her son's behavior and acknowledging her own anger. We wanted to leave her with the clear message that it is normal and healthy to express anger. Sendak's book could be a vehicle for this message. In the final session David played with the "angry wolf" and later with the shark, which turned into a "gentle fish." This material provided a metaphor whereby he and his mother could talk safely about powerful feelings. The therapist suggested to Mrs. X that David had found a good way to talk about and express different parts of himself—and of his mother.

Our format provided an implicit statement that David's play and talk were interesting and of value. We had the feeling that the sessions brought David and his mother closer. They often arrived with a sense of eager anticipation, left chatting happily, and the therapists felt that the sessions had been an intimate project of discovery for both. Mrs. X said good-bye to the co-therapist warmly, with tears in her eyes. Apparently she had been able to experience the sessions as validatory rather than threatening or devaluing.

Discussion

Adam (1982) expressed the hope that the knowledge gained through researching and working in the area of childhood bereavement would provide a sound basis for future preventive work with bereaved children and their families. Given the now well-established grounds for including surviving parents and the wider family network in the assessment and treatment of bereaved children, we have to be ready to fit our approach to the realities of the clinical situation. However, although there is a growing acceptance of the desirability of clinical and conceptual flexibility when working with children and families, and there is increasing acknowledgment that one's effectiveness is enhanced by an ability to integrate individual and family group dynamics (R. Muir, 1975; E. Muir, 1984), some clinical practice still tends to reflect the particular and often restricted orientation of the clinicians. If we accept that our primary task when working with bereaved children and their parents is to preserve or restore family cohesiveness and therefore in particular to ensure the surviving parent's psychological well-being, we have to devise therapeutic strategies to this end; at the same time we cannot ignore the child's individual distress.

When we are confronted with a troubled child in a grieving family, the question of whether to treat the child, the surviving parent, or the whole family can often be answered with a simple "yes"; any or all of these interventions might be indicated depending on the assessed dynamics. Sound therapeutic interventions are dictated by formulations which are derived from a careful and sensitive assessment of individual and family dynamics. In the case of David and his mother, we negotiated the three-generational family session to amplify our initial formulation and to enable us to assess the wider family's supportive capacity. We appreciated how crucial this intervention was when Mrs. X's parents, and in particular her father, revealed family conflicts about loss and the expression of grief. It was clear that in sharing this they were not only providing us with information regarding the source of that difficulty, but were also giving essential permission to their daughter and her children to use our help toward a resolution of mourning.

The therapeutic implications of parents sharing a child's individual therapy (in whatever capacity) must be of considerable consequence.

We are aware that there could be arguments against such a technique and are not suggesting that it has general application. However, there are some recent and some not so recent precedents for such work (Freud, 1909; E. Furman, 1957, 1974, 1981; Winnicott, 1977).

We were also mindful of Winnicott's words, "It is possible for the treatment of a child actually to interfere with a very valuable thing which is the ability of the child's home to tolerate and to cope with the child's clinical states . . . and temporary holdups in emotional development, or even the fact of development itself" (1977, p. 2). The relationship between David and his mother, possibly already vulnerable prior to their bereavement, was endangered because in her state of unresolved mourning, Mrs. X showed a lack of empathy and insight due to her use of projective processes. We were concerned not to interfere with the relationship in such a way as to put it at further risk. We also knew that her lack of objectivity and empathy would prevent her being able to work with him directly; so we had to find a way to permit his mother to share in David's therapy while at the same time not allowing her presence to hamper his need for the free expression of his feelings and fantasies. The question for us was not "Is mourning possible?" but "How can we ensure that mourning is possible for the members of this family?"—more a clinical question than a theoretical one. In our preschool center most of the presenting problems were a reflection of the disturbed relationships between the child and his or her parents; a powerful part of the relationship was characterized by the parents', and in particular our solo mothers', inability to be objective about their children due to a chronic, irreversible use of projective identification (R. Muir et al., 1980). Use of the viewing mirror provides these parents with an opportunity to observe their children, without the normal interpersonal frustrations and stresses they experience when interacting with them directly. It also allows work with the child's individual problems free from the parent's anxious reactions: but the parent shares in the therapeutic process, watching often with surprise and excitement the unfolding of previously inhibited aspects of the child's personality.

In choosing our therapeutic strategy we have been able to blend the rich contributions of child psychoanalysis with the more recent work in family therapy. We might have chosen to take up the challenge to do for David what his mother was at that time unable to do; we could have overlooked the indication to work with her own family of origin; we could have ignored the possibility of helping her to see her son objectively and thus be enabled to help him herself. However, believing as we do that what is important is not so much whether a child can mourn but whether his or her surviving parent can do so, we had no choice but to find a way for her to share safely in her son's therapy.

The last word should come from Mrs. X. In a letter in response to a request from us, she wrote:

> Please find enclosed a little piece on my views from our sessions. David is fine, and seems to be enjoying life tremendously at present, and looking forward to getting back to kindergarten. I have gotten a part-time job, which I think will prove a challenge, and very interesting. Therefore I am facing the new year with a real aim. David will be spending a few hours of the afternoon with a Kindy friend which he is very pleased about, so his care will be no problem. (I hope!) Thank you for your work and help, last year, and I hope my contribution may be of some interest.
>
> Thanks again.
>
> Mrs X.

One of the most interesting experiences of this stage of David's childhood was being able to view him "at play" without his being conscious of my presence. Without the constraints of having me around him, David was visibly different; his conversation and what he was able to talk about with his therapist were really quite surprising to me. He seemed to go on wild flights of imagination giving full reign to his fantasy world, while all the time carefully sidestepping questions which he didn't want to discuss, by ignoring them completely. I found watching him very moving—he was obviously sensitive to a lot of issues relating to death and dying, and rather upsetting at times, being a sensitive issue for me. I began to truly see him as a real personality in his own right, and not just as my son.

It was at times quite frightening to realise the impact of events on him, to see the evidence that he really remembers events which were extremely traumatic to him, but which occurred when he was barely three years old. He witnessed the accident that caused his father's death, and his last sight of his father was seeing him driven away in an ambulance.

Difficult as I realised this was to deal with, it became obvious that he has a great deal of aggression and anger inside of him, which I found very upsetting, of course. One thing which interested me was an almost total lack of any reference to me while I was observing. He made the most of talking about his father. Maybe I wasn't so important to him as I'd liked to think! It certainly brought home the impact of the loss of his father to him, and subsequently presented a new set of problems, of course; dealing with his needs as he grows older and trying to compensate in some ways for being a one-parent family.

A memorable experience in growth for us all.

BIBLIOGRAPHY

ADAM, K. (1982). Loss, suicide and attachment. In *The Place of Attachment in Human Behaviour,* ed. C. Murray Parkes & J. Stevenson-Hinde. New York: Basic Books, pp. 269–294.

ANTHONY, S. (1973). *The Discovery of Death in Childhood and After.* Harmondsworth: Penguin.

BOWLBY, J. (1960). Grief and mourning in infancy and early childhood. *Psychoanal. Study Child,* 15:9–22.

———— (1980). Loss, sadness and depression. *Attachment and Loss,* vol. 3. Harmondsworth: Penguin.

ERIKSON, E. H. (1950). *Childhood and Society.* New York: Norton.

FREUD, A. (1960). Discussion of Dr. John Bowlby's paper. *Psychoanal. Study Child,* 15:53–62.

———— (1963). The concept of developmental lines. *Psychoanal. Study Child,* 18:245–265.

FREUD, S. (1909). Analysis of a phobia in a five-year-old boy. *S.E.,* 10:5–149.

FURMAN, E. (1957). Treatment of under-fives by way of parents. *Psychoanal. Study Child,* 12:250–262.

———— (1974). *A Child's Parent Dies.* New Haven & London: Yale Univ. Press.

———— (1981). Helping children cope with dying. *Child Psychother.,* 10:151–157.

FURMAN, R. A. (1964). Death and the young child. *Psychoanal. Study Child,* 19:321–333.

KLEIN, M. (1946). Notes on some schizoid mechanisms. In *Envy and Gratitude and Other Works 1946–1963.* London: Hogarth Press, pp. 1–24.

MAHLER, M. S., PINE, F., & BERGMAN, A. (1975). *The Psychological Birth of the Human Infant.* New York: Basic Books.

MUIR, E. (1984). On asking what you're not supposed to ask. *Child Psychother.,* 10:239–249.

MUIR, R. (1975). The family and the problem of internalization. *Brit. J. Med. Psychol.,* 48:267–272.

———— MUIR, E., & FLIEGNER, A. (1980). Some developmental hazards of solo parenthood. Unpublished manuscript.

PARKES, M. (1977). *The Place of Attachment in Human Behaviour,* ed. C. Murray Parkes & J. Stevenson-Hinde. New York: Basic Books.

WINNICOTT, D. W. (1954). The depressive position in normal emotional development. *Collected Papers.* New York: Basic Books, 1958, pp. 262–277.

———— (1977). *The Piggle.* London: Hogarth Press.

WOLFENSTEIN, M. (1966). How is mourning possible? *Psychoanal. Study Child,* 21:93–123.

WOLKIND, S. & RUTTER, M. (1985). Separation loss and family relationships. In *Child and Adolescent Psychiatry,* ed. M. Rutter & L. Hersov. Oxford: Blackwell Scientific, pp. 34–57.

APPLIED PSYCHOANALYSIS

Heidi's Metaphoric Appeal to Latency

A Journey through the Oedipus Complex

ALLEN J. PALMER, M.D.

HEIDI, A CHILDREN'S STORY WRITTEN BY JOHANNA SPYRI AND PUBLISHED in 1880, has endured in popularity for over 100 years and has been a favorite of latency-aged and preadolescent girls. *Heidi* contains the universal themes of loss and restitution, separation and reunion, a family romance fantasy, derivative expression of preoedipal and oedipal conflicts, and the resolution of infantile conflicts with concomitant developmental progression. This paper will demonstrate how *Heidi's* preoedipal and oedipal themes appeal to the latency-aged girl reader. The novel's metaphoric appeal will be explored from the standpoint of the concordance of the latency-aged reader's unconscious developmental and dynamic conflicts and the narrative's explication of the same in, more or less, disguised form.

COMMENTS ON THE FUNCTION OF READING FOR CHILDREN

With ego development and cognitive expansion in latency, the child establishes the capacity to read. Many authors have described the host of ways in which a newly acquired skill is used in the service of curiosity and the acquisition of knowledge; the exercise and consolidation of developing ego capacities such as intellectual, perceptual, and fantasy abilities; the reacquaintance with and reworking of old conflicts and

Clinical instructor of psychiatry, Cambridge Hospital, Harvard Medical School; candidate, Boston Psychoanalytic Society and Institute.

I would like to thank Drs. Anton Kris and Steven Ablon for their helpful comments in the preparation of this paper.

anxieties within the safe context of a narrative explicating core conflicts (e.g., birth, death, separation, rivalry, etc.); the recapture of a soothing transitional activity (Freud, 1913; Friedlander, 1942; Peller, 1958, 1959; Goldings, 1968). A child may experience a tale like *Heidi* as a symbolic manifestation of an idealized, sunny childhood upon which to embellish positive reminiscences of her own. From the safe vantage point of maturity, i.e., a subsequent developmental stage, the child may experience nostalgia for a time of infantile gratifications. As Werman (1977) and Castelnuovo-Tedesco (1980) point out, a person may long for a return to a past not only to reexperience gratifications but to rewrite their histories of infantile frustrations with a better outcome. Peller (1959) considers the reader's nostalgic reveries as "daydreams in reverse, i.e., daydreams projected into a mythical past instead of into a rosy future" (p. 421). In addition, fantasies accompanying reading are often used by latency readers to address anxieties about upcoming adolescence, e.g.. by projecting fantasied infantile gratifications into future relationships. As in play and daydreams, safe ego-syntonic excursions into conflictual areas and anticipated developmental events can be made by empathic immersion with the stories' characters or affective resonance with the plot. Wishes and prohibitions are identified with, reality is suspended, and intellectual satisfaction is achieved by seeing personal issues recast in new modes and paradigms and newly developed unconflicted ego capacities put to use. Goldings (1968) noted that an important function of literature for children is "allowing [the child's] temporary exercise of primary process faculties for the ultimate attainment of higher level secondary process integrations" (p. 393).

Where repression of infantile conflicts has set in in latency, a story such as *Heidi* would appeal to young readers by presenting a complex derivative expression of themes unconsciously and dynamically active for a latency child. Yet, symbolic expression must not be too obscure so that the child can experience the pleasure of an "affective harmonic resonance" (Barchilon, 1971) with the subliminal message. Latency requires that if a story is to appeal, its form must be neither too obvious nor too obscure; and, as Peller (1959) has noted, the story's success rests on the presence of a universal daydream woven into the plot and characters' conflicts and motivations through paraphrase and allusion.

THE STORY OF HEIDI: MANIFEST AND METAPHORIC

Heidi is presented as a realistic narrative of an orphan girl's experiences with a variety of caretakers of markedly different quality, spanning the fifth through eighth years of life. The story opens with Heidi being transferred to her hermitlike paternal grandfather in a verdant alpine retreat by a self-interested maternal aunt. Heidi thrives with her grandfather, but two years later the aunt abruptly reclaims Heidi to establish her in a wealthy Frankfurt home to serve as playmate for a hemiplegic preadolescent girl. The separation from her beloved grandfather, friends, and mountain home plus the confinement of the city and the orderly Frankfurt home run by a severe headmistress combine to precipitate homesickness, depression, and somnambulism. Through the perceptiveness of a doctor and the benevolence of her friend's father, Heidi is joyously reunited with her grandfather and proceeds to transform the lives of the people about her. A bitter isolated old man returns to the society of man and God, a blind woman's despair is lifted as she approaches her last days of life with renewed hope, an invalid friend learns to walk, and an oppositional preadolescent goat boy learns to read. With the blessings of her friend's loving grandmother, Heidi, by the end of the story, is assured of a permanent home first with her grandfather and upon his death with the good doctor from Frankfurt who recently lost a daughter of his own.

The absence of Heidi's parents through death casts Heidi in the role of heroine-orphan and sets the stage for Heidi's attachment to surrogate caretakers, the core elements of a family romance fantasy. Whereas the parents are presented as loving, good, and well-liked by others, there is allusion to a deeper ambivalence. The deceased mother by dint of "spells" has a propensity to enter states of unconsciousness and by implication is episodically unavailable to attend to Heidi's needs. The father is sufficiently careless at his work to be felled by a falling beam. Disillusionment with the parents is contained in this preconscious presentation of ambivalence, whereas the manifest story permits the idealization of the parents and the attribution of death to causes completely unrelated to the feelings of the child. The story articulates for a latency-aged reader a fantasy of a guiltless separation and expression of hostility toward both parents by the disappointed oedipal child, launching the heroine-orphan on a search for an incestuous relationship with a father surrogate. Yet, Heidi must traverse through other relationships before achieving a permissible incestuous tie to the father surrogate, her paternal grandfather.

Upon the death of her parents, Heidi lives with her mother's mother and sister, the former characterized as loving and nurturant and the latter as narcissistic and cold. The presentation of two women, directly related to Heidi's mother, diametrically opposite in their attitudes to Heidi and residing under one roof, serves as a representation of the split aspects of an ambivalently held preoedipal mother. The aunt's preoccupation with socioeconomic status, long-feathered hats, and the gratification of her own needs, either to the exclusion of others or through the use of others, serves as a vivid portrayal of an unempathic, phallic-narcissistic mother. She feels little guilt in foisting Heidi onto substitute caregivers, separating the child from an adored man, abandoning her to strangers in a foreign setting, and, in interaction with the child, is concerned with establishing authority over her. The emphasis on control and orderliness over free expression and mobility and the niggardly mode of providing supplies portray Detie, the aunt, as the hostile preoedipal mother. On the other hand, the good grandmother teaches Heidi about God, i.e., permits the child a positive idealization of a fatherlike figure, and tries to influence Aunt Detie to care for Heidi upon her own death. That Heidi lives with both aunt and grandmother for a time illustrates a girl's preoedipal experience of her mother as alternately good and bad, particularly in the experience of oral gratification, bowel control, and separation.

The death of Heidi's grandmother signals the disappearance of the good mother and the movement toward a positive oedipus complex with the girl's predominantly hostile experience of the mother. Heidi's fate at this stage is to live with and be tolerated by a hostile mother. The bad mother is personified by Detie and further embellished by Ursula, an old woman self-absorbed with her bodily state and temperature to the exclusion of Heidi's needs to run and play outdoors. Detie's relinquishment of Heidi to Uncle Alp, i.e., the bad mother's handing over of the girl to the father, is made plausible by presenting the man as bad and the adult woman as too ambitious to be bothered with her daughter. That the woman hands over the child to the man and the girl is cast as passive to the adults' actions serve as a disguise of the girl's active incestuous wishes for the father and wished-for removal of a hostile rival. A forerunner of libidinal expression is illustrated by Heidi's first trek up the mountain and her undressing herself before Peter the goat boy. Uncle Alp's reputation is that of an irascible, forbidding, schizoid man. For some girls the libidinal shift to the father in the positive phase of the oedipus complex may be accompanied by a fearful perception of the father as overpowering in his strength and size. The reader at this stage of the story may fret for Heidi's welfare in the hands of such a man, but this would be short-lived. The reader soon realizes that what is for the bad mother a disinterested abandonment of the girl to a bad man is instead the fulfillment of the child's active feminine wishes for the father. Detie's wariness of Uncle Alp and their thinly veiled hostility for one another serve as an apt illustration for an oedipal girl's fantasy of the parental relationship. By casting their relationship as hostile, the girl can eliminate the mother as a rival, furthering her fantasies in an exclusive relationship with father. Heidi, in meeting Uncle Alp, quickly establishes herself as both an adoring wife and a loving mother. She sets his table, cleans his hut, and tends to his goats, caring for the goats reflecting the feminine-receptive fantasy of the positive oedipal stage of being the mother of the father's children. Thus, the fulfillment of an incestuous wish is achieved in Heidi's relationship to her father's father. Furthermore, Heidi experiences her grandfather not just as a paternal object but as a nurturant maternal object as she thrives on his milk and cheese. The good women are dead, the bad ones removed from the scene, and the positive maternal traits are experienced in relationship with a father surrogate.

Heidi establishes rapport with the goat boy and then with Uncle Alp, then actively engages Peter's grandmother in a relationship colored by the mobilization of Heidi's altruism. Grannie is the only contemporary of Uncle Alp living in close proximity, yet she is rejected by Uncle Alp, as are others. She is blind, helpless, despairing, and feels her faith in God waning in her impoverished state. Thus, we are presented with a paradigm of a suffering, good mothering figure who is seemingly unfairly rejected by a hostile father figure and the girl who actively engages the adult woman in spite of the father figure's position. Heidi presents herself as a vehicle to help Grannie see what she cannot, substituting herself as an organ of perception for Grannie. This constellation can serve as a model for a girl who is conflicted and guilty over positive libidinal cathexis of the father and removal of the "blind" mother rival. The guilty girl invests the mother surrogate with libidinal cathexis, helping her see what is transpiring, empathizing with and rectifying her lonely state of isolation, and attempting to reunite and repair the mother- and father-surrogate relationship.

The incestuous wish is permitted only partial gratification, the tie between Heidi and grandfather being severed by the intrusion of the pastor and Aunt Detie. The pastor declares Uncle Alp's actions (of keeping Heidi to himself, away from society and school) as illegal and immoral, representing the guilty father's and/or child's conscience for breaking a code of civilization, the incest taboo. Aunt Detie, the incarnation of the hostile mother, returns and separates the loving girl from the surrogate father, banishing the girl as punishment for the oedipal crime. Both characters, the pastor and Detie, can evoke a resonance with the girl reader's superego prohibitions of incestuous wishes. Detie's power over Uncle Alp is her veiled accusation that he committed the oedipal crime, of causing his father's death via the impulse-ridden actions of an adolescent, and of trying to abandon his rival infant son soon after birth. That Uncle Alp accedes to Detie's wish to remove Heidi from him and place her in a position of circumstance is a matter of great disillusionment for Heidi. While it would not be in keeping with Heidi's presentation as innocent and good for her to be angry with Uncle Alp, a displaced reference to this can be seen in Heidi's relationship to God while in Frankfurt. At the peak of her despair and homesickness, she is disillusioned with God for allowing her to be sent off to the city, failing to rescue her from her plight and return her to her previous state of bliss. Thus, the invocation of the incest taboo is accompanied by disillusionment at the father's failure to act against the powerful, hostile mother and maintain erotic attachment to the girl. In being removed from the forbidden father-daughter relationship, Heidi's circumstance reflects the latency girl's internalized prohibition against incestuous wishes of the positive oedipal complex.

Detie transports Heidi to the Sesemann household in Frankfurt, a home of wealth, propriety, and incomprehensible rules for social conduct. The city, without grass and trees, is a prison for Heidi. The governess, Miss Rottenmeier, is punitive, controlling, and intolerant of any instinctual expression. While her food may be beautifully prepared, it is devoid of taste. In addition to the governess, the household contains Clara, an invalid prepubertal girl, an ineffectual obsessive-compulsive male tutor, and a caring but powerless adolescent boy servant. Furthermore, the seemingly good father, Mr. Sesemann, is absent and Clara's mother is dead. Thus, the scenario in the Frankfurt home of Clara serves as a paradigm for a helpless, castrated girl living under the dominance of a tyrannical mother and a father who is represented as split: the male figures in proximity being ineffectual and the powerful, adored father being at a distance. The reader's fantasy is of a girl who is tricked away from a father and forced into an early oedipal tie with a hostile mother who indulges the child's passivity and oral gratifications and, indirectly, stands in the way of separation and oedipal progression. Presenting this as the girl's helplessness to the adult woman's actions (Detie to Heidi and Miss Rottenmeier to Clara) disguises the child's disillusionment with the father (Uncle Alp to Heidi and Mr. Sesemann to Clara) who fails to gratify the girl's feminine wishes toward him or the child's defensive retreat to an inverted oedipal position, i.e., the shift of libidinal cathexis from father to mother, due to anxiety and conflict over the positive oedipal progression. Clara's relationship to Miss Rottenmeier and her paternal grandmother connote the conflict inherent in this defensive retreat for the oedipal girl from father to mother. Clara in her invalidism gives ex-

pression to passive, oral, and narcissistic aims, gratified by Miss Rottenmeier, grandmother, and her father. Clara's deep affection for her
loving grandmother represents the gratifying aspects of the inverted
oedipus complex, whereas Clara's relationship with Miss Rottenmeier
signifies a compromise formation where passivity is gratified but at a
cost of maintaining a fixed conflict of control with an anal-compulsive,
phallic-narcissistic mother surrogate and the relinquishment of mobility and active feminine fantasies.

Within this defensive constellation, the father of proximity is conceived of as ineffectual and powerless to challenge the authority of the
hostile mother (e.g., the tutor and servant boy's relationship to Miss
Rottenmeier), whereas the idealized, powerful father of erotic fantasies exists in some distant locale. The episodic return of Clara's father
from business trips represents the experience of intermittent gratification and repeated frustration of positive incestuous wishes. Even Mr.
Sesemann's investing Clara with ultimate authority in the house by his
statement that Clara is not to be displeased in any way by Miss Rottenmeier represents a Pyrrhic oedipal victory, as the girl remains with the
mother and the father is gone. Heidi's seemingly innocent antics,
which set the house on end and drive Miss Rottenmeier to distraction,
signify the (disavowed) breakthrough of aggression and the intermittent usurpation of the tyrannical imposition of strict rules of civilized
conduct. Repeatedly Heidi endears herself to the men in and out of the
house and impulsively introduces kittens and other animals, a sore
point for Miss Rottenmeier who experiences them as frightening bats
and rats to be expelled, while Heidi enacts a maternal role with them. A
latency-aged reader, while consciously holding fast to ideal conduct
and rules, may find pleasure in this play and derivative expression of
aggression at a negative representation of a mother and breakthrough
of positive libidinal cathexis of the men.

The visit of Clara's grandmother to Frankfurt and her avowed love
of her son and faith in God the Father connote not only the gratifying
aspects of the inverted oedipus complex but the girl's shift in experience of the mother. The girl's libidinal investment in the loving mother
becomes a source of identification, as is illustrated when grandmother
lovingly teaches Heidi to read and sew and bestows on Heidi a favorite
book containing a story of a prodigal son's return to his father's alpine
home. Notably, these positive identifications are able to occur when
there is sufficient distance from the incestuous passion for a surrogate
father and in spite of the ongoing ungratified longings, and when the
maternal object invests the paternal object positively. Neutralized libidinal feelings for the grandfather can be seen when Heidi makes the

connection between grandmother's lace flapping gently behind her in the wind and the cool mountain breezes of Uncle Alp's home, infusing the love felt for one into a "new" maternal object. Grandmother's loving relationship with her son and encouragement for Heidi to trust and love God reflect the girl's wish for a good mother who permits the girl a loving adoration of the father, in this instance in a sublimated form of God.

As Clara's grandmother's power supersedes that of Miss Rottenmeier and the weight of ambivalence to the mother shifts to the positive, the stage is set for Heidi's return to her mountain home and a positive oedipal progression. She has begun to neutralize her passionate oedipal longings and can now live with and love her grandfather as a latency-aged girl. Yet, before this occurs, a nighttime scene is enacted with Heidi as an oblivious sleepwalker. Miss Rottenmeier is frightened by the unknown stirrings in the night and ascribes it to some malevolent force from the past overtaking the home. To put an end to such forces, she calls in the good fathers who with guns in hand and alcohol ingested discover the midnight prowler to be Heidi. The scene vividly portrays a girl's wish for intercourse with an idealized, courageous, yet impulse-ridden father and the wished-for removal and engendering of fright in the mother. Additionally, Heidi's somnambulism is a creative device for the disavowal of the positive incestuous fantasy.

Ultimately, Heidi is reinstated to a relationship with her grandfather and through her goodness and moral superiority tames his badness, a theme in juveniles noted by Friedlander (1942). Uncle Alp returns with Heidi and their goats to the society of Man and God and builds a home for them in the midst of others, an illustration of a socially acceptable derivative expression of the incestuous relationship. Heidi's and Uncle Alp's turn to society, education, and religion represent the child's entrance into latency and adaptation to reality, and the external world as oedipal fantasies recede. Nonetheless, the fulfillment of the incestuous fantasy with a father is perpetuated as Uncle Alp, Mr. Sesemann, and Dr. Classen concur that Dr. Classen will serve as Heidi's caregiver upon the death of Uncle Alp. With the grandmother's blessings, Heidi's future with men is assured. The bad mothers are never to return, the good mother gives her blessing and then retreats from the scene, and Heidi is left alone with her grandfather (father) and the goats (babies) within the society of God and Man: an ideal fantasy resolution of the positive oedipus complex. Revenge against the rival is disguised, aggression is denied, a neutralized incestuous relationship is fully permitted, positive maternal identifications are solidified, the ego ideal of goodness and morality is given expression in consciousness, and there is a turn to latency with Heidi's burgeoning intellectual competence in school.

In the context of a gratified derivative form of a socially and intrapsychically acceptable incestuous tie between girl and father surrogate, significant creative metamorphoses are possible: Clara can reach fulfillment as a young girl and face the next developmental period of adolescence by learning to walk; Peter overcomes an opposition to learning to read; and Grannie, through Heidi's altruistic use of new reading skills, is provided a vehicle to "see." That Heidi tames Uncle Alp's antisocial tendency, Peter's aggressiveness, and Clara's invalidism connotes the curative influence of the early latency-aged child's ego ideal of goodness in the service of others, a morally elevated position. Both Peter and Clara are prepubescent and as such represent for the early latency child the future upsurge of impulses of preadolescence: Peter's propensity toward cruelty and destructiveness representing aggression on the one hand, and Clara's invalidism reflecting a masochistic organization of passive libidinal and aggressive aims on the other.

Peter's destruction of Clara's wheelchair and Clara's subsequent successful efforts to walk reflect the theme of destruction of an infantile position of extreme passivity and oral dependence as well as the symbolic murder of a hated rival freeing one to move forward developmentally. The use of the paralysis furthermore indicates the shift from a position of narcissism and phallic (albeit castrated) organization to one of active feminine strivings and developmental progression in object relationships. Heidi, in her altruistic, transformative role, is established as the personification of an all-good superego ideal of an early latency girl. She is innocent of sexuality, lacks any aggression, and is active in the service of others, particularly in a compulsion to replace what is lost or absent.

By the end of the story, Clara, now mobile, can go on vacation with her father and grandmother, a parallel and derivative fulfillment of a positive oedipal fantasy. Thus, the latency-aged reader can vicariously and unconsciously utilize this aspect of the story—the girl's simultaneous turn to the external world and the maintenance of an oedipal success with the approval of all parties while consciously ascribing to their own superego prohibitions. For the girl reader, the narrative serves as a context for a temporary removal from the demands of real life and the vicarious fulfillment of a host of wishes abhorrent to the newly formed superego, but dynamically active in the latency girl's unconscious.

CONCLUSION

I have sought to describe the salient unconscious themes presented in *Heidi,* noting that the story's vast and enduring popularity is based on the explication of important developmental trends for the girl reader, recently arrived in the latency phase of development. The girl reader develops an affective resonance with core themes, engaging in unconscious and preconscious trial, temporary identifications with the characters and the plot line of the narrative. Vicarious, ego-syntonic involvement with the core themes and characters' dilemmas, gratifications, and conflict resolutions, be they in regressions or developmental progressions, provide a context for reminiscing about and mastery of dynamically active earlier conflicts or anticipation of later developmental challenges with newfound ego capacities.

The central emphasis in the tale is the relationship between granddaughter and grandfather, their experiences of separation and reunion, and Heidi's capacity to propel others toward conflict resolution and transformation by dint of her unique personality. The traversal of the vicissitudes of the oedipus complex and the progression to latency underlie the manifest delineation of this endearing girl's experience of loss, substitution, reunion, and metamorphosis. Heidi serves the latency girl as a mythic figure of indomitable spirit and enduring optimism.

A story that articulates the theme of a child emerging from a troubled past and moving toward an uncertain future while simultaneously going through a physical and psychological metamorphosis will appeal to a latency child who is increasingly aware of his or her location in time and space and processes of change. *Heidi,* in its manifest presentation, takes place over several years and informs the reader not only of Heidi's earliest years, but also of the multigenerational history of her family. Within the narrative, unconscious elements of preoedipal and oedipal phases of development are articulated, as is the theme of a latency child anticipating adolescence. *Heidi* is the portrayal of a girl who establishes herself in latency with a stable compromise between the demands of libidinal wishes, superego requirements, and reality factors. Heidi's achievements are the permissible expression of libidinal urges and ego expansion, including newly found cognitive abilities, a wider world view and moral sense, and self-reflective capacities.

BIBLIOGRAPHY

BARCHILON, J. (1971). A study of Camus' mythopoeic tale *The Fall* with some comments about the origin of esthetic feelings. *J. Amer. Psychoanal. Assn.,* 19:193–239.

CASTELNUOVO-TEDESCO, P. (1980). Reminiscence and nostalgia. In *The Course of Life,* vol. 3, ed. S. I. Greenspan & G. H. Pollock. Washington, DC: U.S. Govt. Printing Office, pp. 115–127.

FREUD, S. (1913). The occurrence in dreams of material from fairy-tales. *S.E.,* 12:281–287.

FRIEDLANDER, K. (1942). Children's books and their function in latency and prepuberty. *Amer. Imago,* 3:129–148.

GOLDINGS, C. R. (1968). Some new trends in children's literature from the perspective of the child psychiatrist. *J. Amer. Acad. Child Psychiat.,* 7:377–395.

PELLER, L. E. (1958). Reading and daydreams in latency. *J. Amer. Psychoanal. Assn.,* 6:57–70.

——— (1959). Daydreams and children's favorite books. *Psychoanal. Study Child,* 14:414–433.

SPYRI, J. (1880). *Heidi.* Harmondsworth: Penguin Books, 1956.

WERMAN, D. S. (1977). Normal and pathological nostalgia. *J. Amer. Psychoanal. Assn.,* 25:387–398.

The Power of the Eye in Nature, Nurture, and Culture

A Developmental View of Mutual Gaze

ANNELIESE RIESS, Ph.D.

THE POWERFUL ROLE OF THE EYE AND OF FACE-TO-FACE BEHAVIOR IN daily life is experienced by every being at all times. It affects greatly the formation and the nature of human relationships. Study of ancient monuments, myths, and religions suggests that their creators had also experienced the "power of the eye" and woven this knowledge into their creations.[1]

It is my thesis that ancient beliefs in the function and power of the eye are rooted in universal mutual gaze patterns of childhood. In order to support this thesis, I will describe four developmental phases of childhood and their characteristics in respect to eye experience and assigned eye power. I will use these developmental constructs as a framework to order the data from ancient monuments, myths, and religions.

In addition, I plan to show that the transformation of ancient eye beliefs from more primitive, primary process, magical beginnings to more rational, reality-oriented, secondary process, ethical forms parallels that of the individual child. This process of transformation can be seen most clearly in those cultural works which provide us with continuous evidence over centuries, such as the Bible and the Greek culture.

Formerly assistant clinical professor, department of psychiatry, Albert Einstein College of Medicine, New York; adjunct associate professor, City College, City University of New York.

1. The terms "eye" and "face" are used interchangeably. Eyes are often represented by themselves or as part of faces. A face without eyes, on the other hand, loses the powerful effect, which is the subject of this paper.

The earlier eye beliefs, however, persist side by side with those that evolve later.

There is precedent in Freud's reading certain myths as embodying the characteristics of specific developmental experiences. Both the myth of Oedipus and of Narcissus mirror two specific phases of child development and both contain eye-related elements, which can be translated into developmental language. Narcissus represents the neonate prior to bonding. He loses his life because he can see only himself. He lacks social mutuality. Oedipus reflects the latency child in the stage of forming a conscience and a moral standard (Freud, 1900, 1913).

In this sense cultural creations with eye and looking features are echoes, condensations, and transformations of eye experiences of childhood. It will become apparent that over the millennia humans have retold the story of psychological development in disguise, that is, in the guise of wonderful and colorful inventions.

RESEARCH ON MUTUAL GAZE

The study of interpersonal eye contact has produced massive data as to its important role in social relations (Argyle and Cook, 1976; Ekman et al., 1972). The exchange of a glance with another person may be simply informative, loving or hostile, inviting or threatening, and has been found to evoke highly differentiated responses through its nonverbal but clearly discernible and often powerful emotional message.

Eye power is also exerted between man and animal and between animals. Rhesus monkeys attack or make threats if stared at, even by a human. Gibbons show intense aversion to the human face. Chimpanzees, when frightened, fling an arm across their face and flee (Argyle and Cook, 1976). Schaller (1963) reports that among mountain gorillas the leader of the pack stares his challengers down into submission.

The important role of eyes to influence, affect, and protect can be seen even in the eye designs displayed on various parts of animals. For example, the open wings of certain butterflies and moths (fig. 1) display the design of eyes, whose function is to hold off predators.

Recent findings of neuropsychologists have established a specific neurological reaction to eye and face. Such laboratory work supports the evolutionary character of human sensitivity to eyes and face. In monkeys certain neurons respond selectively to faces as compared to other body configurations (e.g., hand). Human babies appear to prefer faces from birth; it may be that all primates are born with the capacity for the face to stimulate neuronal firing (Desimone et al., 1984).

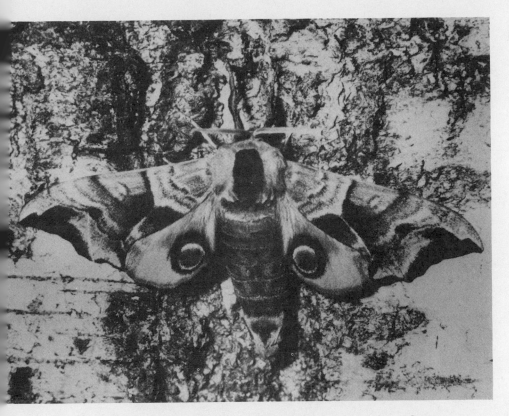

Figure 1. Eyed hawkmoth exposing large eyespots on open wings. Owen, D.: *Camouflage and Mimicry*, p. 91.

In what follows I present developmental and cultural data in four developmental phases. While these behavioral eye patterns unfold in developmental sequence, they also endure side by side throughout life and form part of the human equipment for creating and maintaining human relations.

Phase 1. The World of the Peek-a-Boo Game: The Eye as an Agent of Social-Emotional Bonding

From birth on the human face is the most attractive visual stimulus to the infant (Fantz, 1965). This innate readiness for interpersonal gazing interacts with the child's expanding cognitive skills and the caretaker's mothering, resulting in the infant's increasing sensitivity and responsiveness to the mother's facial messages, which may cover the whole range of the emotional scale from loving to rejecting. Throughout the first year the game of mutual gazing is an important focus of a give-and-take experience between mother and infant, requiring constant mutual attunement and contributing significantly to the nature of their bonding (Spitz and Wolf, 1946; Robson, 1967; Brazelton, 1982; Riess, 1978).

Around one year when the mother's face encourages, cajoles, consoles, supports, threatens, punishes, or disappears, the infant responds with finely differentiated behavior to these facial encounters. When under too much emotional pressure from the mother's eyes or an overload of stimulation, the baby can escape temporarily by averting gaze, or by covering or closing his eyes (fig. 2). Thus with built-in gaze control the baby shows himself a resourceful partner and not helpless. Under severe eye pressure such as staring, the baby may freeze in terror or scream or both (Stern, 1977).

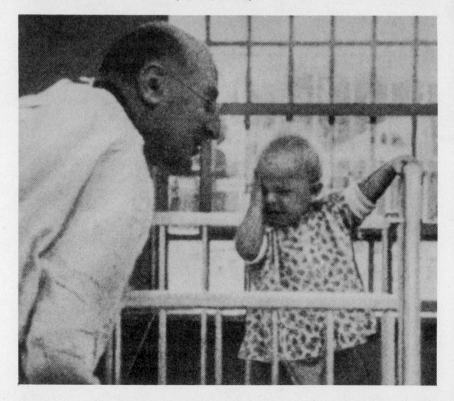

Figure 2. Eight-months anxiety: infant covering eye with protective arm gesture. Spitz, R. A.: *The First Year of Life*, p. 151.

The peek-a-boo game, a universal, evolving over the second half of the first year, is a highlight in this visual mutuality and best characterizes the infant's developmental status around one year of age (Kleeman, 1967). It serves as a paradigm for phase 1. Alternation of appearance and disappearance of the face and joy in recognition and expected reappearance are major elements in its appeal. It offers a view of the infant's developing psychic structure. The slowly expanding short-term memory is seen in the growing ability to recognize, anticipate, and delay. More differentiated visual perception, increased visual-motor coordination, and the beginnings of self and object differentiation also develop.

The image of a face with a message which can be read, as infants and others experience it daily, is found many times in ancient texts and monuments, in which emotionally charged eye messages are sent and are immediately responded to.

The cultural data consist of narrative texts and of figurative materials. The texts show most clearly the interpersonal context of eye behavior. In all instances it is the figure in authority who exerts influence, by eye behavior, on those of lesser rank or on those in a more dependent position, as between parent and child.

NARRATIVE TEXTS

In these myths, written or told in the third millennium, B.C., the eye language is stark. Eyes are believed to possess a truly magical power over life and death. The gods or godlike creatures look at each other or at human heroes with "the eyes of death," whenever they fear transgression on their authority or disregard of the rules of life.

Humbaba, the guardian of the cedar forest, when approached by Gilgamesh (1960), "on him fastened his eye, the eye of death" (p. 81). Gilgamesh came to the gate of the underworld: "At this gate the Scorpions stand guard . . . their stare strikes death into man. . . . When Gilgamesh saw them, he shielded his eyes" (p. 98).

Ultimately and subjectively, being killed by eye power may originate in the infant's experience in the presence of eye threat from the mother, felt as annihilation. The awesome power of the threatening displeased eye is transformed from infant experience into the realm of childhood fantasy and then into culture.

Several myths illustrate the power of the eye as life-giving and life-taking. The sun dies every evening and is reborn every morning. The sun is regarded as the right eye of the sun god Re and also the falcon god Horus. The moon is seen as the left eye of Horus.

In one myth, Seth gouges out the eyes of his brother Horus and buries them on a mountain, where they grow into bulbs and lotuses. The goddess Hathor finds Horus weeping for the loss of his eyes. She catches a female gazelle, milks her, and puts the milk into Horus' eyes, which were thus healed (Watterson, 1984). Clearly, here the eyes are seen as indestructible. The lotus is a symbol of the sun and milk is a metaphor for renewal.

In ancient Egyptian belief, Re created mankind from his tears. When he wanted to destroy mankind, because they plotted against him, Re said, "Summon to me my Eye. . . ." So Re destroyed part of mankind with his eye (Lichtheim, 1976).

In the context of less formal and more personal descriptions Egyptian poems offer a glimpse into the feelings of men and women, often expressed in their faces as shining, beaming, bright, pale, savage, and fierce. For example: "When she opens her eyes, my body is young." "She captures me with her eyes." "When I see you my eyes shine."

Tradition in most, if not all, ancient cultures, forbade eye contact with authority. To transgress was to risk punishment. Veneration of divinity and acknowledgment of defeat required bowing down to the ground with downcast eyes. "Bend your back to your superior." "They were on their bellies before his majesty." "The princes are prostrate saying 'Shalom'" (Lichtheim, 1976).

The Hebrew Bible attributes much power to the eye in the relations between God and "his children, the Israelites." However, this eye power is not killing power; rather God threatens to withdraw his love, to abandon "his children," and to punish them with death by means of his eye power if not obeyed. But he never kills.

There are four different patterns of eye contact between God and the Israelites. In one rare pattern God is visible and may be seen "face-to-face." In Exodus (33:11) it is said, "And the Lord spoke unto Moses face-to-face as a man speaketh to a friend."

In the second pattern God may not be looked at. Only God may do the looking (33:20). "And he said thou canst not see my face, for there shall no man see me and live." And further: "And I will take away mine hand, and thou shall see my backparts, but my face shall not be seen." God is depicted as potentate, a forbidding father, with uncontested authority (33:23).

In the third pattern God appears "in a pillar of a cloud" (13:21) and warns Moses to keep the people from trying to gaze at him. "And the Lord said unto Moses, go down, charge the people, lest they break through unto the Lord to gaze and many of them perish" (19:21).

In the fourth pattern something is interposed between the threatening reflection of God's eye and the people. When Moses came down from Mount Sinai his face was shining. The contact with God had brought radiance over his face, which frightened the Israelites. So Moses put a veil on his face when he spoke with them and took it off when he talked to God.

The common ancient custom of keeping ritual objects covered or behind curtains reflects the belief in the powerful force emanating from them, affecting or even threatening the onlooker. The Torah is traditionally kept behind a curtain. Its opening is a significant part of the ritual. A similar tradition existed in Mesopotamia where the idol of the God is kept from the eyes of the people behind a curtain (Oppenheim, 1977).

Following are some examples of God's promises and threats with his eyes. These examples clearly mirror common interactions between children and parents. "I will instruct and teach thee in the way thou shalt go: I will guide thee with mine eyes" (Psalm 32:8). "Make thy face shine upon thy servant" (Psalm 31:16) or "God has forgotten—he hideth his face" (Psalm 10:11). "And I will hide my face from them and they shall be devoured" (Deuteronomy 31:17).

The Iliad presents the classical world of ancient Greece, a world of violent action, revenge, death, and destruction. The story of the Iliad is a continuous battle scene. Yet its eye language is fundamentally different. The emphasis on the eye continues, but the quality is changed. The eye behavior is tame and remains purely descriptive, without the power over life and death. The magic is gone. Instead there is lively eye communication between the gods of the Olympus. They nod and wink at each other, raising and wrinkling their brows, scowling, smiling, and laughing with pleasure and with scorn. Zeus, the father of them all who ultimately must be obeyed, at times threatens with "his darkened brows" in order to keep control, as parents do with children. It is not stated anywhere that his darkened glance can kill: he only warns.

Homer speaks of the "shining" of the eyes in the same way as the authors of the Gilgamesh and the Bible have done. They address the vitality or aliveness of the eye, the window of the soul, as it has been called.

One naturalistic scene could stand as a paradigm of present-day observation of infant psychological development. Hector approached his infant son with "shining bronze helm topped by a crest of horsehair." When the frightened baby shrank back and screamed at the sight of his father, Hector removed his helm and the infant calmed down and then Hector "tossed him about in his arms and kissed him." Such storytelling comes from observation and understanding of the "real" world, the world of scientific assembly of facts, from which classical Greece evolved. Secondary process is the mode of functioning.

The Odyssey, Homer's other great epic, is similar in eye language to the Iliad. The heroes smile, frown, wink at each other, laugh, and often their eyes shine. The pattern of gaze aversion in the presence of a powerful sight is found here. When Telemachos unexpectedly sees his father Odysseus in youthful appearance, he "turned his eyes in the other direction, fearing this must be a god" (XVI:179).

Medusa is a creature of the preclassical Greek world, a world of cannibalism, murder, and laws of vengeance. The magic of curses, omens, and human sacrifices made individuals into helpless victims of fate. One of three sisters, the Gorgons, Medusa was said instantly to transform into stone anyone who looked at her ugly face. Perseus kills her by cutting off her head while averting his face and then puts her head into a bag so as to avoid being injured by her gaze (Graves, 1960).

Medusa is the embodiment of female deadly eye power. She has all the frightening qualities of an angrily staring and rejecting mother who has a devastating effect on the infant. The common saying "If looks could kill" mirrors the primordial fear of the magic power of the eye. Clearly, in the myth of Medusa, it is the face-to-face encounter which is deadly. Gaze aversion, as Perseus does and as the infant does under eye stress, is a protective maneuver, learned very early in life.

Medusa's head or mask was affixed to Athena's aegis and shield and to the shields of soldiers to evoke horror and fear in the enemy. The Iliad abounds with descriptions of this effect.

The last example of face-to-face looking in the ancient literature comes from a famous poem by Virgil, the Roman poet who wrote the Aeneid. In his fourth Eclogue, a pastoral poem, written in 40 B.C., he addresses the expected birth of a child to a Roman consul. "Begin, then, little boy, to greet your mother with a smile . . . no one who has not given his mother a smile has ever been thought worthy of his table by a god, or by a goddess of her bed" (Verses 60–65). However one may interpret this poem, the significant point is the importance attributed to the infant's smile to his mother, seen as related to his future success and happiness.

The Romans of course, even more than the classical Greeks, had become observers of natural phenomena, in this instance, of the infant's smile and its implications.

FIGURATIVE MATERIAL

The emphasis on the widely staring and disproportionately large eyes is a most striking feature and a common element of much of the early statuary. It is not known whether these works of art were in the service of religious beliefs or represent the worshiper or the worshiped. Whatever their original function, their makers must have intended them to exert eye power, perhaps to have some kind of magic effect, a parallel to what in the texts is often called the shining of the eyes (fig. 3). Clay-modeled skulls, found in tombs, one in Jericho dating from the eighth millennium B.C. and the other in New Guinea, were given eyes made of cowrie shells, which were expected to send eye signals from the grave (Potts, 1981).

Medusa is as prominent in figurative presentations as she is in the written tradition. Her ugly face is found everywhere in Greece and its colonies and in many different contexts. She is often represented as architectural decoration on temples, on Greek vases, or painted on the aegis or shield of Athena (Potts, 1981).

The avoidance of direct gaze at the powerful is vividly represented in several bas reliefs in figures bowing in submission. In one, visiting foreign dignitaries are kneeling before the Egyptian king with heads bowed (Settgast et al., 1976). In another, fan bearers are prostrate before the Egyptian queen (Aldred, 1973). Looking up would have been a punishable transgression.

Another model of eye-protective behavior against a powerful sight is covering of the eyes, as seen in an infant approached by a stranger (fig. 2). It is found on a seal from Cnossos, Crete, where a male worshiper covers his eyes in front of a goddess he is worshiping (Eliade, 1978). Another example is a standing adorant of bronze, also from Crete, who is raising his right arm over his forehead in a typical gesture for Minoan adorants. This gesture also covers the eyes (Marinatos and Hirmer, 1973).

Gaze aversion in the presence of Medusa's killing glance is seen on a black-figured Greek vase of the sixth century B.C., where Perseus is shown in the act of decapitating Medusa with his head averted (Bothmer, 1985). Another instance of gaze aversion is found in a Minoan cult figure on Crete. A worshiper pulls a sacred tree which represents the divinity with averted face (Eliade, 1978).

Summary: In the ancient texts discussed here magic power over life and death in interpersonal encounters is attributed to the eye over several early millennia. The eye is also used by the person in authority to guide, punish, and reward those in a dependent position in order to elicit the desired behavior. This controlling eye interplay is reminiscent of what the preverbal infant may at times experience in his eye games with mother. The infant under intolerable eye pressure can have recourse to gaze aversion, to hiding his face, or to shielding it, patterns

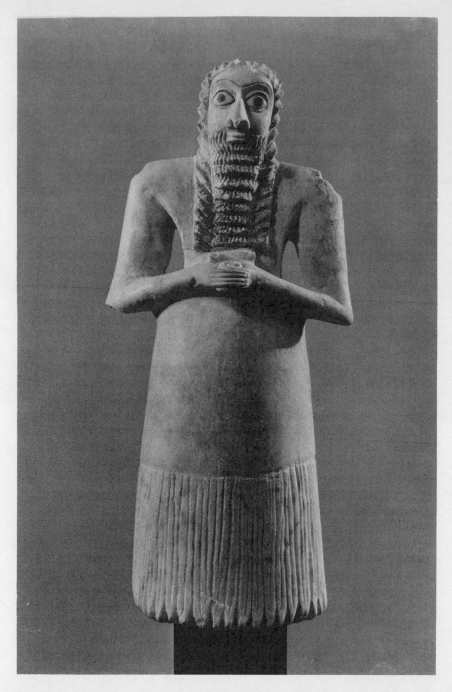

Figure 3. Sumerian gypsum statue from Mesopotamia, ca. 3000 B.C., with strikingly staring eyes. Metropolitan Museum of Art, Fletcher Fund, 1940, 40156.

observed in the texts as well. It may be that the early powerful imprint on the infant's mind of universal mutual gaze experiences with the mother has contributed to the eye beliefs, as they appear in the texts. They often reflect a primitive mentality subject to primary process thinking. This changed only in the classical Greek culture when secondary process thinking began to prevail. Figurative representations of eye power repeat the gaze patterns found in the texts, patterns which originate in infancy.

PHASE 2. THE WORLD OF IMAGINARY CREATURES, GOOD AND BAD: THE EYE AS AN AGENT OF CONFLICT

While the infant's response to the mother depends on her physical presence and their multiple daily encounters, the toddler and young nursery child have begun to develop a more complex psychic structure, in which mental representations of the mother as well as other objects, animate and inanimate, have gradually become intrapsychically available and can be evoked and remembered. An extended sense of time and space and a more long-term memory are some of the building blocks toward this acquired internal world of object constancy. With the acquisition of language and the capacity for symbolic play the nursery-age child can now have a verbal dialogue, can listen to a story, and can spin out one of his own. He can create a whole world of imaginary creatures and events past, present, and future and invest it with his wishful and fearful expectations, which inform us of his internal preoccupations and struggles. Under internal stress he may fear his parents' disapproving or rejecting glances and take recourse in defensive actions, such as repression, denial, and projection. For example, he may populate his world with witches, ghosts, and bogeymen which are the projections of his internal struggles with unacceptable aggressive fantasies. Freud (1913) says, "Spirits and demons . . . are only projections of man's emotional impulses" (p. 92). Mahler (1966) invokes splitting as another early defense. The child's ambivalence toward the parents leads to the splitting of the good from the bad parental images, with the bad images being projected out into the environment and taking the form of threatening creatures. Many of these creatures of the imagination have threatening eyes, a not surprising finding.

I am suggesting that the infant's and young child's real interactions with love objects, including eye-to-eye contact, and their transformation in the fertile mind of the preschooler have resulted in the creative act of inventing whole fantasy worlds, including eye worlds, in the service of his emotional stability and developmental progress. Creative, adaptive, and defensive ego forces have contributed to this accomplishment, as they are always at work in the imagined worlds of writers, poets, and mythmakers.

Freud (1911) recognized early a remarkable affinity between the mental status of the preschooler and that of primitive man. Both are subject to primary process thinking. Both are functioning cognitively on a preoperational level (Inhelder and Piaget, 1958). Primitive man sees nature in animistic terms and believes in the magic power of his thoughts and wishes. Both the young child and early, prelogical man resort to the same means to make their threatening world safer. They invent fantasy beings: the child to ease his internal psychological pressures; early man, to cope not only with internal threats of unacceptable emotions but also with the often destructive forces of nature and the arbitrariness of human events beyond his rational understanding.

It is not surprising to learn that many of these imaginary beings are endowed with prominent eyes—eyes that signal power and destruction; eyes that stare, threaten, hurt, and cause fear. The most universal example of such an eye is the evil eye. It seems that man everywhere created the notion of the evil eye, a universal which illustrates the "invisible unity of the history of the human mind" (Eliade, 1978). The belief in its existence certainly lives on to this day in many cultures and social strata.

What protective means have been invented against the imagined danger emanating from the evil eye? One such countermeasure is the "good" eye. To set a good eye against an evil eye is to assume that the power of the good eye can prevail and eliminate the threat of the evil eye. Of course, the good eye, that is, the amulet or other magic objects, had to be prominently or covertly present to exert its protective power and was (and still is) therefore worn in one way or another as an ornament, as part of clothing or affixed to furniture or walls. The psychological process underlying these beliefs is reminiscent of the young child's splitting the image of mother into a good and a bad mother prior to his being able to integrate the two opposites.

When prelogical man opposes the good eye to the evil eye, he assumes that the good eye can undo the power or intent of the evil eye. Good and evil have been externalized, and the good eye is given an edge over the evil eye so that man can believe in its superior magic power for his salvation from internal stress and from fear of realistic danger. Yet the danger is never completely eliminated. The precautionary measures have to be in force forever. Man cannot ever find a lasting safe haven, just as the young child must continue to defend himself against the unacceptable. He can repress, split, project, and undo, and he can also invent imaginary beings for his salvation.

The evil eye could threaten at any time, but in particular at times of transition. Crucial life events such as birth, pregnancy, puberty, and death needed protective measures against the evil eye. Blessings, such as a good harvest, were also seen as a threat. Entering and leaving holy places or one's own home, travel, and such daily activities as taking meals needed appeasement of the evil spirits. Man needed to pay his dues constantly. The most common such dues were sacrifices of animals and prayers, found in all cultures, and believed to have magic preventive powers. The use of eye magic is another such attempt at warding off the evil eye.

NARRATIVE TEXTS

There are several forms of verbal, not necessarily literary, evidence for the assumed existence of the evil eye. All languages, ancient and contemporary, have a word for evil eye (Seligmann, 1910). A Sumerian-Assyrian text mentions the destructive power of the evil eye (Budge, 1961).

Prophylactic phrases are common in everyday sayings. Among them is the Hebrew phrase, "May no evil eye look upon [or affect, or hurt] you," an expression to protect those to whom it was addressed.

Since the evil eye came to mean not only an evil force that emanates from an individual's eye but also signified, more generally, envy and jealousy of the gods, of the spirits, and of men, its varied meaning was expressed in ancient texts, such as the Bible and Greek tragedies.

FIGURATIVE MATERIAL

Before introducing the figurative evidence I want to address an issue which has to do with the mode of visual presentation of the face. This study clearly and unequivocally shows that full face presentations in two dimensional works such as paintings and bas reliefs were reserved for all those beings which were meant to impress and exert protective or destructive eye power. The conventional way in Egyptian, Babylonian, Assyrian, and Greek art was to present faces in profile. This changed only in late classical Greek style. Profile presentation was chosen not for lack of artistic know-how but because the ancient artists had clearly understood that the full face carried a powerful message which they reserved for special occasions.

Infant observations bear out this fundamental difference in impact between a frontal and a profile presentation of the face. The young infant, even before he can differentiate between faces, smiles at any face or facial likeness, if it is presented frontally, and stops smiling as soon as the face is turned into profile (Spitz and Wolf, 1946).

So when the Egyptians or the Greeks invented creatures which were to exert magic eye power, they showed them full face. Medusa and the Egyptian dwarf god Bes are examples. In Buddhist Asia another solution for the same problem was found. There, conventionally eyes were almond-shaped and half-closed. When they were meant to frighten or protect, they were shown wide open, often bulging to indicate their ferocious nature (figs. 4 and 5).

The figurative evidence to ward off the assumed threat of the evil eye is massive and ubiquitous. I will limit my discussion to those objects representing eyes or figures with prominent eyes and faces.

The dwellings of gods and man were seen in need of protection against evil spirits. Therefore, eyes or faces were put on walls, doorways, and doors to ward off evil spirits.

At the excavation site of an ancient kingdom called Ebla (today's northern Syria), dated in the third millennium B.C., big sculpted limestone eyes were found. They are believed to have been attached to the façades of the palace (Matthiae, 1977).

The winged eye of the god Re decorates the doorway to the Egyptian temple of Dendur (Aldred, 1978).

In Greece, Medusa, the instant killer, was also conceived as guardian of sacred buildings. She is shown as a powerful image in the pediment of a sixth century temple to Artemis in Corfu (Lullies, 1979). Her deadly eye power had become a lasting protective power as well. This interesting transformation of her function from a destructive to a constructive force makes her a representative of phases 1 and 2.

Doors as symbols of transition from the profane to the sacred or from life to death also needed protective images. Their sometimes lavish decorations have been described in ancient texts (Walsh, 1983). No ancient doors are preserved. However, a symbolic door on a Roman sarcophagus of the third century C.E. has two Medusa heads on its panels, an echo of an old tradition (Walsh, 1983).

In the Far East guardian figures with fierce eyes and threatening countenances were set up in front of temples or other buildings. Such figures are still present today in China, Thailand, and Japan.

Furniture and eating and drinking vessels were also decorated with warding-off eyes. A wooden chair of Tutankhamun has the winged eye of Re at its back (Settgast et al., 1976). Another Egyptian chair has the dwarf god Bes carved on its back, Bes seen full face (Scott, 1973).

A magnificent bronze ritual vessel from China dated in the second

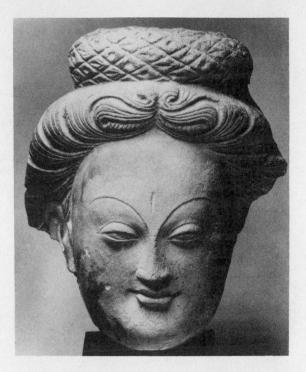

Figure 4.   Head of deity with half-open eyes. Clay, China, 7th century C.E.
Museum for Indian Art, Berlin, 4480.

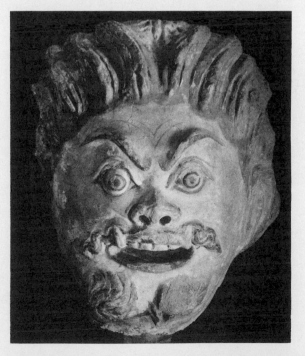

Figure 5.   Head of demon with protruding eyes. Clay. China, 8th to 9th
century C.E. Museum for Indian Art, Berlin, 4527.

millennium B.C. is covered with eyes (Ma Chengyuan, 1980). Face pots
shaped as faces or heads or with face designs on them have been found
in locations as far apart as Jericho, Peru, and New Guinea. The oldest
date from the third millennium B.C. (Potts, 1981). Many Greek vases
have disproportionately huge pairs of eyes painted on them to protect
the drinker against harm (fig. 6).

Jewelry and clothing were also protected by eyes. The pectoral of
Tutankhamun has an eye amidst the colorful stones (Settgast et al.,
1976). They appear on Egyptian sarcophagi to help the dead to a
secure trip to the netherworld (fig. 7). A pair of eyes were painted on
boats to make travel safer. And eyes decorate war implements such as
shields or standards for protection in the most dangerous of enter-
prises. They were found in locations as far apart as Iran and New
Guinea.

Summary: The evil eye belief and the defensive strategies resulting
from it are worldwide phenomena throughout known history, including preliterate history. They are the product of a world of magic make-
believe, which also characterizes a developmental phase of childhood.
The eye experiences of the individual child, based on a combination of
innate and acquired factors, have become common cultural good in the
form of folk beliefs.

PHASE 3. THE WORLD OF CONSCIENCE, CLEAR OR GUILTY: THE EYE AS A MORAL AGENT

As the preschooler matures, his make-believe world yields gradually to
increasingly better reality testing. Imaginary companions are abandoned or discredited. On the other hand, the child's shift in his attachment behavior places added stress on the family. His newly intense
preference for the parent of the opposite sex, accompanied by increased ambivalence toward, and rivalry with, the other parent brings
about a state of excitability, guilt, and internal turmoil. The child's
conflict-ridden frame of mind subsides only gradually, as he approaches school age. Eventually his stressful preoccupations are relegated to the unconscious. Latency then becomes a time of relative calm.

The development of conscience is the major contribution to the
child's psychic structure during latency. The young school-age child,
internally and externally more self-reliant than the preschooler, is
much preoccupied with issues of right and wrong, good and bad, and
rules and regulations. By identification with parental values the latency
child develops his own set of moral standards which help him regulate
his behavior and his self-esteem, with guilt being the price to be paid

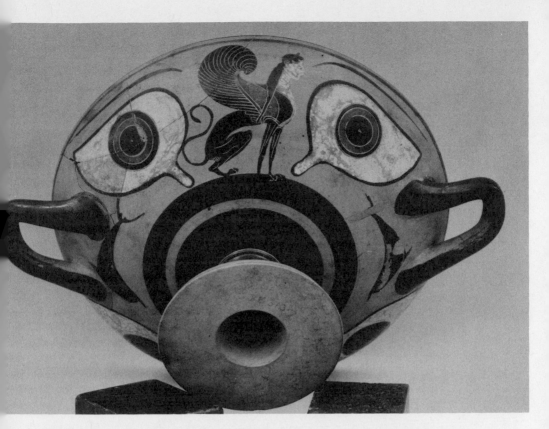

Figure 6. Greek eye cup (kylix) with a pair of huge eyes for protection of the drinker. Attic, 6th century B.C. Metropolitan Museum of Art, Fletcher Fund, 1925, 25.78.6.

Figure 7. Egyptian coffin with a pair of eyes for a secure trip to the netherworld. Painted wood, dynasty 12 (1991-1786 B.C.). Metropolitan Museum of Art, Rogers Fund, 1915, 15.2.2.

for transgressions. According to Freud (1923), early auditory verbal residues become component parts of conscience formation which then contribute to the "inner voice," the conscience. I am suggesting that early preverbal mutual gaze experiences can become component parts of the conscience as well and are reflected in the phenomenon of the "inner eye," a point I am going to illustrate (Riess, 1978).

Karl Abraham (1913) reports of a patient: "as soon as the picture of his father appeared the face became distorted and the eyes took on a fixed stare . . . his death-phantasy directed against his father . . . found utterance in the rigid look of the eyes in his father's image" (p. 221). The late movie maker Luis Buñuel mentions such a vision of his late father's face in his autobiography, *The Last Sigh* (1983). Richard Rodriguez (1981), a Mexican-American, whose level of education led to a clash between his world and that of his Spanish-speaking parents, wrote: "Many mornings at my desk I have been paralyzed by the thought of their faces, their eyes. I imagine their eyes moving slowly across these pages. That image has weakened my resolve. Finally, however, it has not stopped me" (p. 184f.).

Clearly, in these examples, the inner eye acts as a moral agent, an agent signaling superego anxiety. Guilt is projected into the parents' disapproving eyes.

In Egypt the dead had to appear before a tribunal of 42 gods who had to judge their actions in life. The deceased's heart was put on a scale to be weighed against a feather, a symbol of Truth. The deceased had to utter a declaration of innocence about his actions in life. If the gods' verdict was satisfactory, the dead person would be admitted to the joys of the netherworld. If the gods' verdict was negative, the heart of the deceased would be thrown to the waiting "Eater of Hearts," a grotesque animal (Watterson, 1984). Sometimes an eye was substituted for the feather, the eye also being considered a symbol of Truth. Clearly, in this instance, the eye was given the function of moral judge, weighing the dead man's moral behavior in life (Eliade, 1978).

A large part of the Old Testament tells the story of the disobedience of the Israelites to the laws given to them by God at Mount Sinai, of God's wrath and threat of punishment, and of the Israelites' repentance. All moral authority is vested in God who watches over "his children" and judges their adherence to his laws. Again and again he finds them wanting and again and again he uses his eyes as observer, judge, and dispenser of reward and punishment. The Israelites on their part fear his eye when disobedient and repent and atone for their transgressions; when they have been faithful, they bask in the warmth of his eye presence. God's eye serves as an external conscience, as moral guide, so to speak, until the Israelites have made God's moral tenets their own and can live up to his demands.

The classical Greek poets of the fifth century, especially Aeschylus and Sophocles, addressed questions of morality, conscience, guilt and atonement, absent in Homer's world. In their tragedies they used the familiar myths as their vehicles and infused them with the spirit of the current Athenian law, overthrowing the ancient laws of blood ties and vengeance.

The Furies became the embodiment of man's guilty conscience. They persecuted him relentlessly all over the world and chased him to his death, unless prevented from it by the new benign and just government of Athens.

Orestes, the murderer of his mother, and Oedipus, the killer of his father and husband of his mother, are two of the guilt-ridden heroes of Greek tragedy, who are chased by the Furies and cannot find respite from them, that is, from their guilty conscience, until they can find acceptance and forgiveness through the benign laws of Athens.

The eyes of the Furies stand as the unwelcome reminder of man's bad conscience, as a moral agent. In the imagery of the Greek myth the Furies personify guilt, one of their characterizations being their disgusting horrifying eyes.

While Oedipus' self-blinding is commonly interpreted as a symbolic act of self-castration, Sophocles directs our attention to other eye-focused elements motivating Oedipus to deprive himself of his sight. One is his self-reproach for not seeing literally and metaphorically what he should have seen long ago. He is in a way hinting at his own self-deception and denial. He says to himself, "You have . . . failed long enough to know those that you should have known; henceforth you shall be dark" (*King Oedipus*). Sophocles gives another clue for Oedipus' choice of his eyes as the locus of self-punishment. He has him say, "How could I have looked into the face of my father when I came among the dead, aye, or on my miserable mother, since against them both I sinned such things that no halter can punish" (*King Oedipus*). His guilt and fear of a face-to-face encounter with his dead parents in the underworld were additional motivating elements in Oedipus' self-blinding.

Summary: The eye as a moral agent can be a strong internal force in its role as a superego component. It can influence actions, support moral behavior and lawfulness, and signal guilt and the need for punishment. When guilt is projected, the eye can be seen as an external threat emanating from the imagined stern faces of parents.

PHASE 4. THE WORLD OF THE VISIONARY: THE EYE AS SYMBOL AND METAPHOR

The maturation of the adolescent's body and mind endows him with new intellectual and emotional capabilities. His powers of abstraction and symbolization, an extended sense of time—foresight and hindsight—and a capacity for self-reflection are put into the service of his aspirations and wishful thinking. The adolescent is given to formulating ideas and ideals, to setting himself revolutionary goals, and to experiencing messianic fervor. He tries to translate his preoccupation with questions of conscience, justice, and liberty into idealized visions of his future life (Inhelder and Piaget, 1958). It is at this level of adolescent functioning that the eye can be conceived of as metaphor and symbol.

The Books of the Prophets take up more than one fourth of the Old Testament, an indication of their importance to the lives of the ancient Jews. It is in the nature of prophecy—literally meaning prediction—to have visions of the future. Those visions may be cataclysmic or gloriously full of promise. Whatever their nature, they are the product of internal visionary power of an individual's imaginings. This kind of vision can certainly occur at the level of adolescent thinking and projective preoccupation with the future.

The prophets use the eye and seeing again and again as a metaphor for knowledge, understanding, and wisdom, that is, as internalized seeing. This is equally true for other books of the Old Testament and for the New Testament as well.

Isaiah 5:15: ". . . and the eyes of the lofty shall be humbled."

Ezekiel 3:8: "Behold, I have made thy face strong against their faces, and thy forehead strong against their foreheads."

Ecclesiastes 2:14: "The wise man's eyes are in his head; but the fool walketh in darkness."

St. Matthew 6:22–23: "The light of the body is the eye: if therefore thine eye be single, thy whole body shall be full of light. But if thine eye be evil, thy whole body shall be full of darkness."

St. Matthew 13:13: "Therefore I speak to them in parables: because they seeing see not, and hearing they hear not, neither do they understand."

Clearly, parables and metaphors are products of thought processes which correspond to the adolescent's capacity for abstraction and symbolization.

In Greek culture blindness sometimes stands as a symbol for wisdom. Homer is depicted as a blind old man, who created his poetic works from an internal vision, from the "mind's eye" so to speak. Since nothing is known about the historic person Homer, the attribution of blindness to him expresses the Greeks' admiration of his genius as the great creator of epic poems, as a visionary.

Knowledge of the future is ascribed in ancient Greek culture to seers such as Teiresias, the tragic figure in Sophocles' drama *King Oedipus*. As the term "seer" implies, he too has inner visions, he can see the future, a knowledge hidden from the ordinary person.

In *Oedipus at Colonus* blind Oedipus says to a stranger: "All I shall say will be clear-sighted indeed" (verse 74), a statement certainly meant as a metaphor.

The function of the eye and seeing has been totally transformed into an internalized one.

Conclusion

Mutual gaze is a universal form of communication among all humans everywhere and at all times. It has its ancestry in the animal world and has, as is known now, an innate biological component. From birth on the infant is most receptive and responsive to the caretaker's eye signals, an encounter which sets in motion a lively and lifelong social exchange. By the time the child has learned to talk, the eye language, preceding speech by several years, has contributed greatly to everyday social interchange between infant and caretaker and played a prominent role in the forging of their mutual bond. The child, the more dependent and malleable partner in this pair, has had to make adaptation to the mother's eye messages, which can cover the whole gamut of the emotional scale and evoke a wide range of responses in the child.

Mutual eye attunement never ceases to exist as a social force. Due to its very early and intense role in the infant's life it continues to affect the growing child's interpersonal relations and personality development. The impact of the early eye-to-eye contact between infant and caretakers lives on through childhood. It enters into the gradual process of internalization of mutual gaze patterns. Their intrapsychic representation undergoes transformations parallel to the growth of psychic structure and takes on characteristics specific for each phase.

It is no surprise then that the language of the eye as one of the most powerful social communicators among humans would enter the cultural heritage in the multiple forms which I have described above. The eye language of the infant, the preschooler, the school child, and the adolescent has found representation in ancient cultural works.

It has been the goal of this essay to demonstrate the order in which the various phase-specific forms of the eye language evolve successively in the individual child and how they are all absorbed into and preserved in the creations of culture.

BIBLIOGRAPHY

ABRAHAM, K. (1913). Restrictions and transformations of scoptophilia in psycho-neurotics. In *Selected Papers on Psycho-Analysis.* London: Hogarth Press, 1949, pp. 169–234.

ALDRED, C. (1973). *Akhenaten and Nefertiti.* New York & Brooklyn Museum: Viking Press.

––––– (1978). The temple of Dendur. *Metropolitan Mus. Art Bull.,* 36:5–80.

ARGYLE, M. & COOK, M. (1976). *Gaze and Mutual Gaze.* London: Cambridge Univ. Press.

BIBLE (1901). *Old and New Testaments.* Authorized King James Version. Cleveland & New York: World Publishing Company.

BOTHMER, D. VON (1985). *The Amasis Painter and His World.* J. Paul Getty Museum, Malibu, California, New York & London: Thames & Hudson.

BRAZELTON, T. B. (1982). Joint regulation of neonate-parent behavior. In *Social Interchange in Infancy,* ed. E. Tronick. Baltimore: Univ. Park Press, pp. 7–22.

BUDGE, E. A. W. (1961). *Amulets and Talismans.* New York: New Hyde Park.

BUÑUEL, L. (1983). *The Last Sigh.* New York: Knopf.

DESIMONE, R., ALBRIGHT, T. D., GROSS, C. G., & BRUCE, C. (1984). Stimulus-selective properties of inferior temporal neurons in the Macaque. *J. Neurosci.,* 4:2051–2062.

EKMAN, P., FRIESEN, W. V., & ELLSWORTH, P. (1972). *Emotion in the Human Face.* New York: Pergamon Press.

ELIADE, M. (1978). *A History of Religious Ideas.* Chicago: Univ. Chicago Press.

FANTZ, R. L. (1965). Visual perception from birth. *Ann. N.Y. Acad. Sci.,* 118:793–814.

FREUD, S. (1900). The interpretation of dreams. *S.E.,* 4 & 5.

––––– (1911). Formulations on the two principles of mental functioning. *S.E.,* 12:213–226.

––––– (1913). Totem and taboo. *S.E.,* 13:1–161.

––––– (1923). The ego and the id. *S.E.,* 19:3–66.

Gilgamesh, The Epic of (1960). An English version by N. K. Sandars, rev. ed. New York: Penguin Books, 1983.

GRAVES, R. (1960). *The Greek Myths.* New York: Penguin Books.

HOMER (1951). *The Iliad,* tr. R. Lattimore. Chicago: Univ. Chicago Press.

––––– (1975). *The Odyssey,* tr. R. Lattimore. London: Harper & Row.

INHELDER, B. & PIAGET, J. (1958). *The Growth of Logical Thinking from Childhood to Adolescence.* New York: Basic Books.

KLEEMAN, J. A. (1967). The peek-a-boo game. *Psychoanal. Study Child*, 22:239–273.

LICHTHEIM, M. (1976). *Ancient Egyptian Literature*. Berkeley: Univ. California Press.

LULLIES, R. (1979). *Griechische Plastik*, 4th ed. Plate 21. Munich: Hirmer.

MA CHENGYUAN (1980). The splendor of ancient Chinese bronzes. In *The Great Bronze Age of China*, ed. Wen Fong. New York: Alfred Knopf, pp. 1–19.

MAHLER, M. S. (1966). Notes on the development of basic moods. In *Psychoanalysis—A General Psychology*, ed. R. M. Loewenstein, L. M. Newman, M. Schur, & A. J. Solnit. New York: Int. Univ. Press, pp. 152–168.

MARINATOS, S. & HIRMER, M. (1973). *Kreta, Thera und das mykenische Hellas*. Munich: Hirmer.

MATTHIAE, P. (1977). Tell Mardikh. *Archaeology*, 30:244–253.

OPPENHEIM, A. L. (1977). *Ancient Mesopotamia*. Chicago: Univ. Chicago Press.

OWEN, D. (1982). *Camouflage and Mimicry*. Chicago: Univ. Chicago Press.

POTTS, A. M. (1981). *The World's Eye*. Lexington: Univ. Kentucky Press.

RIESS, A. (1978). The mother's eye. *Psychoanal. Study Child*, 33:381–409.

ROBSON, K. S. (1967). The role of eye-to-eye contact in maternal-infant attachment. *J. Child. Psychol. & Psychiat.*, 8:13–25.

RODRIGUEZ, R. (1981). *Hunger of Memory*. Boston: Godine.

SCHALLER, G. B. (1963). *The Mountain Gorilla*. Chicago: Univ. Chicago Press.

SCOTT, N. (1973). The daily life of the ancient Egyptians. *Metropolitan Mus. Art Bull.*, 31:123–172.

SELIGMANN, S. (1910). *Der böse Blick und Verwandtes*. Berlin: Hermann Barsdorf Verlag.

SETTGAST, J. ET AL., eds. (1976). Nofretete—Echnaton. Mainz: Philipp von Zabern.

SOPHOCLES (1947). *King Oedipus*, tr. W. B. Yeats. New York: Dial Press.

———— (1954). *Oedipus at Colonus*, tr. R. Fitzgerald. Chicago: Univ. Chicago Press, pp. 77–155.

SPITZ, R. A. (1965). *The First Year of Life*. New York: Int. Univ. Press.

———— & WOLF, K. M. (1946). The smiling response. *Gen. Psychol. Monogr.*, 34:57–125.

STERN, D. N. (1977). *The First Relationship*. Cambridge, Mass.: Harvard Univ. Press.

VIRGIL (1967). *The Pastoral Poems*, tr. E. V. Rien. Baltimore: Penguin Classics.

WALSH, D. A. (1983). Doors of the Greek and Roman world. *Archaeology*, 36:43–50.

WATTERSON, B. (1984). *The Gods of Ancient Egypt*. New York: Bicester.

Redefining the Revenant

Guilt and Sibling Loss in Guntrip and Freud

PETER L. RUDNYTSKY, Ph.D.

HARRY GUNTRIP'S (1975) RECORD OF HIS ANALYTIC EXPERIENCES WITH
W. R. D. Fairbairn and D. W. Winnicott is at once a moving autobiographical document and an important theoretical discussion of the
nature of therapeutic action in psychoanalysis. Central to Guntrip's
paper, and his motivation for seeking analysis in the first place, is "a
total amnesia for a severe trauma at the age of three and a half years,
over the death of a younger brother" (p. 447), Percy. Recognizing that
it was this trauma which led him to become a psychotherapist, Guntrip
convincingly argued that "it seems that our theory must be rooted in
our psychopathology," and instanced as proof of this interplay between personal suffering and scientific insight "Freud's courageous
self-analysis at a time when all was obscure" (p. 467). Although
Guntrip's was not literally a self-analysis—he had over 1,000 sessions
with Fairbairn in the 1950s and over 150 with Winnicott in the 1960s—
part of his purpose was to investigate the continuing effects of an
analysis after termination in order to assess its therapeutic efficacy.
Emulating Freud's courage, Guntrip distilled the lessons of his encounters with two masters in a luminous piece of self-analysis.

In addition to the self-analytic component of his essay, Guntrip resembled Freud in the biographical accident of sibling loss. As is well
known, Freud was profoundly affected by the death in infancy of his
younger brother Julius, at a time when he himself was just under 2
years of age. Although mentioned in the memory-laden letter to Fliess

Assistant professor of English and comparative literature at Columbia University.
This paper was presented at an International Conference on Literature and Psychology
at Kent State University in August 1987.

of October 3, 1897, and later recalled in a 1912 letter to Ferenczi, the death of Julius was nowhere alluded to in any of Freud's published writings. Max Schur (1972, pp. 153–171) elucidated the importance of the *non vixit* dream in terms of Freud's recurring experience of the "guilt of the survivor"; and Ernest Jones (1955, p. 146) drew upon Freud's own paper, "Some Character Types Met with in Psycho-Analytic Work" (1916), to depict Freud as one who was himself "wrecked by success" through the fulfillment of unconscious death wishes against Julius.

A comparison between the experiences of sibling loss in Guntrip and Freud provides the focal point for the present inquiry. My thesis can be stated relatively simply: whereas in Freud the death of a brother gives rise to the conflict between ambivalent feelings of love and hatred which led to guilt, Guntrip's inability to recall and hence to mourn his brother's death was indicative of arrest at a more primitive stage of emotional development. This contrast between Freud's unresolved ambivalence and Guntrip's "absence of grief" (Deutsch, 1937) is all the more remarkable in that Guntrip was more than 18 months older than Freud at the time of the loss of their respective siblings.

Moreover, the example of Guntrip, who unblocked his amnesia in 1971 after learning of the death of Winnicott, allows us to reconceptualize Freud's persistent struggle with the ghosts or revenants of his unconsciously murdered rivals. Instead of being merely a curse or burden, guilt may be viewed rather as a positive achievement, heralding an arrival at the depressive position (Klein, 1935). The sense of guilt, as Winnicott (1958) remarked, "even when unconscious and even when apparently irrational, implies a certain degree of emotional growth, ego health, and hope" (p. 19).

I

Although Guntrip sought to maintain an evenhanded attitude toward both of his eminent analysts, calling Fairbairn more innovative in theory and Winnicott more spontaneous in practice, and expressing gratitude for what he had received from each, his paper in fact offered a devastating critique of Fairbairn's limitations as a therapist and a corresponding tribute to the genius of Winnicott. Not only were Fairbairn's interpretations excessively intellectualized, but the rigidity of his manner—symbolized by his placement of the patient's couch in front of a large desk, and seating himself on the other side—had the effect of stymieing Guntrip's analysis at the experiences that took place when he was between 3½ and 7 years old, and rendering inaccessible the earlier double traumas of his brother's death and his mother's failures of empathy. In the highly applicable terms of Balint (1968), Fairbairn conducted the analysis at the level of oedipal conflict without reaching to the breakdown of the primary love relationship that defines the area of the basic fault.

I shall summarize the salient details of Guntrip's personal history. His mother, the eldest of 11 children, had already played the part of careworn "little mother" to her younger siblings, and did not want any children of her own when she married Guntrip's father, an eloquent and protective Methodist preacher, in 1898. In his teen-age years, Guntrip was told by his mother that she had breast-fed him because she believed it would prevent her from having another pregnancy; she then refused to breast-feed Percy and was reproached by her husband that Percy would have lived if she had done so. After Percy's death, Guntrip's mother withheld further sexual relations from her husband.

The Kleinian aspects of these issues of breast-feeding, in which the breast becomes consolidated as a "bad" object, and hence no "good" loved object can be installed within the ego, are transparent. Because no good object can be introjected, moreover, the ego remains arrested at the schizoid position and, in Deutsch's words, "is not sufficiently developed to bear the strain of the work of mourning" (1937, p. 13). Both regressive anxiety and a mobilization of defenses—above all, the blocking of affect—are responses to the threat posed by object loss to the immature ego. But a Kleinian analysis purely in terms of internal objects needs to be supplemented by an emphasis on the failure of environmental provision. For, as Winnicott has shown, the infant's attainment of the depressive position "is not so much dependent on the mother's simple ability to hold a baby, which was her characteristic at the earlier stages, as on her ability to hold the infant-care situation over a period of time during which the infant may go through complex experiences" (1958, p. 23). It is precisely the inability of Guntrip's mother to "hold the infant-care situation" which lies at the crux of his difficulties, and for which the struggles over breast-feeding are but the most striking metaphor.

Upon seeing Percy naked and dead on his mother's lap, as he was informed later, the 3½-year-old Harry rushed up and called out, "Don't let him go. You'll never get him back!" He then fell victim to a mysterious illness, from which he would have died had he not been sent temporarily to the family of a maternal aunt. But all memory of his brother's death and his leaving home was totally repressed, though, Guntrip added, "it remained alive in me, to be triggered off unrecognizably by widely spaced analogous events" (p. 455). Both at the ages of

26 and 37, separation from a brother-figure gave rise to an inexplicable exhaustion illness. By the latter occasion, in 1938, Guntrip had studied classical analytic theory and realized intellectually that he lived, as it were, atop the buried memory of Percy's death. He reported a dream: "I went down into a tomb and saw a man buried alive. He tried to get out but I threatened him with illness, locked him in and got away quick" (p. 456). This search for a hidden traumatic scene, "triggered off unrecognizably by widely spaced analogous events," is a paradigm for the psychoanalytic quest, which evokes Oedipus' assembling the clues to his past in *Oedipus the King*.

Upon returning to his parents' home, Guntrip tried to coerce his mother's love, first by various psychosomatic ailments, and then, after the age of 5, by more active defiance. This misbehavior in turn provoked brutal rages and canings from his mother. It was to the dissection of this "world of internalized libidinally excited bad-object relations" (p. 457) that his analysis with Fairbairn was dedicated, and Guntrip derived considerable benefit from it. But, as I have indicated, he came increasingly to realize that he was not making progress on the more important underlying problems of the period before Percy's death, and indeed his conflicted relations with his mother served as a defense against this deeper material. In addition, Fairbairn fell ill—shortly after the death in December 1957 of the friend whose departure 30 years earlier had caused the first adult eruption of the illness modeled on his response to his brother's death—and the analysis was interrupted for 6 months. By 1959, Guntrip reached a crucial insight, though he did not impart it directly to Fairbairn: either remaining in analysis and awaiting Fairbairn's death or losing him by ending the analysis would cause a repetition of the trauma of Percy's death, with no one to help him through it. In view of Fairbairn's declining state of health, Guntrip phased out his analysis during that year.

Part of the courage needed to terminate his analysis with Fairbairn came from Guntrip's decision to seek analysis with Winnicott, with whom he had begun corresponding at Fairbairn's instigation in 1954. Guntrip wrote: "By 1962 I had no doubt that he was the only man I could turn to for further help" (p. 459). In this eminently well-placed confidence in Winnicott's healing powers the 61-year-old Guntrip echoed the distressed plea of the Piggle, 2 years and 4 months old, before her first consultation: "Mummy take me to Dr. Winnicott" (Winnicott, 1977, p. 7). Despite the limited number of sessions, Winnicott allowed Guntrip "to reach right back to *an ultimate good mother, and to find her recreated in him in the transference*" (p. 460). In so doing, and in a way that would only become clear in the fullness of time, he gave Guntrip access to the inner strength needed to face his double traumas of sibling loss and maternal deprivation.

Winnicott's gifts as a clinician are legendary, and readers familiar with any of his case histories or vignettes need not be surprised to find corroboration coming from yet another quarter. Yet Guntrip's account was unusually poignant as it was written from the patient's point of view. As an analogue, I turn to the illustrative case included in "Creativity and Its Origins" (1971). In this paper, Winnicott told of a man who feared to be called mad for thinking himself a girl, to whom Winnicott responded: "It was not that *you* told this to anyone; it is *I* who see the girl and hear the girl talking, when actually there is a man on my couch. The mad person is myself." As a result of enabling the patient "to see himself as a girl *from my position*," Winnicott achieved a break-through: "he and I have been driven to the conclusion (though unable to prove it) that his mother (who is not alive now) saw a girl baby when she saw him as a baby before she came round to thinking of himself as a boy" (p. 74).

Guntrip's symptoms did not include the feature of split-off female elements, but his interaction with Winnicott was otherwise very similar. Essential in both instances was Winnicott's inclusion of his own uncertainty as part of the analytic discourse, while at the same time remaining extraordinarily attuned to the anxieties of the patient. He told Guntrip near the end of their first session, "I've nothing particular to say yet, but if I don't say something, you may begin to feel I'm not here" (p. 460). It was not long before he divined the root of Guntrip's discomfort at silence and his need to talk hard: "You feel silence is abandonment. The gap is not you forgetting mother, but mother forgetting you, and now you've relived it with me. You're finding an earlier trauma which you might never recover without the help of the Percy trauma repeating it. You have to remember mother abandoning you by transference on to me" (p. 461). Winnicott thus took the place of the "good breast mother" at the point where Guntrip's actual mother had failed him. Both in Guntrip's case and in that reported by Winnicott in "Creativity and Its Origins," it is only through the transferential encounter between patient and analyst that it is possible to relive and hence to reconstruct the primordial trauma of maternal madness or abandonment.

In addition to becoming the "good-enough mother" Guntrip never had, Winnicott permitted Guntrip to cultivate his own nurturing powers. Acknowledging his own vulnerability, he went so far as to say, "You too have a good breast. You've always been able to give more than you take. Doing your analysis is almost the most reassuring thing that happens to me. The chap before you makes me feel I'm no good at all. You don't have to be good for me. I don't need it and can cope without it, but in fact you are good for me" (p. 462). By providing a holding environment and refusing to retaliate or be destroyed, Winnicott transformed the meaning of Percy's death and likewise helped Guntrip to resolve his dilemma concerning termination.

In true psychoanalytic fashion, the most enduring results of Winnicott's interventions only manifested themselves after the event, through deferred action. Guntrip last saw Winnicott in July 1969, and in February 1970 Guntrip was told by a physician that he was seriously overworked. But rather than accept retirement, he continued to write feverishly, until in October he contracted pneumonia and spent five weeks in the hospital. Guntrip did not fully realize that his hyperactivity was still a result of his struggle to assert himself as a living being in the face of his mother's apathy. Early in 1971, Guntrip learned that Winnicott had had a flu attack and dropped him a line. Winnicott called soon afterward to thank him for his note. Two weeks later Winnicott's secretary called with the news that he had died.

Winnicott's death precipitated in Guntrip an extraordinary series of dreams. In the first, "*I saw my mother*, black, immobilized, staring fixedly into space, *totally ignoring me* as I stood at one side staring at her and feeling myself frozen into immobility" (p. 463). In previous dreams, his mother had always attacked him. Although he first assumed Winnicott's death to represent a repetition of the loss of his brother, Guntrip soon recognized that he had not dreamed of his mother in this way on the two previous occasions when he had been separated from someone who had reminded him of Percy. Now, moreover, he did not fall ill, as he had both in 1927 and 1938. The dreaming of his mother's indifference was thus a sign that Guntrip was beginning, for the first time, *to remember the events of the period before his brother's death.* In "Dreaming, Fantasying, and Living" (1971), Winnicott makes the unexpected point that "dreaming and living have been seen to be of the same order, daydreaming being of another order" (p. 26). In being able to dream of what he had previously forgotten, Guntrip was making contact with his dissociated past and, as a result, learning to live.

The next two months led Guntrip through a "compelling dreamsequence which went on night after night, taking me back in chronological order through every house I had ever lived in" (p. 463). The climax came in two dreams in which Guntrip clearly saw himself as he was during his brother's life and death. In the first, he was 3, and holding a pram with his 1-year-old brother; their mother was staring vacantly into the distance. The second dream was even more startling:

> I was standing with another man, the double of myself, both reaching out to get hold of a dead object. Suddenly the other man collapsed in a heap. Immediately the dream changed to a lighted room, where I saw Percy again. I knew it was him, sitting on the lap of a woman who had no face, arms, breasts. She was merely a lap to sit on, not a person. He looked deeply depressed, with the corners of his mouth turned down, and I was trying to make him smile [p. 464].

In this dream, Guntrip actually recaptured the memory of trying to reach out to his brother when he beheld him dead on his mother's lap; and in both dreams he also broke through to the earlier period before Percy's death "to see the faceless depersonalized mother, and the black depressed mother, who totally failed to relate to both of us" (p. 464).

Through his death, Winnicott enabled Guntrip to summon his emotionally absent mother and prematurely deceased brother back to life in his mind. As Guntrip wrote, "*He has taken her place and made it possible and safe to remember her in an actual dream-reliving of her paralysing schizoid aloofness*" (p. 464f). Thus, the ghosts of the past, rather than tormentors, became a reassuring sign of the persistence of memory, a confirmation of one's power to grieve over lost objects. In Kleinian terms, Guntrip negotiated the transition from the paranoid-schizoid to the depressive position. Through his belated introjection of Winnicott as a good mother, Guntrip in old age achieved what Freud, likewise confronted by sibling loss but sustained from infancy by his mother's love, struggled with for a lifetime—the ambivalence accompanying the "guilt of the survivor."

II

In his second climactic dream Guntrip referred to standing with "a double of myself." This "double" was, most evidently, a recollected image of himself as a child. But it may also represent his dead brother Percy, no less than the repressed portion of his own past. The consequence of the very idea of the double is to break down distinctions between self and other, or between interpersonal and intrapsychic relations. When, in the *non vixit* dream, Freud made the famous declaration, "My emotional life has always insisted that I should have an intimate friend and hated enemy" (1900, p. 483), he defined his life in terms of a series of encounters with revenants of his nephew John, beneath whom lay the shadowy figure of the dead Julius. As I have argued elsewhere (1987, pp. 44–49), the constant ambivalence in Freud's dealings with male counterparts was paralleled by the oscillation between "delusions of inferiority" and "megalomania" in his own self-esteem.

In thinking about the implications of the common experience of sibling loss in Freud and Guntrip, I find it helpful to invoke Bion's (1950) notion of the "imaginary twin." In the case of a patient whose sister, his elder by 18 months, died when he was 1 year of age,[1] Bion observed the tendency to invent an imaginary figure, a twin, who stood for "the bad part of himself from which he wished to be dissociated" (p. 9). But this menacing Doppelgänger was also that which must be reintegrated, if amnesia was to be overcome and the self was to be made whole.

From the "imaginary twin," it is a short step to a contemplation of the phenomenon of actual identical twins. I rely here on the fascinating autobiographical paper by George L. Engel (1975). Engel's paper is germane in the present context both because it is a venture in self-analysis, displaying courage comparable to that of Guntrip and Freud, and because it turns on the death of a brother.

Unlike the brothers of Guntrip and Freud, however, Frank Engel, George's elder by 5 minutes, died not in early childhood but at 49 years of age. But this difference is of only secondary importance. The Engels' father, like Frank, died unexpectedly of a heart attack, at the age of 58. Freud, as I have tried to document elsewhere (1987, pp. 18–23), though already 40 years of age, was inordinately afflicted by the death of his father in 1896 because it reawakened the "germ of reproaches" implanted by the premature death of Julius. The death of Engel's father preceded that of his brother, as one would expect in the normal course of events, and likewise lacks the infantile factor. But the psychological dynamics of the interplay of survivor guilt toward his sibling and paternal rivals were otherwise closely akin to those found in Freud.

In his paper George Engel describes his mourning process as well as anniversary reactions and parapraxes. He includes some astonishing photographs taken of himself in April 1972 and of his father in April 1928, when each man was 58 years of age, as well as of Frank Engel, on the same day in April 1928, when he was 14 years old. The poses of the

----

1. In his retrospective commentary on the case, Bion states that this information is "factually inaccurate," but that it "approximates closely" (p. 120) the true state of affairs. It should be added that Bion did not develop the theme of sibling loss in his paper.

three men reading are truly uncanny in their likeness. Engel pondered the question: "had I unconsciously begun to fuse the images of my father and my twin? Indeed, had he in my unconscious become my twin?" (p. 29).

One example of a parapraxis committed by Engel must stand for many. When presenting the material orally at the University of Rochester, Engel misspoke and said, "December 10th, 1971, was my ninety-eighth birthday," instead of his fifty-eighth birthday. After being convulsed with "uncontrollable laughter," in which his audience joined wholeheartedly, he interpreted his slip as expressing "my wish to live to a ripe old age, or better still, forever." The age of 58 was, of course, a highly charged milestone because that was the age at which his father had died. But, as a perceptive medical student in the audience pointed out, the slip of 98 was overdetermined by the fact that it represented twice 49, the age at which his brother had died. As Engel sardonically commented, "By doubling his life span I shall live his life for him and enjoy the twinship for both of us. What a triumph! What a marvellous joke! No wonder the uncontrollable laughter and tears" (p. 29).

Very few people have an identical twin, or even a sibling who dies in infancy. But the exceptional individuals to whom such a lot befalls may show us in bolder relief the patterns that likewise shape our own lives. From identical twins, through "imaginary twins," we return to the more general phenomenon of the double. Following Rank, Freud argued that the idea of the double—including belief in an eternal soul—was "originally an insurance against the destruction of the ego," but then "reverses its aspect," and "From having been an assurance of immortality, it becomes an uncanny harbinger of death" (1919, p. 235). The same ambiguity attaches in reverse form to the revenant. The ghost of a loved or hated person who haunts us from beyond the grave, it carries the promise that we, too, may be remembered after death.

III

When the Piggle asked about Winnicott's birthday, he did not hesitate to interpret in terms of opposites: "What about my death day?" (Winnicott, 1977, p. 124). Whether in the analysis of a little girl or an elderly man, the end of life joins up with the beginning. By addressing the hidden anxiety in the Piggle's question, Winnicott was in the most tactful way preparing her not only for the eventual termination of her treatment but also for his own death, which indeed occurred within

432   *Peter L. Rudnytsky*

five years. In the same way, he seemed to have wrought a miracle in the analysis of Guntrip, bestowing in his death the gift of freedom.

Puzzled as to what gave him the strength to face the "basic trauma" of his mother's failure, Guntrip concluded: "It must have been because Winnicott was not, and could not be, dead for me, nor certainly for many others" (p. 464). According to Hans Loewald, "The extended leave taking of the end phase of analysis is a replica of the process of mourning" (1962, p. 259). For Guntrip, this proved to be literally the case. But even those whose contact with Winnicott can only take place through the medium of books may know what it is like to have their lives changed by his. In mourning his loss, we may console ourselves with the thought that, like Freud, Winnicott has become part of our permanent analytic and cultural heritage.

BIBLIOGRAPHY

BALINT, M. (1968). *The Basic Fault.* New York: Brunner/Mazel.

BION, W. R. (1950). The imaginary twin. In *Second Thoughts.* London: Maresfield Reprints, 1967, pp. 3–22.

BUCKLEY, P., ed. (1986). *Essential Papers on Object Relations.* New York & London: New York Univ. Press.

DEUTSCH, H. (1937). Absence of grief. *Psychoanal. Q.,* 6:12–22.

ENGEL, G. L. (1975). The death of a twin. *Int. J. Psychoanal.,* 56:23–40.

FREUD, S. (1900). The interpretation of dreams. *S.E.,* 4 & 5.

———— (1916). Some character types met with in psycho-analytic work. *S.E.,* 14:311–333.

———— (1919). The "uncanny." *S.E.,* 17:219–256.

GUNTRIP, H. (1975). My experience of analysis with Fairbairn and Winnicott. In Buckley (1986), pp. 447–468.

JONES, E. (1955). *The Life and Work of Sigmund Freud,* 2. New York: Basic Books.

KLEIN, M. (1935). A contribution to the psychogenesis of manic-depressive states. In Buckley (1986), pp. 40–70.

LOEWALD, H. W. (1962). Internalization, separation, mourning, and the super-ego. In *Papers on Psychoanalysis.* New Haven & London: Yale Univ. Press, 1980, pp. 257–276.

RUDNYTSKY, P. L. (1987). *Freud and Oedipus.* New York: Columbia Univ. Press.

SCHUR, M. (1972). *Freud: Living and Dying.* New York: Int. Univ. Press.

WINNICOTT, D. W. (1958). Psycho-analysis and the sense of guilt. In *The Maturational Processes and the Facilitating Environment.* New York: Int. Univ. Press, 1965, pp. 15–28.

———— (1971). *Playing and Reality.* London: Tavistock Publications.

———— (1977). *The Piggle.* New York: Int. Univ. Press.

Picturing the Child's Inner World of Fantasy

On the Dialectic between Image and Word

ELLEN HANDLER SPITZ, Ph.D.

CURRENT INTERDISCIPLINARY LITERATURE IN THE HUMANITIES ABOUNDS with fascination for the analysis of signs and sign systems. In particular, there is a resurgence of interest in the distinguishing characteristics of, and relations between, words and images. When these issues are discussed by philosophers, the discourse often turns on questions of representation. Is representation achieved by resemblance or analogy (the modes usually postulated of imagery), by contiguity or convention (the modes associated with language), or by causal connection (as in demonstration)? Functional distinctions such as the density of the image versus the differentiation of the linguistic sign have been noted (Goodman, 1976). Efforts have been made (Gombrich, 1956, 1963, 1981) to tease apart the relative contribution to both verbal and pictorial signs of biology (nature) and convention (culture). Speculation on the effect of experiential differences between the categories of time (associated with words) and space (associated with images) has been linked with the differential reliability attributed to the evidence of the eye (as witness) versus that of the ear (hearsay). Such philosophical discourse, with its venerable tradition extending back into the pages of Platonic dialogue,

Visiting lecturer of aesthetics in psychiatry, Cornell University Medical College.

This paper was written while the author was visiting scholar at the Sigmund Freud Center of the Hebrew University, Jerusalem. Early versions were presented in Jerusalem at the B'nai B'rith Children's Home at the invitation of Dr. Yecheskiel Cohen and at the Ilan Child Guidance Center at the invitation of Dr. Rami Bar Giora. For insights that have found their way into the final version of this paper, the following colleagues are gratefully acknowledged: Gannit Ankori, Bettina Stronach, David Kittron, Amnon Toledano, and Michal Grossman.

reveals recrudescent efforts—both subtle and crude—to foster the hegemony, the preeminence, the superiority, of one type of sign (normally the linguistic, either spoken or written) over the other. However, as W. J. T. Mitchell (1986) has pointed out, the terms of the discourse are not innocent. A "war-torn" border lies between image and text, between picture and word.

My paper offers a modest contribution to this discourse by taking a psychoanalytic developmental perspective on a picture book designed for young children. Picture books, equally neglected in the literature of art, psychoanalysis, and philosophy, are fascinating precisely because they are intended to span this "war-torn" border just at the juncture in the lifespan when such bridges are being constructed. Picture books are artifacts expressly made for use during those unheralded but cataclysmic moments in childhood when gaps between the world of image and verbal language are being negotiated.

Rather than discuss picture books in general, I have chosen in this paper to examine in detail one extraordinary example—a storybook entitled *Where the Wild Things Are,* written and illustrated by Maurice Sendak in 1963. This slender volume, which boasts 19 double unnumbered pages, not only won the coveted Caldecott Medal (awarded to the most distinguished picture book of the year), but has been translated into many languages; though published nearly a quarter of a century ago, it has remained a cherished favorite among young children in the intervening years—so much so that recently, in the United States, soft toy replicas of its characters, in various sizes, have been placed on the market, and it has been used as a basis for children's drama as well as re-created as an opera.

My effort here will be to show that in this picture book word and image reinforce each other to create cross-currents that simultaneously affirm the need for regressive fantasy while gently moving in the direction of more adaptive, integrative function. My claim is that the constituent roles played by picture and text, their collaborative function, their interdependent shares in this extraordinary evocation of, and direct pipeline to, the inner fantasy life of young children, may contribute, at least tangentially, to the philosophical discourse.

Where the Wild Things Are works actively to deconstruct the dichotomies inherent in this discourse while at the same time creating a continuity between words and images that preserves their differences. The picture book not only reveals that the tendency of art (Mitchell, 1986) and play (Winnicott, 1971) is to breach the supposed boundaries between the spatial and the temporal, natural and cultural, inside and outside, self and other, but also and importantly to subtend and elaborate these very dichotomies. In this example, the verbal and pictorial signs serve varying functions with respect to each other: while refusing stereotypy, they maintain their differences, enabling the child to move toward reality testing but without renouncing fantasy and imagination.

I

As Freud (1908) intimated, there is a sense in which, in the case of at least certain artists, theoretical knowledge of psychology is obviated and superseded by intuition. The artist, as he puts it, precedes the scientist in this respect. Although Maurice Sendak, gifted author and illustrator of *Where the Wild Things Are*, was, to all intents and purposes, as innocent of the psychoanalytic theories of, for example, D. W. Winnicott and Melanie Klein as was Wilhelm Jensen, author of *Gradiva*, of Freudian theory (1907), yet the artists, in both cases, demonstrate a subtlety of insight that subsequent psychoanalytic interpretation can serve only partially to unconceal.

Unlike the simplest picture books which juxtapose an image with its name, or, as in alphabet primers, an image with the initial letter of its name, *Where the Wild Things Are* is a picture story in which the images are narrativized and the narrative pictorially represented. Briefly, the narrative concerns a little boy named Max who, after performing "mischief of one kind and another," is called a "WILD THING" by his mother (to whom he retorts, "I'LL EAT YOU UP!") and is sent off to bed without his supper. A forest grows in his bedroom, and Max sails off on an ocean in a "private boat" to "where the wild things are." There he tames the wild things by magic (staring into their eyes) and then participates with them in a "wild rumpus." After making them "stop!" and sending *them* off to bed without *their* supper, Max suddenly feels lonely and wants "to be where someone loved him best of all." He resists the appeals of the wild things (who urge him to stay by protesting that they love him so much they could eat him up) by saying "No!" to them, and finally he sails back "into the night of his very own room," where he finds his supper waiting for him, "and it was still hot."

Addressed to the child of about 3 to 5 years of age, the book is meant, significantly, to be read *to* him rather than *by* him. It creates a transitional space (Winnicott, 1953) between fantasy and reality, which is exquisitely appropriate in that the child of this age actually inhabits a universe of shifting realms in which the boundaries between fantasy and reality are not yet firmly established (Fraiberg, 1959).

Through its acceptance and exploration of the interpenetration of these realms, this work distinguishes itself from other more superficial picture books designed for the same age child that focus on premature adaptation to selected aspects of external reality. *Where the Wild Things Are* openly acknowledges and, in fact, dramatizes the child's subjective state: responsively, it supports his need for regressive fantasy, while unobtrusively reassuring him all the while of a safe return to reality. In doing so, it functions vis-à-vis its child spectator/audience, as do all major works of art on both the highest and deepest levels. And, in parallel with masterpieces of art created for adults, the picture book depends crucially upon the working of convention to secure positive and meaningful experience. Because of the performancelike aspect of the genre (in that it is read *to* the child), its effect depends in large part upon the qualities (self-acceptance, emotional equilibrium, sense of humor) of the reading adult—whose presence and engagement must serve, like that perhaps of conductor and performer of a musical score, to contain, guide, and modify the child's experience. Whereas the images of the picture book are seen essentially without mediation (are "autographic"), its words are both seen and heard, spoken through the voice of another ("allographic") (Goodman, 1976).

Winnicott has given us the evocative and deceptively simple notion of the holding environment, in which mother (and, by analogy, analyst) serves the role of safe and dependable container for the infant's (patient's) fantasies, fears, and hostile impulses. Crucial for the establishment of secure self-object differentiation, reality testing, and therapeutic success is the mother's survival of the infant's aggression. In the arts, various aspects of form and convention serve parallel roles as containers—the frame of the painting, the language, meter, rhyme scheme, and diction of the poem, the established spatial limits, including stage, curtain, lights, and fixed temporal range of a given theatrical performance. When these holding environments are unstable or transgressed, uneasiness and displeasure may ensue: life invades art, therapeutic milieus collapse, and painted monsters emerge from the pages of books to terrorize young minds.

Where the Wild Things Are instantiates a holding environment on several levels. First, in reading it to the child, the mother or mother-surrogate provides a safe and nurturing context for the experience. We can imagine that, quite concretely, in many cases, the child is actually being physically held while read to. Secondly, the design of the book itself (which I shall discuss in detail) creates a sensitive milieu for both fostering and containing the unfolding of the child-listener's own (private) fantasies. On a third level, looking beyond form to content, we perceive another trace, an echo—an invisible character, the off-stage mother of Max, who (in parallel with the reader of the story) provides an attentive, responsive, and dependable medium for the protagonist's play and fantasy. This good-enough mother (Winnicott, 1971) is also a true-to-form Kleinian mother in that she is out of sight, visible only through the perceptions and distortions of her child's psyche. Her voice is heard just once, but she is never seen. Of significance too is the space in which the story unfolds: the child's bedroom, his most familiar and private external space, which is here transformed by fantasy into an arena for the enactment of inner drama.

Freud (1900) spoke about the regressive transformation of thoughts, ideas, and words into pictures. By means of its extraordinary design, *Where the Wild Things Are* almost literally illustrates this concept while simultaneously moving in the opposite direction, that is to say, encouraging its youthful "reader" to progress from the world of the imaginary to the world of the symbolic. The book begins with verbal language, that is, with ordinary communication, as the child-listener hears his mother's reading voice. Words and pictures form coequal partners in conveying the story. Page by page, however, the words (and mother's voice) gradually diminish, and the pictures grow in size relative to the printed text—until, finally, when Max (and the child-listener) are fully transported into their own fantasy worlds, the pictures expand to fill all the available space. Fantasy completely overtakes reality. Mother's voice is no longer heard.

Just as Max has been transported into the world of wild things in "a private boat" (signed in both verbal and pictorial registers), so the child listening is permitted now to fuse with the magical power of fantasy and image. And because these transitions are effected so gradually, almost imperceptibly, the child is not overwhelmed by the world of imagination. Furthermore, since, even at the climax of Max's orgy with the wild things, child and mother are still together, turning the pages of the book, we can conceive the child as experiencing optimally that auspicious state characterized as "being alone in the presence of another" (Winnicott, 1958). Later, as fantasy subsides, the pictures diminish in size. The world of words reasserts itself. With Max, the child-listener returns to consensually validated, intersubjective reality—to the comforting presence of the mother's reading voice, which, like Max's supper, has retained its warmth.

Thus, the very design of the book constitutes a dialectic between image and word, creating what Winnicott has called a facilitating environment. We might also point to the stylistic quality of its drawings. Sendak's style is characteristically linear and precise. His clear, carefully executed graphics convey subtly to the viewer that he is in control—of his medium, surely, and, if that, then perhaps by implication of his message as well. As with other artists whose fantasies are figured with intense linearity (e.g., Bosch, Blake, Dali, Magritte), this quality functions doubly to endow the imagery with a sense of hyperreality while simultaneously marking it as, at least in part, consciously controlled. It is also worthwhile to note that the wild things themselves, the monsters, even in their largest, most frenzied, orgastic incarnations, are not entirely frightening but also silly, humorous, even strangely lovable—rather like parents who become, evanescently, monsters, or children (like Max) who don bestial costumes. With regard to the verbal signs, *Where the Wild Things Are* narrates its plot in the past tense so that implicitly Max has already survived these events—as will, by identification, the child who is listening and looking.

II

The story begins with Max wearing his "wolf suit" and making mischief. We see Max in an enactment of aggression in several registers, and here the images elaborate the verbal text, enriching it, filling it out, offering to it a repleteness (Goodman, 1976), while the words themselves serve mainly as instructions to us for the focus of our gaze. As a costume, Max's wolf suit possesses exaggerated phallic appendages—pointed ears, claws, and an enormous bushy tail—thus reminding us that the symbol of the wolf is redolent of oedipal as well as preoedipal themes, not only threats of devouring and of being devoured (the "I'll eat you up" of "The Three Little Pigs" and of "Little Red Riding Hood") but also the notion of wolf as seducer. The costume, identified via both sign systems, condenses oedipal genitality with preoedipal oral sadism. The pictorial image works doubly, both to deny and to extend the verbal signifier, in that Max's suit looks suspiciously like a baby suit, a sleeper or pajama, mitigating its alleged hostility and revealing the child's aggressiveness to be, in part, an outgrowth of infantile smallness and helplessness.

From the beginning, we can see that the dialectic of word and image functions to forge complex links between preoedipal and oedipal themes, to counterpose and reintegrate them by introducing them into the representational field, even occasionally by distorting, excluding, exaggerating, or foregrounding one over the other. Since the child to whom the picture book is addressed is on the cusp between these developmental curves, the dual registration matches with exquisite fitness his own intrapsychic imperatives.

What is the mischief here? Max has strung up a small animal doll, symbolic perhaps of younger siblings or envied babies. He messes up the house. He ignores the verbal content of two books by stepping on them, proclaiming his emancipation from the rule of language, law, and order. With an enormous hammer, he bangs a nail into the wall. From a Kleinian perspective, it is possible to see the house as signifying the mother, the aggression in general as an attack upon the mother's body in consequence of the child's envy of it as powerful provider (and withholder) of good things. Although from the parental point of view Max's behavior is destructive, we are given pictorial clues that his activities are from his own viewpoint constructive as well. While messing things up inside his mother's house, he seems at the same time to be building himself a sort of tent, a private space, as it were, that will be replicated later in fantasy in terms both of his "private boat" and of the royal tent under which he sits forlornly when he becomes "king of where the wild things are."

On the next page, the mischief continues. Here, in addition to the symbolic attack on the envied body of the mother, we observe an attack with a fork (both oral and phallic) against a little white dog who might almost be taken, at this moment, as a double for Max himself. The doubling of the image suggests a biographical association that is irresistible, though somewhat tangential. Sendak, in choosing "Max" as the name of his naughty protagonist, links this name to his own, Maurice, which is a cognate for the German "Moritz," thus inviting an association to the two devilish young pranksters of the "Max und Moritz" cartoons by Wilhelm Busch—the comic strip being a form closely related to the picture book, in which word and image, temporal and spatial modes, are coupled. In one 1865 "Max und Moritz" drawing especially relevant to *Where the Wild Things Are* (Robinson, 1974), a peasant woman, smiling in anticipation of her dinner, washes a plate in the basement of her house, while on the hearth above a panful of little game hens are roasting. A small white dog, not unlike Sendak's, barks, as do the two naughty boys upon the roof. Max and Moritz gleefully dance around the chimney while, with a fishing rod, they clandestinely extricate the woman's dinner (through the chimney) one roast hen at a time. Thus, the themes of oral aggression, reversal of deprivation, and secret triumph over the mother are here anticipated.

In the second drawing of *Where the Wild Things Are*, oedipal rivalry is adumbrated by the grasping gesture of the child toward the dog's erect tail, and we might remark the understated presence of the shadowy stairway, associated by Freud (1900) with mounting sexual excitement in the oneiric lexicon. Max's mischief then, by dramatizing both oedipal and preoedipal themes, exquisitely taps the developmental imperatives of the child who listens to the story. On the wall hangs a drawing by, and by implication a self representation of, Max as an oral-sadistic monster, bisexual, with plenty of teeth and hair (including a beard), eyes like breasts, and a horn as a displaced phallus. Gleefully, the child's aggression is fused with his polymorphous sexuality and exuberant narcissism. In the background, unseen, the mother in a double sense as reader (performer) and character allows, permits, continues (goes on being, Winnicott, 1958) unthreatened.

On the third page, however, Max's aggression calls forth a response. He has, as it were, projected his own badness into the offstage mother, and now he must experience her counteraggression. As mentioned, it is significant that the mother never appears visually in the book, that she lives entirely through the experience of the child, again, in the double sense—both for Max and for the child-listener. In a classic dramatization of projective identification, the child, having done mischief and provoked the mother into calling him a "wild thing," now feels the need to incorporate her orally—to eat her up (as he says quite literally).

The principal dynamic here, projective identification, has been described as the forceful entry into an external object which is then compelled to acquire unacceptable characteristics. Subsequently, as the external object becomes threatening and persecutory, a need arises to control and (orally) destroy the now-threatening object (Segal, 1964). Max is bad (implicitly, to the mother); mother is bad (to Max). Max wishes to devour and destroy her (i.e., to destroy the consequences of his own aggression).

But now Max *loses* her. He loses food; and food equals mother. In the picture, the expression on Max's face conveys more clearly than words the response he is making to this painful consequence of his own hostility. His face proclaims: "I'll show you!" To avoid pain and anxiety, he must deny the loss. Through the medium of Sendak's graphics, we can almost see him resorting unconsciously to the defense of splitting—as he prepares to triumph in fantasy over this "bad" mother who has sent him to his room and refused him his supper. Here the image does not illustrate or expand upon the text but rather responds to it in a kind of counterpoint: word contra image (child versus mother).

In the fourth picture, we witness the proliferation of fantasy, as Max magically transgresses the boundary set by the mother. As the forest grows in his bedroom, we see, marvelously portrayed in Max's face and pose, his triumph over any feelings of anxiety and loss. Again, words and image form a contrapuntal ensemble, as in the next duo of pages where Max's covering of his mouth with the paw to hide his smile betokens and betrays the secret sadism of his victory. Finally, the room completely disappears, and the forest takes over. In this next picture (the sixth), the many-treed forest may be read as emblematic not only of mystery and the feminine (as in "The Sleeping Beauty" and "Hansel and Gretel," for example) but, more deeply, as the forbidden inside of the mother's body, with all its treasures, including the phallic treasure, multiply represented. It is also interesting to note the presence and changing shape, size, and position of the moon in each of the pictures in which it appears, beginning with Max's banishment and loss therefore of his mother. Here, for example, the moon is ambiguously both crescent and full, and Max prances directly under it. It is hard to resist interpreting these ever-changing, omnipresent moons as displacements, fantasy evocations of the absent yet ever-present maternal object.

As fantasy overtakes reality in this sixth picture, only Max's back is shown. Thus, the child can supply and project his own affect and expression, for, as possibilities for reading-in multiply, so the potentiality for identification increases. Max assumes the posture of a necromancer, a shaman casting a spell.

Having created and entered an alternative world, Max in the seventh picture faces fully toward us and smiles with a pose and expression unmistakably smug and self-satisfied. He sails on an ocean of rhythmical waves—soothing, womblike perhaps, betokening new birth as well as return to the place of no loss and without boundaries. This is the first time in the book that the illustration exceeds its limits, transgressing the space previously reserved for written text. From this point on, image will increasingly encroach upon the domain of words until, at the height of fantasy, printed words are crowded out altogether.

It is significant that Max is provided with a "private" boat, since a focal aspect of his fantasy is his denial of dependence on the "bad," withholding mother. Here, with sails rigged, floating independently in his private sailboat, he is free—captain, literally, of his fate. The notion of privacy is also relevant, as I have indicated, to the relationship between the child-listener and the reader of the story, in that it gives license, so to speak, for a certain kind of independence as well—encouraging the child to create *his* own private fantasies while listening to the story.

As image gradually gains hegemony over word, space prevails over linear temporality. Max travels "in and out of weeks and almost over a year"—an evocation of the timelessness of the unconscious. As loss is denied, with the transcendence of both temporal and spatial boundaries and the increasing invasion of the world of words by pictorial image, it is possible to interpret a confluence of narrative and intrapsychic time, so that the fantasy of the wild things, narrativized by the text, is taken as occurring simultaneously with the mischief-making. In other words, the dialectic of signs makes possible a reading that privileges synchronic rather than diachronic time—subjective over historic or narrative time. According to this alternative reading, Max does not do mischief and *then* fantasize the wild things; rather, Max does mischief and simultaneously fantasizes his journey and his return.

Now, however, in the eighth and ninth pictures, Max must meet the persecutory objects he has introjected—creatures of his own (disowned) aggression. In terms of the cyclical syndrome described by Klein, these persecutory introjects are now reexperienced and appear as monsters, "wild things." Just as Max's mother called *him* a "wild thing," so he projects his wild thing-ness into these fanciful creatures.

Interestingly, there are several wild things and not just one. Bion (1967) has developed a notion of what he has called "bizarre objects," which refers to just such a maneuver, namely, the secondary splitting of persecutory objects for defensive purposes. The strategy, a variation on the theme of "divide and conquer," splits the enemy into fragments; like the brooms of the sorceror's apprentice, these become multiple potential persecutors which then need, of course, all the more urgently to be controlled.

The monsters themselves are marvelous illustrations of the fantasy of the combined parental imago. They possess secondary sexual characteristics of both sexes and represent at the same time a warding off of castration anxiety by their superabundance of phallic appendages, including horns, claws, teeth, tails, and hair. That they resemble in these details Max's portrait at the beginning of the story betokens an underlying identification of the child with them. As the parents become increasingly differentiated for the child at the oedipal stage, and their sexual intercourse arouses both envy and jealousy, he may regress to a fantasy of the combined parental imago which both denies their coveted and exclusive partnership while at the same time providing a vehicle for the expression of his aggression against them. Max's wild things thus serve as exquisitely elaborated instances of the rather typical monsters dreamed up by children on the cusp of preoedipal and oedipal development.

In the tenth picture, Max tames the wild things. By this time, image has literally superseded text, the latter being placed here, as on the preceding page, not insignificantly, beneath it. Max defends against his persecutory objects by a counterphobic omnipotent act of mastery and control. By this act, he instantaneously reverses the young child's helplessness with respect both to his drives and to his parental objects.

Bypassing the slower, more difficult path of true reparation which acknowledges loss and guilt, Max secures his omnipotence by means of magic—the act of magic being that he stares into the monster's eyes.

In a classic paper on the symbolism of the eye, Ferenczi (1913) pointed out that, because of their extreme sensitivity, vulnerability, movability, changeability of size, and the extraordinarily high value which we accord to them, the eyes serve as apt symbols for the genitals. We also note the frequency of equations in verbal language of the visual with the oral ("he devoured her with his eyes"), so that the magical staring may be related both to notions of oral incorporation and of phallic attack. Staring may betoken a potential violent intimacy—a condensation, as with the wolf suit, of oral sadism and genital rape.

It is extremely important that Max *does* triumph over his wild things—that, even in fantasy, the child is not destroyed by his monsters. From an object relations perspective, the survival of this (fictional) child despite his ravaging introjects is indicative of the abiding virtual presence of the good maternal object who is perhaps figured, as mentioned above, in the various new, half, crescent, and waning moons.

As, in the eleventh picture, Max becomes king, gaining crown and scepter, and, to use the classical psychoanalytic terminology, ego achieves supremacy over id, we see that Max does not have any further need to squelch or destroy his introjects. Instead, he can now permit himself to *enjoy* them! Because his ego is intact, and he is in control, he can afford to take pleasure in regression. In a vibrant illustration of the notion of regression in the service of the ego (Kris, 1952), Max gives his permission for frenzied frolic, crying, "And now, let the wild rumpus start!"

The next three pages form the centerpiece of the book. With Max, pictorial signs now reign triumphant. Narrative sequencing is suspended. Transported into the realm of pure play, pure daydream, pure wish fulfillment, words fall away. Words are, for the child, at a greater remove from drive than images. Therefore, these scariest moments of the storybook are experienced by the child in silence through imagery alone, as he is both permitted and compelled to be alone with his (private) fantasies. At the height of the orgy, however, Max is still king; the pages of the book itself provide a tangible boundary, and, as suggested above, the child is alone *within* a holding environment jointly created by imagery, text, reader's presence, and the contribution of his own psyche—alone now in Winnicott's sense, as an achievement—alone securely in the presence of another.

On the fifteenth page, a major shift occurs. The silence is broken as Max tells the wild things to "stop!" In sending them off to bed without their supper, he does precisely to them what was done to him by his mother. He not only turns passive into active but identifies with the maternal object. In replicating her (speech) act, he reinvokes her in her absence. Having attacked and banished his persecutory objects, he feels depleted and begins to experience loneliness. The wild, frenzied activity, the imaginative projection, has left him empty, yearning for the love object—whose loss he only now begins to suffer. His oral dependent needs reassert themselves: he smells food.

As he allows himself for the first time to experience sadness and separation, he is shown sitting, pondering, wondering whether per-haps—as a consequence of his own aggression—he has in fact de-stroyed the beloved mother. As the pictorial sign figures little Max, still crowned, pining, at the door of his regal tent (a fantasy fulfillment and visual quotation of the abortive efforts made on page 1), it is hard to avoid associations to images of the Biblical Saul (I Samuel:16) who, like Max, is tormented by evil spirits and for whom, by analogy, the sweet sounds of David's lyre might be likened to the soothing sounds of the mother's voice. In silence, the evil spirits may terrify, but, with the return of a gentle voice, melancholy ensues.

Accepting his need and his lack, Max gives up being king of where the wild things are. He relinquishes the fantasy of omnipotence and complete independence. He begins to go back. Verbal language reas-serts itself, and the pictures begin to recede.

The wild things, however, will not let him go so easily. By repeating to Max exactly what he had said to his mother ("we'll eat you up"), they inadvertently betray the double entendre of this expression. The de-sire to incorporate the loved object in order to possess it and the desire to destroy the loved object in order to possess it both stem from the paradigm of the infant feeding at the breast: both betoken a denial of the independent existence of the beloved.

Max, however, says "No!" Here, the child's negative constitutes a powerful positive assertion of self. As Spitz (1965) points out, the child must learn to say no to himself, and the negative therefore possesses enormous power in defining the boundaries of self. By saying "No!" Max returns to the realm of boundaries—he moves toward reality and away from fantasy. Winnicott would stress that it is the very presence of a good internal object that renders the child capable of saying no. We see in this picture (#16) the reintroduction of Max's boat. Going back, interestingly, it does not present the side marked with his name—an indication, possibly, that the boat no longer needs to be quite so "private." As the pictures diminish in size and the domain of verbal language reasserts itself, the young child is borne along on its waves, traveling onward, developmentally, from the land of private image to the realm of public word. We also see the child's strength and pleasure in his capacity to say no and to stop his play and, not only to stop, but even to wave good-bye, and to do so with a smile.

As Max slowly and gradually sails back through the timeless land of make-believe, the child-listener also is eased back; in the eighteenth and next-to-last picture, the safe boundaries of Max's bedroom are reinstated. We notice that his wolf's hat is beginning to slip off his head. The picture is a replication of page 3: familiarity has been restored. And, best of all, his supper is waiting for him. The invisible mother has survived his assaults. She still loves him; she is still feeding him. And Max too, and the child who has heard and seen the story, have lived through it and survived. Visually, it is interesting to note that the table, bowl, and moon in this image may for the child-spectator evoke another beloved picture book, *Goodnight Moon* (Brown, 1947), which is addressed to a slightly younger child and tenderly deals with the issue of bedtime separation. Parenthetically, *Goodnight Moon* also addresses with unusual sensitivity the child's developmental dialectic between image and word as the magical recurrence of its images is mirrored by the rhymes of its verbal text.

On the last page of *Where the Wild Things Are* there is no picture. The child listening to the story hears his mother utter the final words, "and it was still hot." Love is ongoing and warm; it occurs in the intersubjective realm of language and consensual reality. As the child has experienced, through the vehicle of this deeply empathic and exquisitely constructed work, the vicarious enactment of splitting, projective identification, manic triumph, omnipotence, and, finally, loss and separation, he may take steps toward gradually learning that both he and his objects can and will survive the ravages of his destructive impulses. It probably takes, however, a mother who is quite comfortable with her own wild things to be able to read this story again and again and enjoy it fully with her child.

III

My effort has been to demonstrate, by the analysis of just one picture book, the treasure trove constituted by this genre, not only for our understanding of the fantasy life and developmental imperatives of young children, but for the philosophical discourse on word and image. Because the child of picture-book age is not yet fully assimilated into the realm of verbal language, spoken or written, this genre functions on the boundary, the divide, between two great sign systems. It must travel, as we have seen, dialectically between them, sometimes translating verbal into visual signs and vice versa, sometimes supplementing one code with the other, at other times employing the different modes as opposing voices in a dialogue. For the child, at least two major agendas are operant—the push toward language and socialization, toward acceptance of differentiation, limit, loss, diachronic time, and pari passu the pull toward image, wish, and fantasy.

From a psychoanalytic perspective, the border zone here is better described as criss-crossed in highly complex paths than as "war-torn," for although the developmental trajectory leads ineluctably toward the mastery and refinement of verbal language, it does not lead away from image. The wizened ideology of mother/earth/space/picture versus father/time/story/name is partially deconstructed by a genre that is impelled by the naïveté of its clientele to play freely with both sign systems in unorthodox, highly original ways. Representation is achieved via all three modes—analogy, contiguity, and indexicality, the latter largely through its performance aspect. What Sendak's beautiful book and others like it demonstrate is the awesome power of images to inform as well as deform, to inspire as well as derail, the inevitable trajectory.

BIBLIOGRAPHY

BION, W. R. (1927). *Second Thoughts.* London: Heinemann.
BROWN, M. W. (1947). *Goodnight Moon.* New York: Harper & Row.
FERENCZI, S. (1913). On eye symbolism. *First Contributions to Psychoanalysis.* New York: Brunner/Mazel, 1952, pp. 270–276.
FRAIBERG, S. (1959). *The Magic Years.* New York: Scribner's Sons.
FREUD, S. (1900). The interpretation of dreams. *S.E.,* 4 & 5.
——— (1907). Delusions and dreams in Jensen's *Gradiva. S.E.,* 9:3–95.
——— (1908). Creative writers and day-dreaming. *S.E.,* 9:142–153.
GOMBRICH, E. H. (1956). *Art and Illusion.* Princeton: Princeton Univ. Press.
——— (1963). *Meditations on a Hobby Horse and Other Essays on the Theory of Art.* New York: Phaidon Press.
——— (1981). Image and code. In *Image and Code,* ed. W. Steiner. Ann Arbor: Univ. Michigan Studies in the Humanities, no. 2.
GOODMAN, N. (1976). *Languages of Art.* Indianapolis & Cambridge: Hackett.
KLEIN, M. (1957). Envy and gratitude. In *Envy and Gratitude and Other Works, 1946–1963.* New York: Delacorte Press/Seymour Lawrence, 1975.
KRIS, E. (1952). *Psychoanalytic Explorations in Art.* New York: Int. Univ. Press.

MITCHELL, W. J. T. (1986). *Iconology*. Chicago & London: Univ. Chicago Press.

ROBINSON, J. (1974). *The Comics*. New York: Berkeley Windhover Books.

SEGAL, H. (1964). *Introduction to the Work of Melanie Klein*. New York: Basic Books.

SENDAK, M. (1963). *Where the Wild Things Are*. New York: Harper & Row.

SPITZ, R. A. (1957). *No and Yes*. New York: Int. Univ. Press.

WINNICOTT, D. W. (1953). Transitional objects and transitional phenomena. In *Collected Papers*. New York: Basic Books, 1957, pp. 229–242.

_____ (1958). The capacity to be alone. In *Maturational Processes and the Facilitating Environment*. London: Hogarth Press, 1979, pp. 29–36.

_____ (1971). *Playing and Reality*. New York: Basic Books.

Index

449